Clinical Endodontics

Dedication

To John Dresser, whose continued commitment to excellence and the pursuit of knowledge sets the highest bar for what it means to provide exceptional patient-centered care.

One book, one tree: In support of reforestation worldwide and to address the climate crisis, for every book sold Quintessence Publishing will plant a tree (https://onetreeplanted.org/).

Library of Congress Cataloging-in-Publication Data
Names: Blicher, Brooke, author. | Lucier Pryles, Rebekah, author. | Lin, Jarshen, author. | Li, Alice, author.
Title: Clinical endodontics / Brooke Blicher, Rebekah Lucier Pryles, Jarshen Lin, Alice Li.
Description: Batavia, IL : Quintessence Publishing Co. Inc., [2023] | Includes bibliographical references and index. | Summary: "This manual equips clinicians with all the best protocols and knowledge for administering general endodontic care"-- Provided by publisher.
Identifiers: LCCN 2023027796 | ISBN 9781647241759 (spiral bound)
Subjects: MESH: Endodontics--methods | Periodontal Diseases | Dental Pulp Diseases
Classification: LCC RK351 | NLM WU 241 | DDC 617.6/342--dc23/eng/20230726
LC record available at https://lccn.loc.gov/2023027796

A CIP record for this book is available from the British Library.
ISBN: 9781647241759

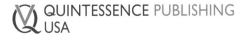

QUINTESSENCE PUBLISHING
USA

Quintessence Publishing Co, Inc
411 N Raddant Road
Batavia, IL 60510
www.quintessence-publishing.com

5   4   3   2   1

Editor: Kristen Clark
Design: Sue Zubek
Production: Angelina Schmelter

Printed in China

Clinical Endodontics

Brooke Blicher, DMD

Private Practice Limited to Endodontics
White River Junction, Vermont

Lecturer
Department of Restorative Dentistry
and Biomaterials Sciences
Harvard School of Dental Medicine

Assistant Clinical Professor
Department of Endodontics
Tufts University School of Dental Medicine
Boston, Massachusetts

Jarshen Lin, DDS

Director of Predoctoral Endodontics
Department of Restorative Dentistry and
Biomaterials Sciences
Harvard School of Dental Medicine

Clinical Associate
Department of Surgery, Division of Dentistry
Massachusetts General Hospital
Boston, Massachusetts

Rebekah Lucier Pryles, DMD

Private Practice Limited to Endodontics
White River Junction, Vermont

Assistant Clinical Professor
Department of Endodontics
Tufts University School of Dental Medicine

Lecturer
Department of Restorative Dentistry
and Biomaterials Sciences
Harvard School of Dental Medicine
Boston, Massachusetts

Alice Li, DMD

MMSc Candidate
Advanced Graduate Program in Endodontics
Harvard School of Dental Medicine
Boston, Massachusetts

Chief Content Officer
My Dental Key, LLC

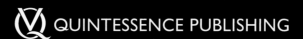

QUINTESSENCE PUBLISHING

Berlin | Chicago | Tokyo
Barcelona | London | Milan | Mexico City | Paris | Prague | Seoul | Warsaw
Beijing | Istanbul | Sao Paulo | Zagreb

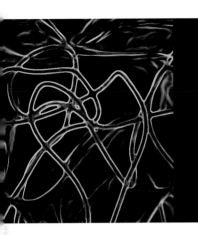

Contents

QUICK GUIDE
Booklet insert located in pocket of back cover.

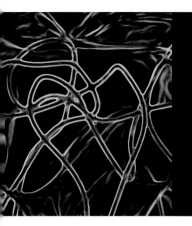

Preface

Endodontic care is integral to the practice of dentistry. Sadly, however, many practitioners are intimidated by endodontic diagnosis and treatment planning. This text aims to cover the full breadth of endodontic diagnosis and care to bring an evidence-based perspective to clinical practice. The vast swath of endodontic literature offers clinicians both classic wisdom and new information that can be applied directly to patient care, and readers will find literature references throughout the text to support evidence-based practice.

Though the origins of this book were in the development of predoctoral endodontics curricula, its comprehensive scope renders it useful for practitioners of all levels, including dental students, residents, general practitioners, and specialists alike. Even providers who do not perform the full scope of endodontic procedures should be knowledgeable about their existence and availability.

The main text is dedicated to the overall theory and biologic basis of diagnosis and treatment, including detailed procedure guides. The Quick Guide, found at the back of the book, is modeled on cookbooks and includes tray setups and step-by-step procedural instructions, making this guide useful for not only practitioners but also clinical staff tasked with operatory setup.

We hope you enjoy our illustrated and evidence-based guide to clinical endodontic practice and that it promotes both your learning and the delivery of excellent clinical care.

PART I

Establishing a Diagnosis

The practice of endodontics is grounded in the management of orofacial pain and infection. Pain and infection, however, are not exclusive to endodontic pathology. Furthermore, not all endodontic diagnoses warrant endodontic treatment. The establishment of an accurate and complete diagnosis is an essential prerequisite for any endodontic treatment. This section of the text discusses the materials and techniques for detecting and diagnosing endodontic pathology, as well as its differential diagnosis.

Examination Protocols

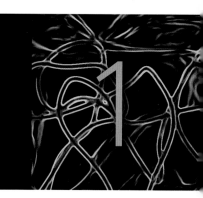

Diagnosis is the foundation of endodontics. The diagnosis of endodontic pathology and orofacial pain requires gathering a careful patient history and performing both clinical and radiographic examinations. These components are referred to as the subjective and objective exams. Taken together, the exam findings are used to establish the patient's diagnosis and direct the selection and provision of appropriate treatment modalities. This chapter reviews the components of the diagnostic exam.

Subjective Examination

As is true of all medical and dental encounters, a thoughtful and thorough patient interview, also known as the subjective examination, is both foundational to the development of a trusting patient-clinician relationship and provides necessary information to direct the objective examination that follows. This interview can take place either in person or, when in-person encounters are not possible, as a telehealth encounter via phone or video as permitted by local practice laws. The components of the subjective exam are (1) the chief complaint, (2) the history of the present illness (HPI), (3) the past dental history (PDH), and (4) the medical history (Fig 1-1).

Chief
complaint

History of present
illness: timeline, intensity,
localization, exacerbating factors,
alleviating factors

Past dental history

Medical history

FIG 1-1 The components of the subjective examination.

The chief complaint is the reason the patient is seeking care. This should be recorded in the patient's own words, not only to demonstrate to the patient that their concerns are understood but also to ensure that treatment plans address the patient's explicit and individualized needs.

The HPI should further develop the clinician's understanding of the patient's chief complaint. If not immediately volunteered, the timeline of symptoms (ie, the onset and duration) and their trajectory over time (increased, decreased, or steady) should be established. Furthermore, clinicians must inquire about symptom intensity, localization, and exacerbating and alleviating factors. If analgesic use is reported, the timing of the last dosage should be established because medications may directly affect responses to clinical testing.

Because endodontic pathology develops as a result of pulpal irritation, the PDH provides clues to the etiology of the chief complaint, including but not limited to restorative care, endodontic treatment, fractures, and trauma. The setting, type, and timing of prior dental care should be ascertained. If trauma is included in the history, the specifics surrounding the traumatic injury must be understood. Deep restorative care may result in the development of endodontic pathology years after treatment.[1] Teeth with a history of deep restorations face a lifetime of elevated risk for requiring nonsurgical root canal therapy (NSRCT), with the risk being further increased for teeth serving as abutments for partial dentures than for those supporting single crowns.[2–6]

As with all dental examinations, a thorough medical history, including past and present illnesses, medications, and allergies, should be obtained. The medical history can alert clinicians to medications and conditions that may interfere with endodontic diagnosis. Ibuprofen taken to treat the chief complaint or another painful condition can directly mitigate responses to clinical testing, including responses to percussion, palpation, and cold testing.[7] Additionally, a history of head/neck radiation may lessen the expected responses to pulp sensitivity testing.[8]

The medical history may also alert clinicians to other medications or conditions that could impact the delivery of care. Blood thinners warrant consideration both because of their direct effects in increasing bleeding in cases of planned surgical care and because they contraindicate the use of nonsteroidal anti-inflammatory drug (NSAID) family pain relievers.[9,10] Antiresorptive medications, including bisphosphonate and RANKL inhibitors, or a history of head/neck radiation therapy affect treatment planning because they increase the risk of osteonecrosis following invasive dental procedures, including surgical endodontic care and extractions.[11–13] Patients with poorly controlled diabetes or other systemic or drug-related immune system compromise may have difficulty healing from infections, and consideration might be made for antibiotic coverage in consultation with their physicians.[14] Cardiac conditions warranting antibiotic premedication for endodontic procedures should be documented.[15,16]

Measurement of vital signs should also be included in the review of a patient's medical history. This should include measurement of the patient's blood pressure and body temperature. An oral or temporal temperature is important for detecting systemic effects of infection. A high-quality thermometer should be used and the measurement recorded in the patient's chart whenever infection is suspected.

The results of the subjective exam should be recorded in the patient's chart. From a medico-legal perspective, this ensures that patient needs and desires are being communicated and addressed. Most importantly, the patient interview should develop the clinician's differential diagnosis. The interview and differential diagnosis should then be utilized to guide the objective examination that follows.

Objective Examination

The objective examination includes both a clinical and radiographic examination. The clinical exam consists of a careful extraoral and intraoral inspection of the hard and soft tissues, as well as clinical testing. The radiographic examination should include both 2D and 3D radiographs, when relevant. The standard armamentarium for the objective endodontic exam is shown in Fig 1-2, and the clinical components are detailed in Fig 1-3.

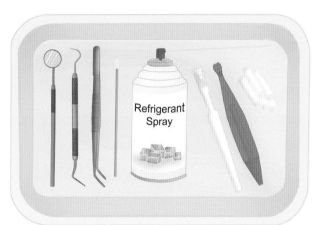

FIG 1-2 The standard armamentarium for the clinical examination includes a clean mirror, an explorer, a periodontal probe, cotton-tipped applicators or pliers with a no. 2 or no. 4 cotton pellet, refrigerant spray, and bite testing implements including cotton rolls and/or commercially available bite testers, such as a Tooth Slooth (Professional Results) or Fracfinder (Denbur).

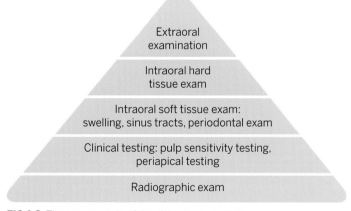

FIG 1-3 The components of the objective examination.

Extraoral examination

The extraoral examination of the head and neck should assess for swelling, asymmetries, and lymphadenopathy (Fig 1-4). The quality of any swelling should be assessed as fluctuant or firm. Palpation of submandibular and cervical lymph nodes can be used to detect lymphadenopathy resulting from infections of the head and neck region, though not necessarily specific to the dentition. Extraoral sinus tracts, though rare, should also be documented. These represent a means of drainage from an infected tooth. As with intraoral sinus tracts, they should be radiographically traced with gutta-percha to confirm the source.

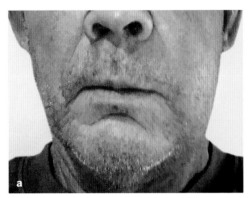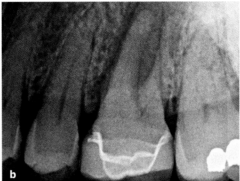

FIG 1-4 Extraoral swelling (a) may indicate an endodontically derived cellulitis, such as this case that occurred secondary to pulpal necrosis with acute apical abscess of the maxillary left first molar (b).

The muscles of mastication and the temporomandibular joint should also be inspected during the extraoral examination (Fig 1-5). Palpation of the masseter and temporalis muscles, particularly in patients with a history of bruxism, is essential to evaluate whether a patient's chief complaint is the result of myofascial pain as opposed to endodontic pathology.

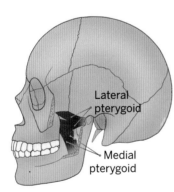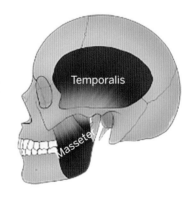

FIG 1-5 The muscles of mastication and the temporomandibular joint should be examined during the extraoral exam to rule out myofascial pain or a temporomandibular joint disorder as the etiology of the chief complaint.

Adjunctive trauma examination

When evaluating traumatic dental injuries, the objective examination should be expanded if the clinician is the first to examine the patient following the injury. A primary patient survey should be conducted following the mnemonic **ABCDE**. Clinicians must ensure a patent **airway** and stabilized cervical spine. They should also ensure that there is adequate **breathing** and ventilation and intact **circulation** without evidence of shock. Clinicians must assess for neurologic **disability**, and the patient should be fully undressed to achieve **exposure** of the full body for examination.[17] Additionally, because dental trauma carries the risk of concomitant head trauma, a neurologic screening tool, such as the Glasgow Coma Scale,[18,19] should be used to rule out neurologic compromise or decompensation, which would warrant immediate EMS referral (Table 1-1).

TABLE 1-1 The Glasgow Coma Scale

Behavior	Response	Score
Eye Opening Response	Spontaneously	4
	To speech	3
	To pain	2
	No response	1
Best Verbal Response	Oriented to time, place, and person	5
	Confused	4
	Inappropriate words	3
	Incomprehensible sounds	2
	No response	1
Best Motor Response	Obeys commands	6
	Moves to localized pain	5
	Flexion withdrawal from pain	4
	Abnormal flexion (decorticate)	3
	Abnormal extension (decerebrate)	2
	No response	1
Total Score	Best response	15
	Comatose client	8 or less
	Totally unresponsive	3

Intraoral examination

Hard tissue examination

A comprehensive examination of the dentition is crucial to establish both a potential etiology for endodontic pathology and to evaluate the restorability of the tooth or teeth in question. New or recurrent carious lesions should be identified. Assessment of the lesions with a dental explorer not only discloses caries depth but also reveals any associated sensitivity indicative of near or frank exposures of the adjacent pulp. The overall quality of existing restorations should be evaluated because poorly sealed restorations can permit coronal leakage even in the absence of frank caries.

Cracks or fractures should be visualized and explored for loss of tooth structure and separation or mobility between fractured segments. Cracks and fractures may be better visualized with the use of a fiber optic light to transilluminate the fracture line itself; the fracture will stop transmission of the light, delineating a clear break.[20,21] Certain dyes, including vegetable-based versions (eg, To Dye For, Roydent) and methylene blue, can also be used to more clearly delineate coronal fracture lines[21] (Fig 1-6). It can be difficult to assess the depth of unseparated fracture lines running mesiodistally in posterior teeth due to extensions into interproximal spaces. That said, this assessment is crucial to determine the prognosis for a tooth (see chapters 11 and 14 for more on fractured teeth).

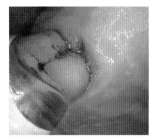

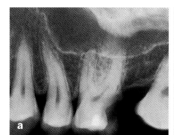

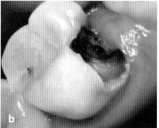

FIG 1-6 Dyes such as methylene blue or vegetable-based dyes can be used to better visualize fracture lines.

FIG 1-7 *(a and b)* The assessment of restorability should begin during the examination process because restorability dictates whether endodontic treatment can or should be provided in the presence of pulpal and periapical pathology. (Photo courtesy of Dr Alicia Willette.)

Whether caries or fractures are noted, clinicians must carefully evaluate restorability (Fig 1-7). Deep caries may violate biologic width, warranting consideration of adjunctive procedures, including crown-lengthening surgery or orthodontic extrusion. Cracks and fractures may similarly violate periodontal structures, warranting adjunctive procedures or extraction.

Just as caries and fractures must be assessed, so too must the color of the tooth or teeth in question. Discoloration of a tooth as compared to neighboring controls can indicate transient pulpal pathology or necrosis. Other discolorations may be present because of endodontic or restorative materials within the crown of the tooth, and although these may not create biologic issues, esthetic concerns may warrant management (Fig 1-8). The patient's level of concern about such discoloration will impact treatment planning, including the potential need for internal bleaching following endodontic treatment. Gray or brown discolorations suggest staining secondary to an infected pulp, whereas pink discolorations suggest resorptive etiologies.[22]

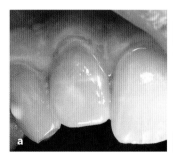

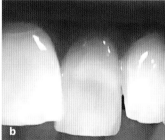

FIG 1-8 Discoloration of the dentition should be assessed as part of every endodontic evaluation. Pink discoloration *(a)* may indicate the development of a resorptive defect, whereas yellow, gray, or brown discoloration *(b)* points to pulpal necrosis or dental materials as the cause of discoloration.

A basic examination of occlusal patterns and contacts can be performed to check for alternative sources of pain as well as potential risk factors for fractures. Bruxism and parafunctional habits can both cause initial endodontic pathology when fractures develop and may cause posttreatment failures if not corrected. The presence of wear facets can similarly indicate parafunction and potential occlusal trauma.

It should be noted that there is a clear etiology for most cases of endodontic pathology. That said, spontaneous pulp necrosis may rarely occur due to adjacent nonodontogenic masses or tumors or surgical care leading to devitalization of roots. Case reports have additionally suggested that pulp necrosis might occur secondary to medical conditions including herpes zoster[23] and sickle cell anemia.[24]

Soft tissue examination

The intraoral soft tissues should be examined during every dental examination. The endodontic exam specifically aims to visualize any signs of intraoral swelling, sinus tracts, or periodontal defects.

- **Swelling:** Acute endodontic infections are associated with the development of swelling (Fig 1-9). Many intraoral swellings are visible, and manual palpation can also help to detect subtle swellings, especially when making comparisons to contralateral tissues. The location of the swelling must be carefully documented. Swelling associated with endodontic pathology is often detectable buccal or facial to the tooth, but palatal or lingual swellings may also develop. Endodontically derived swelling is most often located adjacent to the root apex of the affected tooth. Swelling located closer to the gingival margin raises suspicion of periodontal pathology, fractures, or resorptive defects but may also result from periodontal-endodontic infections.[25] As with extraoral swellings, the quality of the swelling as fluctuant or firm should be noted, as well as its dimensions and extension.

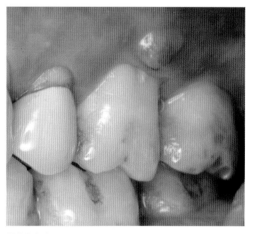

FIG 1-9 Localized swelling associated with endodontic pathology typically occurs adjacent to the apices of the teeth involved. This patient presented with an acute apical abscess associated with the maxillary left first molar. The fluctuant swelling was noted apical to the tooth. (Case courtesy of Dr Coco Lin.)

- **Sinus tracts:** Chronic endodontic infections are associated with sinus tracts. These sinus tracts present as an opening through the alveolar mucosa and may develop on the buccal or lingual/palatal aspects of teeth (Fig 1-10). Like swellings, sinus tracts of endodontic origin are typically located adjacent to the root apex of the affected tooth.[26] Coronally positioned sinus tracts raise suspicion of vertical root fractures or periodontal-endodontic infections. Because sinus tracts may not always present directly adjacent to their source, radiographic tracing with gutta-percha is essential. CBCT imaging represents an alternative radiographic means of assessing sinus tracts; the pathway of bone loss can be followed from the radiographic lesion to the sinus tract opening as visualized clinically.

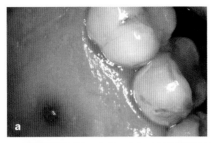
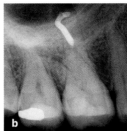
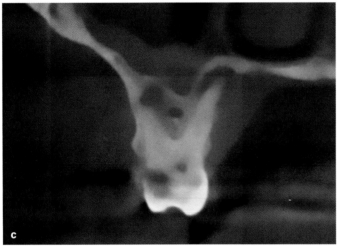

FIG 1-10 Sinus tracts indicate a draining infection, and radiographs must be used to confirm their source. Both periapical imaging utilizing a gutta-percha cone for tracing or CBCT imaging to accurately show the pathology and its tract through bone to soft tissue are acceptable options. In the case shown, a palatal sinus tract (a) was traced to the maxillary right first molar first with gutta-percha and periapical imaging (b) and then via CBCT imaging without tracing (c).

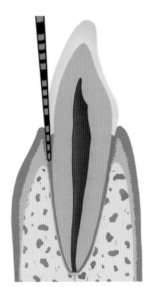

FIG 1-11 A limited periodontal exam, including an assessment of probing depths and mobility, should be performed on all teeth undergoing endodontic evaluation.

- **Periodontal exam:** The soft tissue exam should include a limited periodontal exam, incorporating measurement of circumferential probing depths, detection of associated bleeding or purulence, assessment of mobility, and checking for recession (Fig 1-11). Localized narrow and deep probing measurements are associated with both periodontal-endodontic infections and vertical root fractures.[26] Wider defects or generalized probing depths, on the other hand, are more frequently associated with periodontal disease. Bleeding or purulence on probing can indicate inflammation or infection, respectively. Mobility of a single tooth may indicate severe periodontal disease or a larger endodontic infection with loss of bone support. Mobility of several teeth together suggests alveolar fracture.

Clinical testing

The diagnosis of endodontic pathology requires an accurate replication of the patient's chief complaint. This is accomplished through clinical tests referred to as pulp sensitivity and periapical tests. These tests act as conduits to determine the health of the dental pulp and to detect signs of inflammation of the adjacent periodontal ligament (PDL).[27] The results should be considered as a whole. It is rare that the results of a single test can be used to confer the absolute diagnosis for a tooth. The results of two or more of these tests will confirm the presence or absence of endodontic disease.

As with all types of diagnostic tests, control testing is essential. These results must also be recorded in the patient's chart. Referred pain from endodontic pathology is common, and confirming the source of pain via clinical and radiographic exam findings is essential. Referral patterns include pain originating in neighboring teeth or even teeth in the opposing arch.[28] When the pain is difficult to localize, testing should be completed on all teeth in the suspected arch as well as the opposing arch. Contralateral teeth may be used as controls when neighboring controls are unavailable or perhaps have been previously endodontically treated. Consideration should be given to the type of restoration on control teeth because teeth with indirect restorations or metallic restorations may globally exhibit stronger responses to thermal testing than those with full-coverage restorations, particularly ceramic restorations. Clinicians must never ignore the possibility that more than one tooth may be the source of symptoms. Figure 1-12 provides an example of control selection.

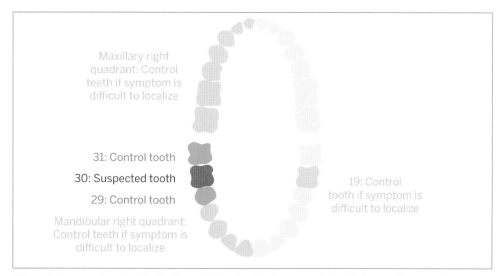

FIG 1-12 An example of control teeth used when testing for suspected pathology in the mandibular right first molar. At the very least, the adjacent second molar and second premolar should be tested as control teeth. In patients with poorly localized pain, the area of testing should be expanded to include the remaining teeth in the quadrant (teeth 25 to 28), as well as teeth in the opposing arch (teeth 2 to 8) to rule out referred pain. The mandibular left first molar can also be used as a control tooth; pulp sensitivity tests and PDL tests should provoke similar responses in the contralateral tooth.

PULP SENSITIVITY TESTS

Testing modalities that can be used to ascertain the health or disease of the pulp tissue include cold testing, heat testing, and electric pulp testing. Pulp sensitivity testing measures a response to conduit measures of nerve sensibility. Presently, no assessment methods for the true measures of pulp vitality are available for use in routine clinical

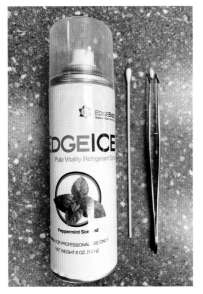

FIG 1-13 The armamentarium for pulp sensitivity testing should include a refrigerant spray (eg, EdgeIce, EdgeEndo) and either a cotton-tipped applicator or cotton pellet.

practice, but modalities are under investigation in laboratory settings. For now, the term "pulp sensitivity testing" is more accurate than "pulp vitality testing."

As a result of testing limitations and the fact that the presence of vital tissues does not always correspond to a response to tests, false positive and false negative results are possible. Limitations in accuracy must be considered whenever inconsistent test results arise, and a diagnosis should never be made based solely on the results of sensitivity testing. Pulp sensitivity tests are notoriously inaccurate in immature teeth[29] and immediately following traumatic dental injuries.[30] Consequently, extra care must be taken when making a diagnosis with these comorbidities.

Cold testing is the most accurate pulp sensitivity test currently available.[31] Refrigerant sprays are considered the safest and most convenient and effective means of cold testing.[31,32] These can be delivered to the surface of the tooth using either cotton-tipped applicators or a cotton pellet held with cotton pliers (Fig 1-13). Because the buccal or facial surface balances the needs for accessibility and proximity to the pulp chamber, it is the surface of choice for cold testing. That said, the occlusal and lingual or palatal surfaces can be tested when an initial response is not detected. A common issue with cold testing is insufficient application of the refrigerant spray to the cotton, which may not elicit a response. Thus, it is important to ensure that the delivery device is sufficiently soaked in cold spray, which may require several seconds of spraying to enhance test accuracy.

Patients should be instructed to raise their hand to communicate the sensation of cold or pain resulting from the test and to keep their hand raised until the sensation diminishes to allow for detection of both the presence and duration of the response. Additionally, patients should be asked to compare the intensity of the sensation felt after each tooth is tested in order to determine if a tooth exhibits a heightened or reduced response compared to controls. Although cold testing may be less accurate on teeth restored with full-coverage restorations,[33] testing should still be completed because many heavily restored teeth will continue to exhibit a response.[34] Ultimately, comparison with similarly restored controls allows for the best assessment of what is normal for the individual patient.

Although heat testing is not as accurate as cold testing,[31] it is useful when heat sensitivity is part of the patient's chief complaint. Heat sensitivity is most commonly reported in teeth with symptomatic irreversible pulpitis or necrosis and has also been reported in previously treated teeth due to the presence of untreated anatomy.[35] Heated gutta-percha is the safest and most effective means for heat testing.[36] This can be done by heating gutta-percha over a flame on a plastic instrument or by using a commercially available heat testing tip with an obturation downpack device. The commercially available tips are considered the safest means for heat testing at this time (Fig 1-14).

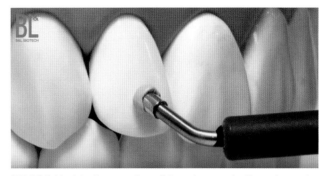

FIG 1-14 Heat testing may be safely and conveniently performed with a commercially available welled tip attached to an obturation downpack device. (Photo courtesy of B&L Biotech.)

Electric pulp testing (EPT) is an adjunctive pulp sensitivity test that is best used to confirm the presence or absence of sensitive, and presumably vital, tissue in a tooth (Fig 1-15). EPT should not be used in teeth without exposed enamel or cementum because the electrical impulse will be impeded by any foreign material barriers, including restorative materials.[31] Historically, it was advised not to use EPT in patients with pacemakers, but there is no published evidence that EPT units interfere with pacemaker devices.[37] That said, as with all medical devices, confirmation of safety with the pacemaker manufacturer is advised.

EPT units display a readout corresponding to the electric current, ranging from 0 to 80. If a response is felt in that range, especially if it is similar to that of a control tooth, the presence of vital tissue is inferred. If no response is detected during the full duration of the test up to a readout of 80, the absence of vital pulp tissue is inferred. Specific numbers for readouts are not indicative of normal or inflamed tissue, underscoring the need for careful comparison with control teeth.

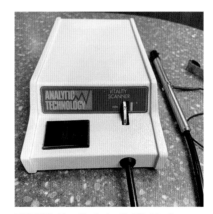

FIG 1-15 Kerr Endodontic Vitality Scanner 2006. Electric pulp testing is a useful and safe pulp sensitivity test to confirm the presence or absence of sensitive tissue within a tooth.

In applying EPT, an electric circuit is created by use of a ground and an electrode. The electrode end of the unit, coated in toothpaste to maximize conduction, should be applied to the cusp tip or incisal edge of the exposed enamel, while the opposing ground component should be rested on the contralateral commissure of the lip to complete the circuit. The electrode applies electric current, increasing on a logarithmic scale, to the exposed tooth structure; it should be removed once the patient reports a response. Patients should be advised to raise their hand to indicate the sensation as soon as it is felt so that the electrode can be removed.

False positives and negatives are common with EPT.[31] The test may be wholly unreliable in that no tooth is responsive in an individual patient. Other patients may report a late sensation of "vibration" in a nonvital tooth, which differs from the responses in presumed

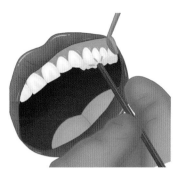

FIG 1-16 Percussion tests can be performed with a mirror handle as depicted. In symptomatic teeth, digital pressure can be used to assess percussion response. (Image courtesy of My Dental Key.)

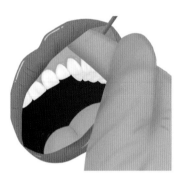

FIG 1-17 Palpation testing can be used not only to assess symptoms resulting from apical inflammation but also to detect swelling and other anatomical abnormalities. (Image courtesy of My Dental Key.)

normal controls. EPT is generally not a reliable test in immature teeth because the nerves responsive to the test develop around the time of root maturation.[29] EPT may, however, be more reliable than thermal tests in teeth exhibiting pulpal canal obliteration or calcification because it relies on ionic changes in nerves rather than dentinal tubular fluid movement, which is the basis for thermal responses.[38]

PERIAPICAL TESTS

Periapical tests represent the gold standard for assessing inflammation within the periodontium. Typical testing modalities include percussion testing, palpation testing, and bite testing. Positive findings for periapical testing must be considered alongside pulp sensitivity tests. Although abnormalities are common with endodontic disease extending into the periapex, abnormal periapical test results may derive from non-endodontic pathology, including periodontal disease, acute traumatic injuries, and occlusal trauma.[39]

Percussion testing is classically performed with a metal mirror handle struck firmly on the surface of the tooth. For extremely sensitive teeth, testing should begin with light manual pressure with the clinician's finger before moving to the more noxious metal instrument (Fig 1-16). Because percussion sensitivity can differ depending on the surface tapped, a suspected tooth can be percussed on the occlusal, facial/buccal, and palatal/lingual surfaces. Teeth without inflammation of the periapical tissues should not exhibit pain on percussion. Teeth with positive percussion tests are said to have mechanical allodynia, or a painful response to a normally non-painful stimulus.[40] This test allows for localization of periapical inflammation because, unlike bite testing, it allows for testing one arch at a time. That said, the teeth adjacent to a very percussion-tender tooth may also exhibit mild sensitivity if inflammation has spread to adjacent structures.

Manual palpation of the soft tissues overlying root structure can not only reveal sensitivity of the periapical structures caused by inflammation but can also facilitate the detection of swelling, bony expansion, or other asymmetries (Fig 1-17). Because the root apices most often sit proximally to the buccal or facial cortical plates, palpation tenderness is most often noted in these areas. That said, examination of the lingual or palatal mucosa is also advisable to rule out pathology in these areas.

Bite sensitivity can be associated with periapical inflammation or cracked or fractured teeth.[39] Testing is performed using either a cotton roll, a cotton-tipped applicator, or a commercially available plastic tester such as the Tooth Slooth (Professional Results) or Fracfinder (Denbur), which allows for testing of individual cusps (Fig 1-18). Unlike percussion testing, bite testing cannot reliably localize symptoms to the maxilla or mandible.

Documentation of clinical findings is a crucial part of clinical practice both for medicolegal reasons and to consolidate information for diagnosis and follow-up. Creating a system for documentation that organizes numerous data points is essential. Depending on the established protocols in a practice setting, recordkeeping may take the form of a narrative, a table (Table 1-2), or a hybrid of both. Regardless of the means utilized, shorthand characters like "+" and "-" are often used to record clinical findings.

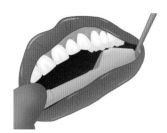

FIG 1-18 Biting tests should replicate a patient's biting sensitivity complaints. Commercially available bite sticks can be used for this test, but cotton rolls and cotton-tipped applicators may also be used. (Image courtesy of My Dental Key.)

TABLE 1-2 Example compilation of diagnostic testing results for the mandibular right quadrant

Tooth	29	30	31
Cold	+	−	+
Percussion	−	+	−
Palpation	−	+	−
Biting	−	+	−

"+" signs indicate positive test results, whereas "−" signs indicate negative responses to tests. An alternative shorthand narrative for the same results would state: 30 exam: Perc +, Palp +, Biting +, Cold −; results for 29 and 30 WNL.

Radiographic examination

The final portion of the objective examination is the radiographic exam. Radiographs should adequately visualize both crown and root structures. Radiographic findings should provide further clues as to the etiology of endodontic disease. Standard imaging in endodontics includes bitewing and periapical radiographs, though CBCT is becoming increasingly relevant in endodontic diagnosis.[41,42]

2D imaging

2D radiography, including periapical, bitewing, and panoramic radiographs (Fig 1-19), remains the standard in dentistry and in endodontic diagnosis. Images must be of sufficient quality to provide accurate diagnostic information.

- **Periapical radiographs:** These images represent the gold standard radiograph for endodontic diagnosis. High-quality images should depict the full crown and root of the tooth in question. If apical periodontitis is present, the entirety of the radiolucency must be visible within the image. When relying on periapical imaging alone for endodontic diagnosis, multiple images taken from varying horizontal and vertical angulations are recommended for improved diagnostics, visualization, and localization.[43]

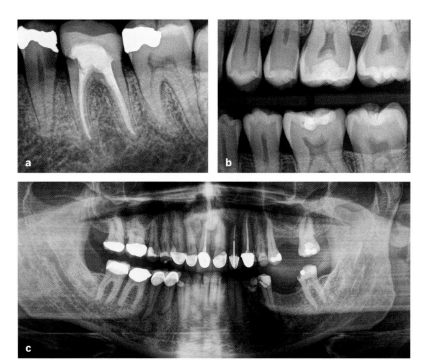

FIG 1-19 2D radiographs include *(a)* pericapical, *(b)* bitewing, and *(c)* panoramic radiographs. Periapical images remain the standard of care in endodontic diagnosis.

- **Bitewing radiographs:** These images are a useful adjunct to periapical images in endodontic diagnosis. They more accurately depict the proximity of caries, restorative margins, and coronal fractures to the pulp. This assessment is critical both to predict carious exposures and to assess the restorability of the tooth in question. Bitewings also provide a more accurate representation of periodontal bone heights. Furthermore, they may uniquely show external cervical resorption when it presents on the mesial or distal aspects of a tooth. Bitewings are especially useful in endodontic assessment because they present the accurate size, shape, and localization of the pulp chamber.[44]
- **Panoramic radiographs:** Panoramic radiographs have limited utility in endodontic diagnosis given issues with poor resolution and anatomical noise. Their utility lies in the work-up of traumatic dental injuries, particularly in evaluating for alveolar, mandibular, and condylar fractures.[45] That said, clinicians who routinely take panoramic radiographs for their patients should examine them for evidence of endodontic pathology.

2D images are limited by structural overlap, particularly of adjacent anatomy,[46] geometric distortion,[47] and challenges in localization of findings. Lesions must either be large[48] or extend through cortical bone in order to be visualized.[46] Localizing findings can be challenging with 2D radiographs and requires use of the Buccal Object Rule (also known as Clark's Rule or the Same Lingual Opposite Buccal [SLOB] Rule), which employs multiple angled radiographs.[49] With this technique, pathology on the lingual or palatal aspects of the tooth will move in the same direction as the x-ray tube head, whereas pathology on the buccal aspect will move in the opposite direction (Fig 1-20).

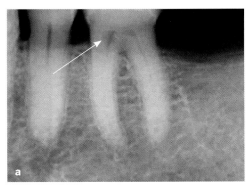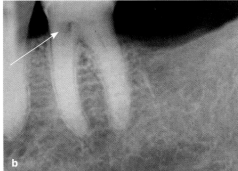

FIG 1-20 The use of multiple angled radiographs can help localize findings to the buccal or lingual aspect of a tooth. This is referred to as Clark's Rule or the SLOB Rule. Pathology on the lingual aspect of the tooth will move in the same direction as the x-ray tube, whereas pathology on the buccal aspect will move in the opposite direction. In this instance, the coronal radiolucency noted in a shifted mesially in image b when the x-ray tube was moved distally, indicating that the pathology is located on the buccal aspect because it moved in the opposite direction of the tube.

3D imaging

CBCT imaging is not yet the standard of care in endodontic diagnosis, but its utility has become more apparent with broader usage. Ultimately, 3D imaging overcomes the myriad limitations of 2D radiography, including structural overlap, geometric distortion, and the limited ability to localize pathology in space (Fig 1-21). CBCT imaging possesses greater sensitivity than periapical films and can be used to detect pathology in earlier stages of development.[50–52] CBCT images are also dimensionally accurate,[52] eliminating the geometric and spatial distortion associated with 2D images and allowing for accurate visualization of anatomical relationships. CBCT imaging does, however, have limitations. The increased cost and reduced availability of the technology can limit its use. Furthermore, capturing images takes between 20 and 40 seconds, and patients with special needs, pediatric patients, and those with tremors may have difficulty keeping still long enough for image capture.

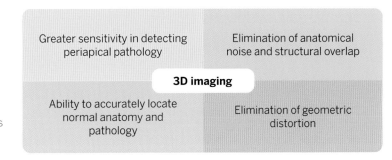

FIG 1-21 Advantages of 3D imaging over 2D imaging.

Greater sensitivity in detecting periapical pathology

Elimination of anatomical noise and structural overlap

3D imaging

Ability to accurately locate normal anatomy and pathology

Elimination of geometric distortion

Many patients have concerns regarding radiation dosage with CBCT imaging because they are aware of the high radiation doses associated with medical CTs. Generally speaking, although doses may vary among models, the limited field of view CBCT machines used routinely in endodontics impart radiation dosages that are only nominally more than the dosages from multiple 2D images often used for endodontic diagnosis.[53–55] That

Examination Protocols

said, not every case requires multiple periapical images, and following the principles of ALARA (as low as reasonably achievable), the lowest radiation dosage appropriate for diagnosis and treatment should be utilized.[56]

CBCT images provide radiographic data in three orthogonal planes: the axial, the coronal, and the sagittal. The axial plane is viewed from the patient's toes to their head, the coronal from anterior to posterior, and the sagittal from the patient's lateral side (Fig 1-22). Images must be interpreted in their entirety, including all soft and hard tissues depicted. Consequently, clinicians must be familiar with normal soft and hard tissue anatomy as visualized in three dimensions, including extragnathic structures. Depending on the area of exposure, CBCT imaging has the potential to showcase both normal anatomical structures and potential pathology that may be outside the routine scope of dental practice. Inexperienced clinicians should consider additional training and, in certain cases, consult with an oral and maxillofacial radiologist for an image overread, particularly when aberrant findings are found.

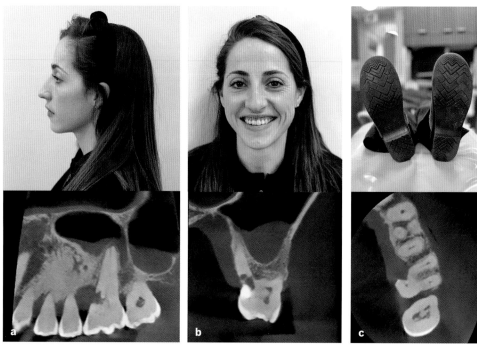

FIG 1-22 CBCT images are evaluated in three planes: the sagittal, the coronal, and the axial. (a) The sagittal plane is a lateral view of the patient, (b) the coronal plane is an anteroposterior view of the patient, and (c) the axial view is from the patient's feet.

The indications for CBCT imaging are wide ranging (Box 1-1). When available, CBCT imaging can be considered routine in the diagnosis of traumatic dental injuries, suspected resorption, root fractures, and in previously endodontically treated teeth, particularly when retreatment or apical microsurgery is being considered.[41,42,57] CBCT imaging is also recommended when existing clinical and radiographic means are insufficient to make a definitive diagnosis.[41,42] Furthermore, images are useful intraoperatively to address challenging anatomical configurations or suspected complications like perforations or instrument separation.[41,42,57,58] Lastly, CBCT can be considered for follow-up imaging, particularly when it was utilized during the diagnostic workup[41,42] (Fig 1-23).

BOX 1-1 Indications for CBCT imaging in endodontics[41,42]

- When existing clinical and radiographic means are insufficient to make a definitive diagnosis
- Assessment of previously endodontically treated teeth, particularly when considering retreatment or apical microsurgery
- Assessment of traumatic dental injuries
- Evaluation of root resorption
- Evaluation for fracture pathology
- Intraoperative location of calcified canals or complication assessment (eg, perforations, separated instruments)
- Follow-up, particularly when CBCT imaging was utilized during the diagnostic work-up

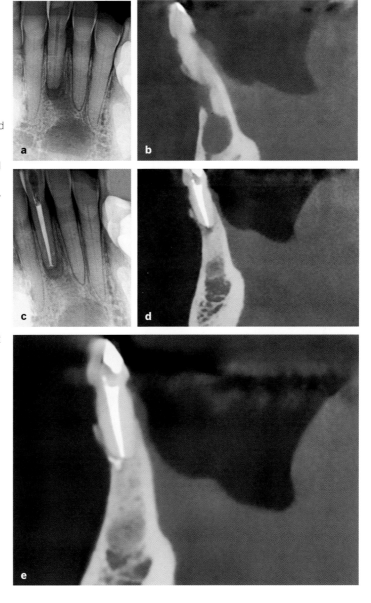

FIG 1-23 CBCT imaging can prove useful in radiographic follow-up after endodontic treatment, particularly when it was employed during diagnosis. (a and b) This patient presented with a large and unusually shaped periapical radiolucency associated with a necrotic tooth, as seen on the periapical radiograph and the sagittal section of CBCT imaging. (c) NSRCT was completed, and close follow-up was warranted to determine if surgical intervention would be needed. (d) The early CBCT follow-up at 3 months demonstrated signs of bone fill that would not likely have been apparent with 2D periapical imaging. (e) Complete apical healing was noted at the 1-year follow-up.

Although useful, CBCT images have several limitations. They are subject to artifacts creating scatter and distortion, particularly around dense, and especially metallic, restorative materials. As a result, their utility is limited in the detection of recurrent caries and especially the detection of lateral root pathology or suspected root fractures when metal posts are present.[59,60] The application of filters and artificial intelligence are active areas of research to improve upon these limitations.[61]

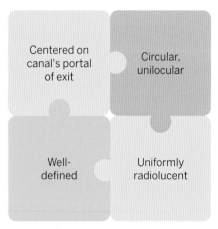

FIG 1-24 Radiographic characteristics of endodontic pathology.

Centered on canal's portal of exit

Circular, unilocular

Well-defined

Uniformly radiolucent

Radiographic interpretation

In describing any radiographic lesion, attention should be paid to the lesion's localization, periphery and shape, internal structure, and effects on surrounding structures.[62] Lesions of endodontic origin (LEOs) have a characteristic appearance in both 2D and 3D imaging (Figs 1-24 and 1-25). Most LEOs are radiolucent. LEOs will be centered on the canal's portal of exit, which may coincide with the radiographic apex or be off center, depending on canal anatomy. LEOs are well-defined, unilocular, and uniformly radiolucent. Early LEOs present as PDL widening localized to the apical portion of the PDL. Less commonly, LEOs may present as radiopacities. This is referred to as condensing osteitis, wherein a localized sclerotic reaction develops in response to chronic pulpal inflammation or infection (Fig 1-26), and is distinct from other periradicular radiopacities not associated with endodontic disease, including cemento-osseous dysplasia, dense bone islands, hypercementosis, and cementoblastomas.

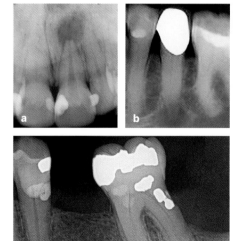

FIG 1-25 (a to c) Examples of radiolucent lesions of endodontic origin. They present as well-defined, unilocular, and uniform radiolucencies centered around the canal's portal of exit.

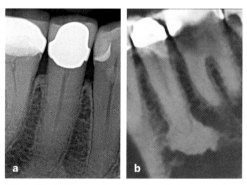

FIG 1-26 While most lesions of endodontic origin are radiolucent, condensing osteitis represents a radiopacity of endodontic origin and can be seen in periapical (a) and CBCT (b) images. In these cases, a localized sclerotic reaction develops in response to chronic pulpal inflammation or infection.

Radiographs cannot differentiate between the histologic diagnoses of cysts, granulomas, or other pathology.[63-65] Therefore, radiographic findings must be taken together with clinical test results to establish a diagnosis.[66] When clinical findings do not line up with pathology of endodontic origin, clinicians should consider the possibility of nonendodontic sources of pathology, including radiolucencies and radiopacities. Questionable radiographic findings, in particular, may be reviewed by an oral radiologist who can provide expertise in radiographic diagnosis of nonendodontic pathology.

Another dental finding that must be documented if visualized is pulp canal obliteration (PCO), often referred to as *calcification* (Fig 1-27). This can develop secondary to pulpal injury or irritation, systemic disease, or dental trauma.[67-72] PCO is not pathologic in and of itself but should be documented. If endodontic treatment is needed, PCO can significantly increase case complexity.[73] Because modern endodontic care with either magnification and ultrasonics or apical microsurgery can accommodate treatment of even the most calcified cases, preventive root canal therapy is not justifiable.

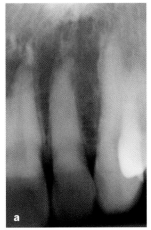 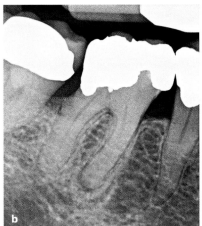

FIG 1-27 PCO, often referred to as *calcification*, is radiographically visible but does not require treatment in the absence of other pulpal or periapical pathology. It may develop in response to trauma (*a*) or pulpal irritation secondary to restorative care (*b*).

Radiographs can also be used to visualize both resorption and fracture pathology. These entities are discussed in more detail in chapters 11, 12, and 14.

Intraoral photography

Intraoral photography is a useful tool for documentation and for communication between clinicians and patients. Patients presenting with swelling or a sinus tract may benefit from "seeing" their infection. Furthermore, clinicians can benefit from documentation to which they can compare healing at future visits (Fig 1-28). Coronal fractures and caries can be well visualized by high-quality photography. Additionally, coronal discoloration may be detected and monitored. Any patient considering nonvital bleaching should be photographed so that treatment progression can be monitored. Intraoral photography can similarly monitor for re-eruption of intrusively luxated teeth or intrusion of teeth undergoing replacement resorption.

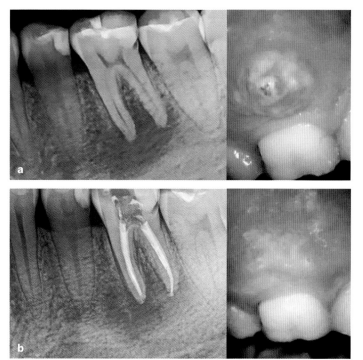

FIG 1-28 Intraoral photography allows clinicians to communicate dental findings, such as the presence *(a)* and healing *(b)* of a sinus tract, to both patients and other clinicians alike.

Adjunctive Examination Tools

When traditional means of diagnosis, including the patient history and clinical and radiographic exams, are insufficient to make a definitive diagnosis, adjunctive methods exist to aid in the diagnostic process.

Selective anesthesia

When clinical testing alone cannot be used to pinpoint the origin of pain, selective anesthesia can be utilized.[25,74] Additionally, selective anesthesia can effectively rule out endodontic sources of pain, allowing for consideration of referral from nonodontogenic sources. Local anesthetic agents should be administered following usual methodologies (namely, infiltration and block anesthesia) with careful strategies to maximize the information gained. Ultimately, the result of effective selective anesthesia is the elimination of a patient's pain from anesthetic effects. Because PDL injections have the effect of anesthetizing neighboring teeth, they are considered inappropriate for selective anesthesia.[75]

Selective anesthesia should begin in the maxilla (Fig 1-29). Local infiltration methods in the maxilla should move mesial to distal because the anesthesia provided by posterior infiltration in the maxilla is more widely distributed. As teeth are ruled out as the source of pain, the injections can proceed posteriorly, moving to infiltrations on the most mesial suspected tooth in the mandible. Mandibular block anesthesia should be the last means utilized given the potential for a broader anesthetic effect.

| Anterior maxillary infiltration | Posterior maxillary infiltration | Anterior mandibular infiltration | Inferior alveolar nerve block |

FIG 1-29 For the greatest effect, selective anesthesia techniques should start narrow with localized methods of anesthesia and then widen sequentially, with block anesthesia techniques last.

Once a patient confirms that their pain has been resolved, findings may be combined with hypotheses based on the prior subjective and objective findings, and a definitive diagnosis can be made. Selective anesthesia itself is palliative beyond these diagnostic effects, and its use as a diagnostic aid is often appreciated by the patient in terms of pain relief. It may even immediately precede delivery of definitive care. When treatment must be delayed, long-acting anesthetic agents like bupivacaine may be employed for selective anesthesia to give a greater duration of analgesia. A selective anesthesia case is presented in Fig 1-30.

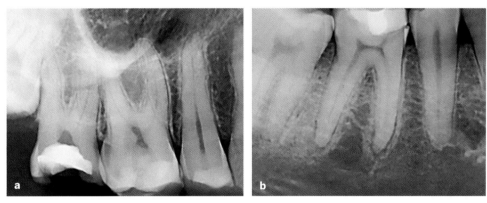

FIG 1-30 Selective anesthesia was used to determine the source of pain in a patient presenting with poorly localized, radiating pain on the right side. Both teeth 2 and 30 were tender to percussion, and neither were responsive to cold; however, testing of both teeth failed to replicate the patient's symptoms. Administration of local infiltration adjacent to tooth 2, with a prior history of pulpotomy, had no effect on the pain. Secondary administration of mandibular block anesthesia relieved pain, allowing the clinician to deliver emergent nonsurgical root canal therapy on tooth 30 as a means of definitive pain relief.

Testing on another day

Clinicians should never feel pressured to make a definitive diagnosis without replication of a patient's symptoms. Occasionally, the intermittent nature of endodontic symptoms in early stages of disease or the use of ibuprofen by a patient prior to presentation[7] will prevent replication of symptoms during an exam. Endodontic symptoms typically localize and become more consistent with time, and instructions can be given to avoid the use of interfering analgesics to better allow for accurate testing. The timing of the follow-up appointment should reflect the severity of symptoms; follow-up may be the following day or up to several weeks later depending on the situation. In certain cases, reimaging may be undertaken, but considering the principles of ALARA, a reasonable interval of time should pass before exposing the patient to additional radiation to confirm likely radiographic changes.

References

1. Abou-Rass M. The stressed pulp condition: An endodontic-restorative diagnostic concept. J Prosthet Dent 1982;48:264–267.
2. Yavorek A, Bhagavatula P, Patel K, Szabo A, Ibrahim M. The incidence of root canal therapy after full coverage restorations: A 10-year retrospective study. J Endod 2020;46:605–610.
3. Valderhaug J, Jokstad A, Ambjørnsen E, Norheim PW. Assessment of the periapical and clinical status of crowned teeth over 25 years. J Dent 1997;25:97–105.
4. Saunders WP, Saunders EM. Prevalence of periradicular periodontitis associated with crowned teeth in an adult Scottish subpopulation. Br Dent J 1998;185:137–140.
5. Kontakiotis EG, Filippatos CG, Stefopoulos S, Tzanetakis GN. A prospective study of the incidence of asymptomatic pulp necrosis following crown preparation. Int Endod J 2015;48:512–517.
6. Cheung GSP, Lai SCN, Ng RPY. Fate of vital pulps beneath a metal-ceramic crown or a bridge retainer. Int Endod J 2005;38:521–530.
7. Read JK, McClanahan SB, Khan AA, Lunos S, Bowles WR. Effect of ibuprofen on masking endodontic diagnosis. J Endod 2014;40:1058–1062.
8. Gupta N, Grewal MS, Gairola M, Grewal S, Ahlawat P. Dental pulp status of posterior teeth in patients with oral and oropharyngeal cancer treated with radiotherapy: 1-year follow-up. J Endod 2018;44:549–554.
9. Lin S, Hoffman R, Nabriski O, Moreinos D, Dummer PMH. Management of patients receiving novel antithrombotic treatment in endodontic practice: Review and clinical recommendations. Int Endod J 2021;54:1754–1768.
10. Kaplovitch E, Dounaevskaia V. Treatment in the dental practice of the patient receiving anticoagulation therapy. J Am Dent Assoc 2019;150:602–608.
11. Katz H. Endodontic implications of bisphosphonate-associated osteonecrosis of the jaws: A report of three cases. J Endod 2005;31:831–834.
12. Ruggiero SL, Fantasia J, Carlson E. Bisphosphonate-related osteonecrosis of the jaw: Background and guidelines for diagnosis, staging and management. Oral Surg Oral Med Oral Pathol Oral Radiol Endod 2006;102:433–441.
13. Chrcanovic BR, Reher P, Sousa AA, Harris M. Osteoradionecrosis of the jaws—A current overview—Part 1. Oral Maxillofac Surg 2010;14:3–16.
14. Fouad AF, Burleson J. The effect of diabetes mellitus on endodontic treatment outcome: Data from an electronic patient record. J Am Dent Assoc 2003;134:43–51.
15. Otto CM, Nishimura RA, Bonow RO, et al. 2020 ACC/AHA Guideline for the management of patients with valvular heart disease: A Report of the American College of Cardiology/American Heart Association Joint Committee on Clinical Practice Guidelines. Circulation 2021;143:e72–e227 [erratum 2021;143:e229].
16. Wilson WR, Gewitz M, Lockhart PB, et al. Prevention of Viridans group streptococcal infective endocarditis: A scientific statement from the American Heart Association. Circulation 2021;143:e963–e978.
17. Steelman R. Rapid physical assessment of the injured child. J Endod 2013;39(3 Suppl):S9–S12.
18. Teasdale G, Jennett B. Assessment and prognosis of coma after head injury. Acta Neurochir (Wien) 1976;34:45–55.
19. Teasdale G, Jennett B. Assessment of coma and impaired consciousness. A practical scale. Lancet 1974;2:81–84.
20. Friedman J, Marcus MI. Transillumination of the oral cavity with use of fiber optics. J Am Dent Assoc 1970;80:801–809.
21. Wright HM Jr, Loushine RJ, Weller RN, Kimbrough WF, Waller J, Pashley DH. Identification of resected root-end dentinal cracks: A comparative study of transillumination and dyes. J Endod 2004;30:712–715.
22. Heithersay GS. Clinical, radiologic, and histopathologic features of invasive cervical resorption. Quintessence Int 1999;30:27-37.
23. Rauckhorst AJ, Baumgartner JC. Zebra. XIX. Part 2. Oral herpes zoster. J Endod 2000;26:469–471.
24. Costa CPS, Thomaz EBAF, Souza SFC. Association between sickle cell anemia and pulp necrosis. J Endod 2013;39:177–181.
25. Berman LH, Rotstein I. Diagnosis. In: Berman LH, Hargreaves KH (eds). Cohen's Pathways of the Pulp, ed 12. St. Louis: Elsevier, 2020:1–33.
26. Rivera E, Walton RE. Cracking the cracked tooth code: Detection and treatment of various longitudinal tooth fractures. Chicago: American Association of Endodontics, 2008.

27. Ricucci D, Loghin S, Siqueira JF Jr. Correlation between clinical and histologic pulp diagnoses. J Endod 2014;40:1932–1939.
28. Bender IB. Pulpal pain diagnosis—A review. J Endod 2000;26:175–179.
29. Fulling HJ, Andreasen JO. Influence of maturation status and tooth type of permanent teeth upon electrometric and thermal pulp testing. Scand J Dent Res 1976;84:286-290.
30. Bhaskar SN, Rappaport HM. Dental vitality tests and pulp status. J Am Dent Assoc 1973;86:409–411.
31. Mainkar A, Kim SG. Diagnostic accuracy of 5 dental pulp tests: A systematic review and meta-analysis. J Endod 2018;44:694–702.
32. White J, Cooley RL. A quantitative evaluation of thermal pulp testing. J Endod 1977;3:453–457.
33. Hazard ML, Wicker C, Qian F, Williamson AE, Teixeira FB. Accuracy of cold sensibility testing on teeth with full-coverage restorations: A clinical study. Int Endod J 2021;54:1008–1015.
34. Miller SO, Johnson JD, Allemang JD, Strother JM. Cold testing through full-coverage restorations. J Endod 2004;30:695–700.
35. Keir DM, Walker WA 3rd, Schindler WG, Dazey SE. Thermally induced pulpalgia in endodontically treated teeth. J Endod 1991;17:38–40.
36. Bierma MM, McClanahan S, Baisden MK, Bowles WR. Comparison of heat-testing methodology. J Endod 2012;38:1106–1109.
37. Wilson BL, Broberg C, Baumgartner JC, Harris C, Kron J. Safety of electronic apex locators and pulp testers in patients with implanted cardiac pacemakers or cardioverter/defibrillators. J Endod 2006;32:847–852.
38. Ketterl W. Age-induced changes in the teeth and their attachment apparatus. Int Dent J 1983;33:262–271.
39. Seltzer S, Bender IB, Nazimov H. Differential diagnosis of pulp conditions. Oral Surg Oral Med Oral Pathol 1965;19:383–391.
40. Owatz CB, Khan AA, Schindler WG, Schwartz SA, Keiser K, Hargreaves KM. The incidence of mechanical allodynia in patients with irreversible pulpitis. J Endod 2007;33:552–556.
41. AAE and AAOMR joint position statement: Use of cone beam computed tomography in endodontics 2015 update. Oral Surg Oral Med Oral Pathol Oral Radiol 2015;120:508–512.
42. AAE and AAOMR joint position statement: Use of cone beam computed tomography in endodontics 2015 update [editorial]. J Endod 2015;41:1393–1396.
43. Brynolf I. Roentgenologic periapical diagnosis. II. One, two or more roentgenograms? Sven Tandlak Tidskr 1970;63:345–350.
44. Robinson D, Goerig AC, Neaverth EJ. Endodontic access: An update, Part I. Compendium 1989;10:290–292, 294–296, 298.
45. American Association of Endodontists. Recommended Guidelines of the American Association of Endodontists for the Treatment of Traumatic Dental Injuries. 2013. https://www.aae.org/specialty/wp-content/uploads/sites/2/2019/02/19_TraumaGuidelines.pdf. Accessed 16 March 2023.
46. Bender IB, Seltzer S. Roentgenographic and direct observation of experimental lesions in bone: II. 1961. J Endod 2003;29:707–712.
47. Vande Voorde HE, Bjorndahl AM. Estimating endodontic "working length" with paralleling radiographs. Oral Surg Oral Med Oral Pathol 1969;27:106–110.
48. Chang L, Umorin M, Augsburger RA, Glickman GN, Jalali P. Periradicular lesions in cancellous bone can be detected radiographically. J Endod 2020;46:496–501.
49. Gutmann JL, Endo C. Clark's Rule vis a vis the buccal object rule: Its evolution & application in endodontics. J Hist Dent 2011;59:12–15.
50. Patel S, Dawood A, Mannocci F, Wilson R, Pitt Ford T. Detection of periapical bone defects in human jaws using cone beam computed tomography and intraoral radiography. Int Endod J 2009;42:507–515.
51. Lofthag-Hansen S, Huumonen S, Gröndahl K, Gröndahl HG. Limited cone-beam CT and intraoral radiography for the diagnosis of periapical pathology. Oral Surg Oral Med Oral Pathol Oral Radiol Endod 2007;103:114–119.
52. Low KMT, Dula K, Bürgin W, von Arx T. Comparison of periapical radiography and limited cone-beam tomography in posterior maxillary teeth referred for apical surgery. J Endod 2008;34:557–562.
53. Ludlow JB, Ivanovic M. Comparative dosimetry of dental CBCT devices and 64-slice CT for oral and maxillofacial radiology. Oral Surg Oral Med Oral Pathol Oral Radiol Endod 2008;106:106–114.
54. Ludlow JB, Timothy R, Walker C, et al. Effective dose of dental CBCT—A meta analysis of published data and additional data for nine CBCT units. Dentomaxillofac Radiol 2015;44:20140197.
55. Pauwels R, Beinsberger J, Collaert B, et al. Effective dose range for dental cone beam computed tomography scanners. Eur J Radiol 2012;81:267–271.
56. Farman AG. ALARA still applies. Oral Surg Oral Med Oral Pathol Oral Radiol Endod 2005;100:395–397.
57. Patel S, Brown J, Semper M, Abella F, Mannocci F. European Society of Endodontology position statement: Use of cone beam computed tomography in endodontics: European Society of Endodontology (ESE) developed by. Int Endod J 2019;52:1675–1678.

58. Fayad MI. The impact of cone beam computed tomography in endodontics: A new era in diagnosis and treatment planning. American Association of Endodontics, 2018. https://www.aae.org/specialty/newsletter/the-impact-of-cone-beam-computed-tomography-in-endodontics-a-new-era-in-diagnosis-and-treatment-planning. Accessed 16 March 2023.

59. Costa FF, Gaia BF, Umetsubo OS, Cavalcanti MGP. Detection of horizontal root fracture with small-volume cone-beam computed tomography in the presence and absence of intracanal metallic post. J Endod 2011;37:1456–1459.

60. Scarfe WC, Levin MD, Gane D, Farman AG. Use of cone beam computed tomography in endodontics. Int J Dent 2009;2009:634567.

61. Setzer FC, Shi KJ, Zhang Z, et al. Artificial intelligence for the computer-aided detection of periapical lesions in cone-beam computed tomographic images. J Endod 2020;46:987–993.

62. Lam EWN, Mallya SM. White and Pharaoh's Oral Radiology: Principles and Interpretation, ed 8. St Louis: Mosby, 2018.

63. Brynolf I. A Histological and Roentgenological Study of the Periapical Region of Human Upper Incisors [thesis]. Stockholm: Almqvist and Wiksell, 1967.

64. Peters E, Lau M. Histopathologic examination to confirm diagnosis of periapical lesions: A review. J Can Dent Assoc 2003;69:598–600.

65. Lalonde ER. A new rationale for the management of periapical granulomas and cysts: An evaluation of histopathological and radiographic findings. J Am Dent Assoc 1970;80:1056–1059.

66. Weissman J, Johnson JD, Anderson M, et al. Association between the presence of apical periodontitis and clinical symptoms in endodontic patients using cone-beam computed tomography and periapical radiographs. J Endod 2015;41:1824–1829.

67. Sener S, Cobankara FK, Akgünlü F. Calcifications of the pulp chamber: Prevalence and implicated factors. Clin Oral Investig 2009;13:209–215.

68. Pettiette MT, Wright JT, Trope M. Dentinogenesis imperfecta: Endodontic implications. Case report. Oral Surg Oral Med Oral Pathol Oral Radiol Endod 1998;86:733–737.

69. Pettiette MT, Zhong S, Moretti AJ, Khan AA. Potential correlation between statins and pulp chamber calcification. J Endod 2013;39:1119–1123.

70. Gold SI. Root canal calcification associated with prednisone therapy: A case report. J Am Dent Assoc 1989;119:523–525.

71. Sayegh FS, Reed AJ. Calcification in the dental pulp. Oral Surg Oral Med Oral Pathol 1968;25:873–882.

72. Edds AC, Walden JE, Scheetz JP, Goldsmith LJ, Drisko CL, Eleazer PD. Pilot study of correlation of pulp stones with cardiovascular disease. J Endod 2005;31:504–506.

73. Robertson A, Andreasen FM, Bergenholtz G, Andreasen JO, Norén JG. Incidence of pulp necrosis subsequent to pulp canal obliteration from trauma of permanent incisors. J Endod 1996;22:557–560.

74. Blicher B, Pryles RL. The use of selective anesthesia in endodontic diagnosis. Compend Contin Educ Dent 2021;42:498–575.

75. White JJ, Reader A, Beck M, Meyers WJ. The periodontal ligament injection: A comparison of the efficacy in human maxillary and mandibular teeth. J Endod 1988;14:508–514.

The Definitive Diagnosis

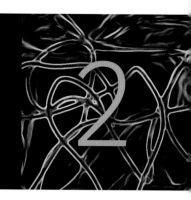

The data collected from the subjective and objective examinations is what directly facilitates the development of a definitive diagnosis. While the great majority of pain and infection in the orofacial region relates to endodontic pathology, clinicians must also be aware of nonendodontic diseases that may present similarly. This chapter reviews the diagnosis of endodontic pathology and its adjuncts, as well as common differential diagnoses.

Diagnosis of Endodontic Pathology

Every endodontic diagnosis consists of two parts: the pulpal diagnosis and the periapical diagnosis (Fig 2-1).[1] These diagnoses are developed based on the results of the clinical and radiographic examinations. The diagnostic terminology for both the pulpal and periapical diagnosis is defined in the glossary of this book, and the clinical test results used to establish these diagnoses are organized in Tables 2-1 and 2-2. The pulpal and periapical diagnoses are separate but related entities. Certain pulpal diagnoses correlate with certain periapical diagnoses (Fig 2-2), and typical patterns emerge in diagnosis.

Pulpal diagnosis

- Normal pulp
- Reversible pulpitis
- Asymptomatic irreversible pulpitis
- Symptomatic irreversible pulpitis
- Necrosis
- Previously treated
- Previously initiated

Periapical diagnosis

- Normal
- Asymptomatic apical periodontitis
- Symptomatic apical periodontitis
- Chronic apical abscess
- Acute apical abscess
- Condensing osteitis

FIG 2-1 Pulpal and periapical diagnoses.[1]

Though diagnosis-specific clinical and radiographic findings are generally well defined, the chief complaint may be variable, particularly for teeth with necrotic pulps or teeth that were previously endodontically treated or where endodontic treatment was initiated.

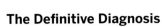

TABLE 2-1 Subjective and objective findings corresponding to pulpal diagnostic categories

Pulpal diagnosis	Chief complaint	Thermal testing	Electric pulp testing	Radiographic findings (apex)
Normal	NA	+	+	Normal
Reversible pulpitis	Cold sensitivity	++	+	Normal
Asymptomatic irreversible pulpitis	NA	+ or ++	+	Normal or widened PDL
Symptomatic irreversible pulpitis	Cold and/or heat sensitivity, spontaneous pain, radiating pain	++ with lingering pain	+	Normal, widened PDL, or PARL
Pulp necrosis	Variable	−	−	Normal, widened PDL, or PARL
Previously treated	Variable	− (potential + if untreated anatomy present)	−	Normal, widened PDL, or PARL
Previously initiated	Variable	− (potential + if untreated anatomy present)	−	Normal, widened PDL, or PARL

+ = response similar to controls; ++ = heightened response; − = no response; PDL = periodontal ligament; PARL = periapical radiolucency.

TABLE 2-2 Subjective and objective findings corresponding to periapical diagnostic categories

Periapical diagnosis	Chief complaint	Percussion	Palpation	Radiographic findings (apex)
Normal	NA	−	−	Normal
Symptomatic apical periodontitis	Sensitivity to chewing or pressure	+	+	Normal, widened PDL, or PARL
Asymptomatic apical periodontitis	NA	−	−	Widened PDL or PARL
Chronic apical abscess	Intermittent discharge of pus through sinus tract, minimal discomfort	−	−	PARL
Acute apical abscess	Swelling, rapid onset of pain	+	+	Widened PDL or PARL
Condensing osteitis (rare)	Variable	+/−	+/−	Apical radiopacity

+ = greater sensitivity than controls; − = similar to control responses; PARL = periapical radiolucency; PDL = periodontal ligament.

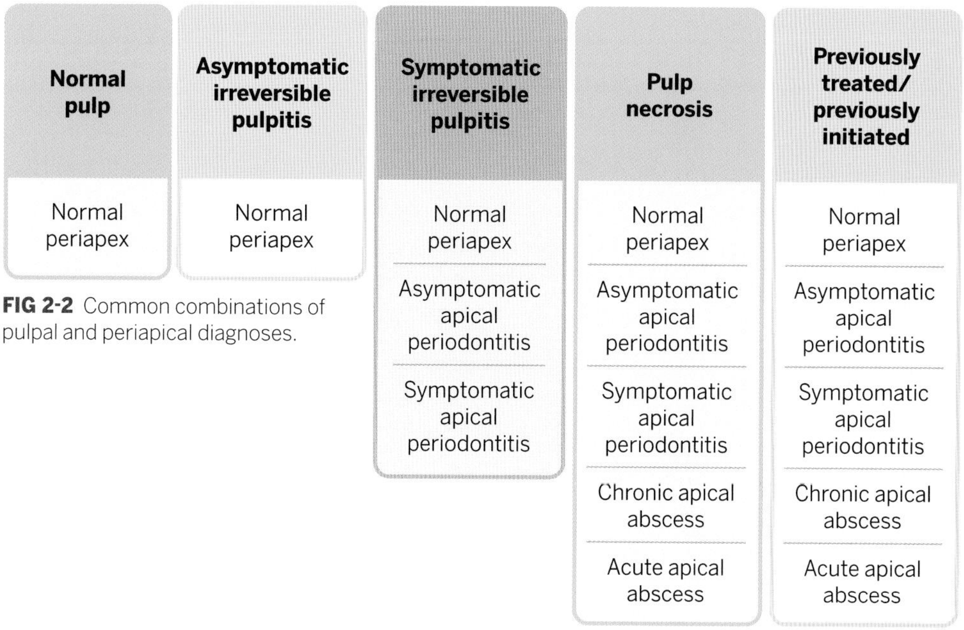

Normal pulp	Asymptomatic irreversible pulpitis	Symptomatic irreversible pulpitis	Pulp necrosis	Previously treated/ previously initiated
Normal periapex	Normal periapex	Normal periapex	Normal periapex	Normal periapex
		Asymptomatic apical periodontitis	Asymptomatic apical periodontitis	Asymptomatic apical periodontitis
		Symptomatic apical periodontitis	Symptomatic apical periodontitis	Symptomatic apical periodontitis
			Chronic apical abscess	Chronic apical abscess
			Acute apical abscess	Acute apical abscess

FIG 2-2 Common combinations of pulpal and periapical diagnoses.

For example, a previously treated tooth containing untreated anatomy may present with a history of heat sensitivity as well as biting tenderness (Fig 2-3). Teeth with vital pulp tissue can similarly present in a myriad of symptomatic and asymptomatic states. Additionally, radiographic findings may be limited by anatomical noise when 2D imaging is used,[2] though CBCT imaging will overcome these limitations to showcase apical pathology whenever present.[3] For example, although periapical radiolucencies in the posterior maxilla are difficult to visualize with periapical imaging due to overlap with the maxillary sinus, CBCT removes this obstruction[4] (Fig 2-4).

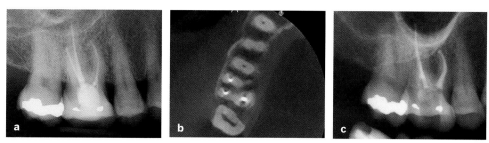

FIG 2-3 Heat sensitivity may develop in previously endodontically treated teeth with untreated canals. *(a)* This patient presented with a chief complaint of heat sensitivity in the right maxilla that was localized to the maxillary right first molar during testing. *(b)* Preoperative CBCT imaging revealed an untreated second mesiobuccal canal. *(c)* Retreatment of the tooth resolved symptoms.

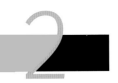

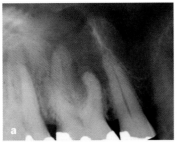 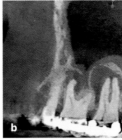

FIG 2-4 Periapical pathology is often much more apparent on CBCT imaging than periapical imaging due to anatomical noise, particularly in the posterior maxilla. In this case, periapical pathology was suspected only in the maxillary right first molar when studied with periapical imaging (a) but confirmed to extend also to the second molar in the sagittal section of CBCT imaging (b).

Adjunctive endodontic diagnoses

Beyond the pulpal and periapical diagnoses defined for each endodontically involved tooth, certain teeth have comorbid conditions either causing the endodontic pathology or increasing its complexity. These adjunctive diagnoses include fractures, resorption, periodontal-endodontic infections, and traumatic dental injuries, described in detail in part III. It is important for the diagnosing clinician to understand and define these conditions because they greatly impact management strategies. Each condition involves its own nuanced diagnostic methodology and criteria and management strategy.

Maxillary sinusitis of endodontic origin

Not only can nonodontogenic sinus pathology produce dental symptoms including thermal sensitivity and pressure discomfort, but dental pathology also has the ability to produce unilateral sinus disease. The latter effect has long been recognized by the medical community. Otolaryngologists often refer patients with unilateral sinusitis for dental evaluation.[5,6] This pathologic extension of endodontic disease into the maxillary sinus, referred to as maxillary sinusitis of endodontic origin (MSEO), should be considered in the context of adjunctive endodontic pathology.[7]

Whenever sinus pathology is present secondary to endodontic disease, patients will often volunteer a history of symptoms including low-grade nasal drainage, congestion, or headaches. Although 2D images rarely depict obvious signs of MSEO given the limitations of this modality in visualizing the sinus,[2] CBCT images readily depict sinus pathology.[4] The earliest and most common sign of MSEO is periapical mucositis, a thickening of the sinus mucosa greater than 2 mm often creating a dome-shaped appearance adjacent to the apex of an infected tooth.[8,9] Later stages of MSEO present with periapical osteoperiostitis, an osteogenic reaction that elevates the sinus periosteum into the sinus. This creates a corticated border superior to the periapical lesion that may close around the lesion or open and drain into the adjacent sinus cavity. MSEO may also present as unilateral opacification of the entire maxillary sinus adjacent to the diseased tooth (Fig 2-5).

Endodontic treatment represents first line therapy for MSEO. It will typically resolve both mild sinonasal symptoms and radiographic sinus pathology[7] (Fig 2-6). If symptoms remain or radiographic findings persist at follow-up, referral to otolaryngology specialists is advised. Patients with severe or chronic sinonasal symptoms or disease should be informed of the potential need for concomitant medical management of sinus disease, usually by way of saline irrigation and topical corticosteroids[10] and possibly surgical interventions to facilitate drainage.[7]

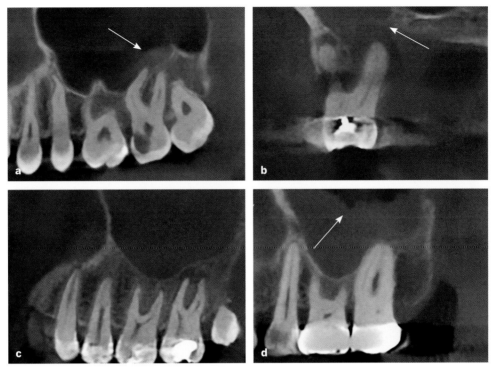

FIG 2-5 *(a)* Endodontic pathology in the posterior maxilla is often associated with periapical mucositis, even before pulp necrosis develops and apical radiolucencies are apparent. *(b)* Late stage MSEO is associated with periapical osteoperiostitis. *(c)* Severe MSEO is associated with unilateral opacification of the sinus. *(d)* Air bubbles may also be noted in the mucosa, suggestive of MSEO.

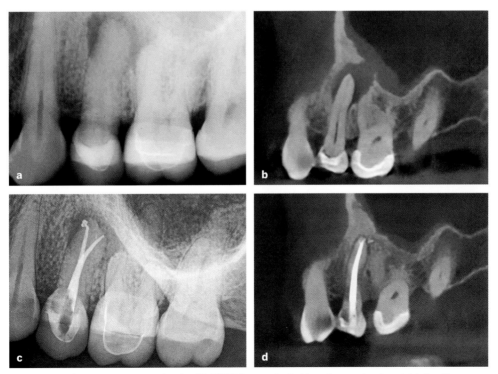

FIG 2-6 MSEO, seen much more clearly with CBCT than periapical imaging, can heal completely with endodontic interventions. *(a and b)* Periapical and CBCT images of MSEO associated with a necrotic maxillary left second premolar. *(c)* The immediate postoperative radiograph. *(d)* The 1-year follow-up CBCT image.

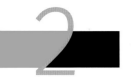

Diagnosis of Nonendodontic Pathology

Inconsistencies in clinical and radiographic findings that do not permit categorization into one of the common pulpal and periapical diagnoses warrant consideration of nonendodontic pathology. This section reviews the common differential diagnosis of the odontogenic and nonodontogenic sources of infection, pain, and radiographic pathology outside of endodontics.

Odontogenic infections

Not all odontogenic infections are endodontically derived. Generally, if the tooth in question exhibits normal responses to pulp sensitivity testing, nonendodontic sources of infection should be suspected. Acute periodontal infections (abscesses) may present with swelling and drainage similar to infections of endodontic origin. In these patients, generalized signs of periodontal disease are often present, including probing depths and radiographic bone loss, in addition to the swelling adjacent to a vital tooth (Fig 2-7). Acute periodontal infections generally present with milder symptoms than infections of endodontic origin and rarely result in extraoral swelling.[11]

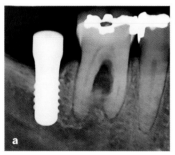 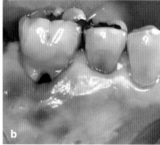

FIG 2-7 *(a and b)* Acute periodontal abscesses are a common odontogenic infection. Swelling of periodontal origin is associated with obvious periodontal disease, as evidenced here by attachment loss and furcal bone loss around the mandibular right first molar and, most notably, by the presence of vital pulp tissue.

Of note, acute or chronic periodontal conditions are distinct from periodontal-endodontic infections. These latter infections constitute chronic endodontic infections either draining through or communicating with concomitant periodontal pathology. Other odontogenic sources of infection include those entities involving only the root surface, such as infected cemental tears, vertical root fractures, or areas of root resorption. Detailed discussions of periodontal-endodontic infections, fractures, and resorption are discussed in part III.

Nonodontogenic infections and swelling

Infections and swelling in the oral cavity may also be nonodontogenic in origin. In these instances, swelling and/or drainage will be noted in the presence of vital or previously endodontically treated teeth. These include infections of the alveolar bone, including osteomyelitis, and infections secondary to osteonecrosis (Fig 2-8). Notably, infection in these cases is not typically derived from apical periodontitis. Furthermore, swelling noted in the oral cavity may be both nonodontogenic and noninfectious. Entities associated with noninfectious swellings include bony cysts and tumors and soft tissue pathologies. Because some of these can be associated with aggressive nonmalignant or even malignant tumors, care in making a complete diagnosis is crucial (Fig 2-9). In most cases, this involves multispecialty referral for biopsy and surgical management.

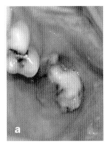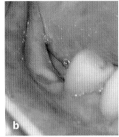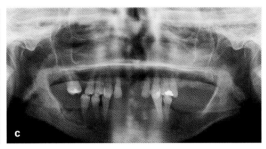

FIG 2-8 Though it is a nonodontogenic infection, medication-related osteonecrosis of the jaw (MRONJ) can present similarly to endodontic pathology with pain and infection in the alveolar bone. This patient presented with infected MRONJ lesions in both the maxillary left *(a)* and mandibular right *(b)* quadrants, secondary to recent extractions *(c)*. The lesions were attributed to her history of Xgeva (Amgen) use secondary to metastatic breast cancer. (Courtesy of Dr Rocco Addante.)

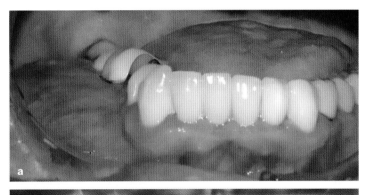
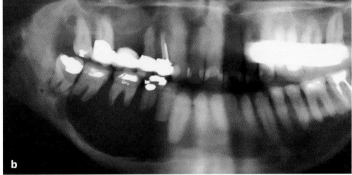

FIG 2-9 *(a and b)* Intraoral swellings may derive from nonodontogenic sources, such as this lower right quadrant swelling relating to an ameloblastoma that was revealed upon excision and biopsy. (Courtesy of Dr Rocco Addante.)

Odontogenic pain

While a large percentage of odontogenic pain is of endodontic origin, other nonendodontic and even nonodontogenic sources of pain exist (Fig 2-10) Typically, nonendodontic odontogenic pain is less intense than pulpally mediated pain. Pain due to dentinal hypersensitivity, shallow fractures, or caries may present with signs and symptoms of reversible pulpitis, namely, cold and/or biting hypersensitivity of short duration. Dental trauma may cause pain representative of inflammation resulting from the acute injury with or without active endodontic involvement. Many of these nonendodontic conditions, including caries, fractures, and pain from acute dental trauma, will progress to endodontic pathology if unaddressed. These lesions exist on a continuum wherein endodontic involvement may become apparent over time, sometimes immediately following interventions meant to treat them (eg, crown preparations) or in the following months or years. Acute periodontal infections, discussed previously, may be associated with sensitivity to cold and pressure and will always present with both obvious signs of periodontal disease and pulp tissues that exhibit normal responses.

Other odontogenic sources	Nonodontogenic sources
• Dental hypersensitivity • Caries • Fracture • Trauma • Occlusal pain • Acute periodontal abscess	• Myofascial pain • Sinus pain • Neurovascular pain (ie, headaches) • Neuropathic pain • Persistent idiopathic facial pain/persistent dentoalveolar pain disorder • Vascular/cardiac pain • Psychogenic pain

FIG 2-10 Common sources of nonendodontic pain.

Nonodontogenic pain

Nonodontogenic sources of pain have a wide variety of presentations and include myofascial pain, sinus pain, neurovascular pain (eg, headaches), neuropathic pain, idiopathic facial pain, vascular and cardiac pain, and psychogenic pain, among others. Typically, these sources of pain cannot be replicated with dental clinical testing and will not be relieved with administration of local anesthetic agents. Additionally, radiographs will present inconsistencies with dental pathology. Whenever nonodontogenic sources of pain are suspected, referral should be made to the appropriate dental or medical specialists.

Myofascial (muscular) pain is characterized by referred pain from the muscles of mastication to the dentition or other orofacial structures. It most commonly involves the masseter muscles, with pain referred to the mandibular molars.[12] Myofascial pain may occur at rest or with movement and can be clinically replicated by palpation of localizable trigger points in the affected muscles.[13] Myofascial pain can be managed by dental professionals familiar with the condition. Therapies may include trigger point injections, injection with botulinum toxin, splint therapy, isometric exercises, pharmacologic treatment with muscle relaxers, and complementary treatments, including massage, acupuncture, and biofeedback.[14,15]

Sinusitis of bacterial, viral, or allergic origin may refer pain to the maxillary posterior dentition.[16,17] Patients with sinusitis characteristically report a sensation of fullness or pressure as well as congestion or nasal drainage. Clinically, these patients will present with pressure tenderness of multiple posterior teeth with normal pulp sensitivity responses. If CBCT imaging is used to make the diagnosis, findings may include mucositis, fluid within the sinus, or generalized opacification, and the absence of periapical changes. Intraoral administration of local anesthetics is ineffective to relieve pain of sinus origin, but decongestants may alleviate symptoms. Patients with nonodontogenic sinusitis should be referred for medical management.[16]

Neurovascular pain (headaches) is another common source of nonodontogenic orofacial pain. This category includes migraines, tension-type headaches, trigeminal autonomic cephalalgias, and other primary headaches.[18,19] These entities can be confused with dental diseases that create referral patterns beyond the dentition. Migraine headaches often present as unilateral, pulsatile pain of moderate to severe intensity lasting anywhere between 4 and 72 hours. They are often preceded by a visual, sensory, or dysphasic aura and may be accompanied by nausea and vomiting, photophobia, and phonophobia.[18] Tension-type headaches tend to present as bilateral tightening in the head and face and are of milder intensity than migraines.[18] They can be differentiated from migraines by their lack of aura, nausea, vomiting, photophobia, and phonophobia. The trigeminal autonomic cephalalgias include cluster headaches and the paroxysmal and continuous hemicrania. They are characterized by autonomic symptoms of the eyes, nose, and face, occurring either episodically or chronically.[18] These and other unmanageable headaches should be immediately referred for medical assessment. The diagnosis and management of neurovascular pain may be complex and warrants the care of physicians.

Neuropathic pain, classically referred to as *trigeminal neuralgia*, is yet another nonodontogenic source of orofacial pain. Neuropathic pain presents as episodic and sudden sharp, shooting, electrical, or stabbing pain following a dermatomal distribution, such as the trigeminal nerve.[19–21] Notably, neuropathic pain does not resolve with anti-inflammatory or narcotic analgesics, which may aid in diagnosis. Causes of neuropathic pain include nerve compression by vascular lesions or tumors, so suspected neuropathic pain warrants medical consultation, both to evaluate for serious underlying causes[22] and for pharmacologic management of its severe symptoms via neurologic mediators.[23]

Persistent idiopathic facial pain (PIFP), also called atypical facial pain, atypical odontalgia, and phantom tooth pain, is a group of nonanatomically distributed painful conditions for which local anesthetic is typically ineffective.[19] Pain is typically of a burning quality and may change location. PIFP is a diagnosis of exclusion made by orofacial pain specialists or neurologists. Persistent dentoalveolar pain (PDAP) disorder describes a similar condition arising either spontaneously or at an extraction site in the absence of clinical or radiographic evidence of other hard or soft tissue pathologies.[24] PDAP is generally unaffected by dental treatment or may represent a new postoperative pain that is distinct from the preoperative symtoms. Both PIFP and PDAP are managed pharmacologically by orofacial pain or neurology experts.

Vascular pain can include temporal arteritis and pain of cardiac origin. Temporal arteritis can cause referred pain to the dentition, along with the classical temporal headache, ocular symptoms, and burning tongue.[25] It is a systemic granulomatous disease often associated with polymyalgia rheumatica. Because this condition can progress to blindness, prompt medical referral is warranted.[25] Similarly, cardiac pain due to angina or myocardial infarction may cause pain in the left mandible experienced upon exertion that may or may not improve with administration of nitroglycerin. Suspected pain of cardiac origin warrants immediate referral to emergency medical services.[26–28]

The final type of nonodontogenic orofacial pain to include in the differential diagnosis is psychogenic pain. Psychogenic pain is a somatoform disorder in which pain somatization occurs independent of other mental health conditions.[29] It differs from malingering in that the patient is not reporting false or grossly exaggerated physical and/or psychological symptoms with the goal of receiving a reward. The psychogenic toothache is a diagnosis of exclusion that can only be made by a psychiatric professional.[30]

Nonendodontic radiographic pathology

Radiographic changes located at the apices of teeth are frequently the result of endodontic pathology, namely, the spread of necrotic pulp tissue remnants and bacteria into the periapical tissues. When clinical finding suggest the presence of normal pulp tissue in teeth with radiographic pathology, consideration of pathology of nonendodontic origin is warranted. Figure 2-11 shows the differential diagnosis for jaw radiolucencies and radiopacities that may mimic endodontic pathosis. Clinical examples of nonendodontic radiolucencies are provided in Fig 2-12, with radiopacities presented in Figs 2-13 and 2-14.

Radiolucencies	Radiopacities
• Ameloblastoma • Aneurysmal bone cyst • Brown tumor of hypoparathyroidism • Cemento-osseous dysplasia (early) • Central giant cell granuloma • Dentigerous cyst • Hemangioma • Langerhans cell histiocytosis • Malignancies (lymphoma, metastatic lesions) • Nasopalatine duct cyst • Odontogenic keratocyst • Odontogenic myxoma • Stafne defect • Traumatic bone cyst	• Ameloblastic fibro-odontoma • Calcifying epithelial odontogenic tumor • Cementifying ossifying fibroma • Cemento-osseous dysplasia (late) • Cementoblastoma • Condensing osteitis • Enostosis • Exostosis • Fibrous dysplasia • Idiopathic osteosclerosis • Odontoma • Osteoma • Osteosarcoma • Osteitis deformans

FIG 2-11 Differential diagnosis for radiolucent and radiopaque jaw lesions.

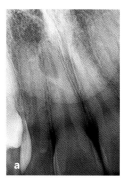 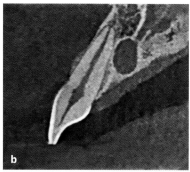

FIG 2-12 *(a)* A radiolucency was noted at the apex of the maxillary right central incisor. The tooth responded normally to pulp sensitivity testing. *(b)* CBCT imaging revealed that the radiolucency was located within the nasopalatine canal and was not confluent with the apex of the tooth. The pathology report indicated that the lesion was a nasopalatine duct cyst. (Courtesy of Dr Stephanie Jue.)

FIG 2-13 *(a)* Although the differential diagnosis included apical periodontitis due to the apical radiolucency, the mandibular left central incisor exhibited a normal response to pulp sensitivity testing. *(b)* The mixed radiolucent-radiodense appearance on CBCT imaging was consistent with periapical cemento-osseous dysplasia.

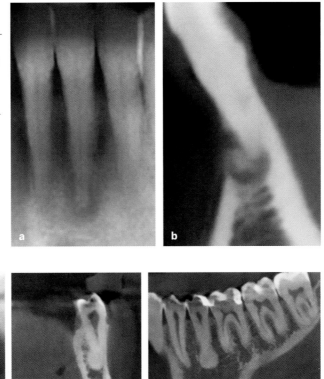

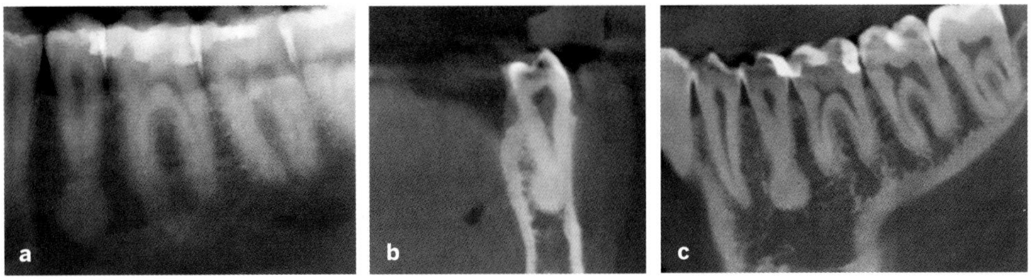

FIG 2-14 *(a)* A radiopacity was noted at the apex of the mandibular right first premolar with periapical imaging, and the tooth exhibited normal responses to pulp sensitivity testing. *(b and c)* CBCT imaging revealed an intact PDL consistent with cementoblastoma, although the differential diagnosis included condensing osteitis, as well as periapical cemento-osseous dysplasia and hypercementosis. Biopsy of the lesion confirmed cementoblastoma as the definitive diagnosis, and extraction of the tooth along with the lesion was indicated.

Radiographic pathology must also include consideration of sinus pathology. While mucositis or sinus opacification is a common finding associated with maxillary sinusitis of endodontic origin, it must be differentiated from nonodontogenic sinus pathology when endodontic pathology is absent in the adjacent teeth. This opacification may be obscured in limited field of view images that fail to show the entirety of the ipsilateral sinus or contralateral structures but should prompt careful diagnostics because the differential *diagnosis* for unilateral opacifications of the sinus includes potentially serious conditions, such as fungal infections and malignancies.[7]

Conclusion

Diagnosis is the foundation of endodontic care. A complete and accurate diagnosis ensures that patients receive the care needed to alleviate their symptoms, whether by endodontic treatment or by appropriate referral to manage nonendodontic conditions. An accurate and complete diagnosis must precede any discussion of the interventions described in part II of this manual.

References

1. American Association of Endodontists. Glossary of Endodontic Terms, ed 10. Chicago: American Association of Endodontists, 2020.
2. Brynolf I. Roentgenologic periapical diagnosis. II. One, two or more roentgenograms? Sven Tandlak Tidskr 1970;63:345–350.
3. Patel S, Dawood A, Mannocci F, Wilson R, Pitt Ford T. Detection of periapical bone defects in human jaws using cone beam computed tomography and intraoral radiography. Int Endod J 2009;42:507–515.
4. Low KMT, Dula K, Bürgin W, von Arx T. Comparison of periapical radiography and limited cone-beam tomography in posterior maxillary teeth referred for apical surgery. J Endod 2008;34:557–562.
5. Patel NA, Ferguson BJ. Odontogenic sinusitis: An ancient but under-appreciated cause of maxillary sinusitis. Curr Opin Otoloaryngol Head Neck Surg 2012;20:24–28.
6. Longhini AB, Branstetter BF, Ferguson BJ. Otolaryngologists, perceptions of odontogenic maxillary sinusitis. Laryngoscope 2012;122:1910–1914.
7. American Association of Endodontists. Maxillary Sinusitis of Endodontic Origin: AAE position statement, 2018. https://www.aae.org/specialty/wpcontent/uploads/sites/2/2018/04/AAE_PositionStatement_MaxillarySinusitis.pdf. Accessed 20 March 2023.
8. Sakir M, Yalcinkaya SE. Associations between periapical health of maxillary molars and mucosal thickening of maxillary sinuses in cone-beam computed tomographic images: A retrospective study. J Endod 2020;46:397–403.
9. Shanbhag S, Karnik P, Shirke P, Shanbhag V. Association between periapical lesions and maxillary sinus mucosal thickening: A retrospective cone-beam computed tomographic study. J Endod 2013; 39:853–857.
10. Fokkens WJ, Lund VJ, Mullol J, et al. EPOS 2012: European position paper on rhinosinusitis and nasal polyps 2012. A summary for otorhinolaryngologists. Rhinology 2012;50:1–12.
11. Berman LH, Rotstein I. Diagnosis. In: Berman LH, Hargreaves KH (eds). Cohen's Pathways of the Pulp, ed 12. St. Louis: Elsevier, 2021:1–33.
12. Wright EF. Referred craniofacial pain patterns in patients with temporomandibular disorder. J Am Dent Assoc 2000;131:1307–1315.
13. Fricton JR, Kroening R, Haley D, Siegert R. Myofascial pain syndrome of the head and neck: A review of clinical characteristics of 164 patients. Oral Surg Oral Med Oral Pathol 1985;60:615–623.
14. Wright EF, Schiffman EL. Treatment alternatives for patients with masticatory myofascial pain. J Am Dent Assoc 1995;126:1030–1039.
15. Khalifeh M, Mehta K, Varguise N, Suarez-Durall P, Enciso R. Botulinum toxin type A for the treatment of head and neck chronic myofascial pain syndrome: A systematic review and meta-analysis. J Am Dent Assoc 2016;147:959.e1–973.e1.
16. Law AS, Nixdorf DR, Mattscheck D. Diagnosis of the nonodontogenic toothache. In: Berman LH, Hargreaves KM (eds). Cohen's Pathways of the Pulp, ed 12. St Louis: Elsevier, 2021:115–138.
17. Shueb SS, Boyer HC, Nixdorf DR. Nonodontogenic "tooth pain" of nose and sinus origin. J Am Dent Assoc 2016;147:457–459.
18. Headache Classification Committee of the International Headache Society (IHS). The International Classification of Headache Disorders, 3rd edition. Cephalalgia 2018;38:1–211.
19. International Classification of Orofacial Pain, 1st edition (ICOP). Cephalalgia 2020;40:129–221.
20. Zakrzewska JM. Diagnosis and differential diagnosis of trigeminal neuralgia. Clin J Pain 2002;18:14–21.
21. De Toledo IP, Conti Réus J, Fernandes M, et al. Prevalence of trigeminal neuralgia: A systematic review. J Am Dent Assoc 2016;147:570.e2–576.e2.
22. Goh BT, Poon CY, Peck RH. The importance of routine magnetic resonance imaging in trigeminal neuralgia diagnosis. Oral Surg Oral Med Oral Pathol Oral Radiol Endod 2001;92:424–429.
23. Tody S, Merrill RL, Matthews J. Intracranial tumor manifesting as mandibular pain: A case report. J Am Dent Assoc 2018;149:481–484.
24. Malacarne A, Spierings ELH, Lu C, Maloney GE. Persistent dentoalveolar pain disorder: A comprehensive review. J Endod 2018;44:206–211.
25. Friedlander AH, Runyon C. Polymyalgia rheumatica and temporal arteritis. Oral Surg Oral Med Oral Pathol 1990;69:317–321.
26. Natkin E, Harrington GW, Mandel MA. Anginal pain referred to the teeth. Report of a case. Oral Surg Oral Med Oral Pathol 1975;40:678–680.
27. Kreiner M, Falace D, Michelis V, Okeson JP, Isberg A. Quality difference in craniofacial pain of cardiac vs dental origin. J Dent Res 2010;89:965–969.
28. Kreiner M, Okeson JP, Michelis V, Lujambio M, Isberg A. Craniofacial pain as the sole symptom of cardiac ischemia: A prospective multicenter study. J Am Dent Assoc 2007;138:74–79.
29. Diagnostic and Statistical Manual of Mental Disorders: DSM-5. Arlington, VA: American Psychiatric Association, 2013.
30. Dworkin SF, Burgess JA. Orofacial pain of psychogenic origin: Current concepts and classification. J Am Dent Assoc 1987;115:565–571.

PART II

Management of Endodontic Pathology

With an established diagnosis, treatment planning and management can begin. Several available treatment options exist for each endodontic diagnosis. The chosen treatment strategy must address the endodontic pathology and restore the affected tooth. This section of the text discusses both endodontic and restorative treatment considerations and protocols.

Diagnosis-Driven Treatment Planning

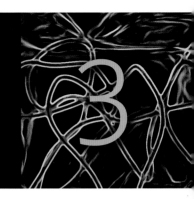

Endodontic treatment planning must be grounded in an understanding of the anticipated prognosis of the proposed treatment. The restorability of a tooth with endodontic pathology is the single most pertinent treatment planning concern. An exception to this rule is found only in patients presenting with significant medical comorbidities, such as exposure to intravenous bisphosphonate medications, other immunologic drugs, or radiation to the head and neck. In these cases, nonsurgical root canal therapy (NSRCT) or nonsurgical retreatment may be considered to avoid extraction and the associated risk of osteonecrosis (Fig 3-1). In all other cases, clinicians must determine whether the tooth with endodontic pathology can support an adequate restoration to provide functionality to the patient. Similarly, clinicians must also assess and inform the patient whether adjunctive restorative procedures are necessary to retain the tooth in question, namely, crown-lengthening surgery or orthodontic extrusion.

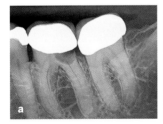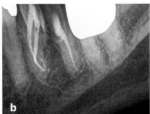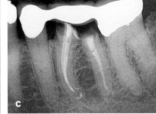

FIG 3-1 Patients with a history of intravenous bisphosphonate or other immunologic drug use or radiation to the head and neck warrant consideration for maintaining a tooth with NSRCT or nonsurgical retreatment, even in the presence of unrestorable caries, in order to avoid the risk of osteonecrosis. (a) This patient presented with unrestorable recurrent caries on the mandibular left first molar. (b) Because of her history of intravenous zoledronic acid (Zometa, Novartis) exposure, NSRCT and decoronation were performed to avoid extraction. (c) The area remained asymptomatic at the 2-year follow-up, with an absence of radiographic pathology.

For anterior teeth in a patient with sufficient posterior support and no history of bruxism, either direct or indirect intracoronal restorations are appropriate.[1] That said, if significant tooth structure is missing or if a patient is missing a significant portion of their posterior dentition such that greater occlusal forces would be rendered on the restored tooth, full-coverage restorative care may be indicated. For posterior teeth, adequate restorative care involves providing full-coverage restorations because the

Diagnosis-Driven Treatment Planning

predictability of root canal therapy in the posterior dentition decreases significantly in the absence of cuspal-coverage restorations.[2] Clinicians must also ensure that an adequate ferrule is present to support the restorations required for both anterior and posterior teeth. For more information on restoring endodontically treated teeth, refer to chapter 5.

In addition to an assessment of restorability, endodontic treatment planning must consider both the pulpal diagnosis and the stage of root maturation. As shown in Fig 3-2, a multitude of treatment options exist for every diagnosis, as well as the option to delay care in the short or longterm. Treatment selection should reflect both the patient's and the clinician's understanding of the prognosis of the treatment option and the associated risk factors. Success following treatment is defined in the literature as the absence/resolution of clinical signs and symptoms and radiographic findings of apical periodontitis (Fig 3-3). A summary of success rates for the procedures described in detail in the following chapters is available in Table 3-1.

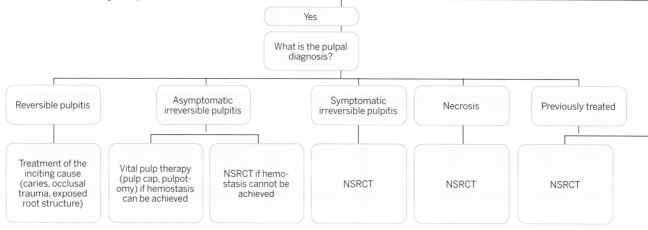

FIG 3-2 A decision tree for endodontic treatment. For each diagnosis, extraction, no treatment, and delayed treatment also represent acceptable management alternatives.

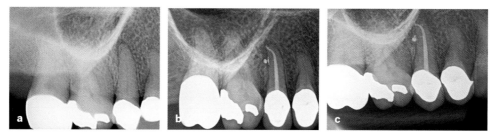

FIG 3-3 NSRCT offers patients a predictable means to maintain their dentition. Success following treatment is defined as the absence of clinical signs and symptoms and radiographic findings of apical periodontitis. Pretreatment (a), immediate postoperative (b), and 1-year follow-up (c) radiographs depicting successful NSRCT on the maxillary right second premolar.

Irrespective of the status of root maturation, a diagnosis of reversible pulpitis should be treated by removing the inciting cause. Potential causes of reversible pulpitis include occlusal trauma,[3] exposed root structure, or caries without pulp exposure. Addressing the cause of reversible pulpitis should resolve symptoms without the need for endodontic intervention.

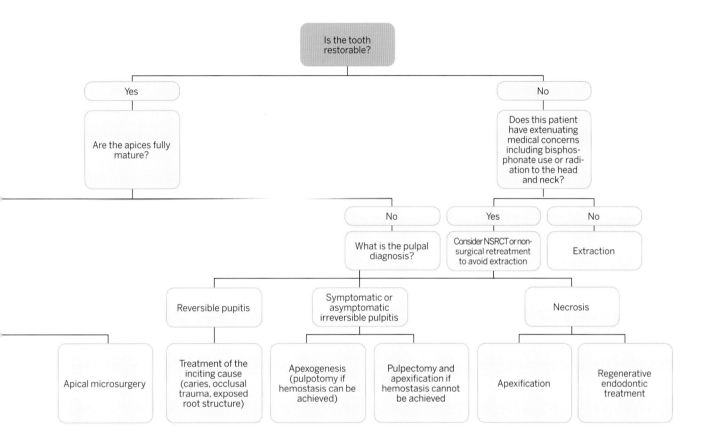

TABLE 3-1 Success rates for endodontic therapies	
Treatment modality	**Success rate**
NSRCT	86–95%
Nonsurgical retreatment	82–94%
Apical microsurgery	79–95%
Pulp cap	95%
Partial pulpotomy	91%
Full pulpotomy	95%
Apexification	77% (CH) 95% (BC)
Regenerative endodontic treatment	95%

CH = calcium hydroxide; BC = bioceramic.

Also irrespective of the root maturation status, the treatment of choice when asymptomatic irreversible pulpitis is diagnosed is vital pulp therapy.[4] Vital pulp therapy treatment modalities include direct pulp caps and full or partial pulpotomies. The success of vital pulp therapy in mature teeth depends both on the clinician's ability to obtain hemostasis of the exposed pulp tissue after caries removal and on the use of bioceramic materials to cover the exposed pulp.[4] The results of vital pulp therapy when using bioceramic materials are quite favorable, including when it is used to treat mature permanent teeth, with reported success rates at 95% for direct pulp caps, 91% for partial pulpotomies, and 95% for full pulpotomies.[5] Success rates when using calcium hydroxide materials are significantly less favorable.[6]

Pulpal diagnosis of symptomatic irreversible pulpitis or necrosis warrants consideration of NSRCT. NSRCT offers patients a predictable means to maintain their dentition, with 5 to 10 year success rates reported as 86% and survival rates as 95%.[7] Several factors outside the scope of the quality of endodontic treatment can, however, negatively impact outcomes following NSRCT. These include the presence of apical periodontitis,[8] periodontal attachment loss,[9] and fractures.[10] Conversely, several factors under operator control can improve outcomes following treatment. These include the use of dental dam isolation,[11] magnification,[12] and excellent and timely posttreatment restorative care.[13,14]

A pulpal diagnosis of previously treated teeth warrants consideration of nonsurgical retreatment or apical microsurgery. When deciding between options, greater consideration for nonsurgical retreatment should be given when the source of pathology is a leaking restoration resulting in coronal leakage, when correctible issues are noted with the initial NSRCT (namely, undertreated or untreated root canal spaces), and when prior treatment was performed under questionable conditions.[15] Consideration should be given to the pursuit of apical microsurgery versus retreatment if prior NSRCT or nonsurgical retreatment appears adequate upon clinical and radiographic evaluation; coronal disassembly is overly complex, such as when removing posts in the canal spaces would represent a significant risk of perforation or fracture; or prior treatment complications render nonsurgical approaches impossible.[16] Furthermore, if the prior endodontic treatment was completed under favorable conditions (with dental dam isolation) and is of excellent quality but symptoms or pathology remains, clinicians should first consider apical microsurgery. That said, both nonsurgical retreatment and apical microsurgery are predictable treatment modalities.

Nonsurgical retreatment offers a predictable means to maintain the natural dentition. Reported success rates are 82%, and survival rates are 94%.[17] Preoperative factors that can negatively impact outcomes include preoperative apical periodontitis and untreated perforations.[17] The quality of the initial treatment has a significant impact on the outcomes following nonsurgical retreatment. The outcomes following retreatment of cases with deficiencies in the initial therapy are more predictable than outcomes for cases treated well at the outset.[17] Factors under operator control that can improve outcomes include the use of modern techniques and equipment, namely the surgical operating microscope and ultrasonic instrumentation,[18] dental dam isolation,[11] and quality postendodontic restorative care.[19]

Apical microsurgery is a predictable means to maintain teeth affected by recurrent or persistent endodontic pathology. With modern techniques and technology, the prognosis for apical microsurgery is favorable, with reported success rates between 79% and 95%.[20,21] Modern technologies such as microscopy, ultrasonics, and bioceramic retrofillings are associated with positive outcomes following surgery.[20]

Treatment planning options differ for teeth with immature apices. For these teeth, a diagnosis of symptomatic irreversible pulpitis warrants consideration of vital pulp therapy.[4] When vital pulp therapy is employed in the presence of immature roots, it is referred to as *apexogenesis* because treatment facilitates the continued deposition of root dentin and, ultimately, the continued maturation of the root apex. Again, vital pulp therapy treatments fall on a spectrum and include direct pulp caps and partial or full pulpotomies. The success of vital pulp therapy, irrespective of root maturity, depends on the clinician's ability to obtain hemostasis of the exposed pulp tissue as well as the use of bioceramic materials.[4] As in mature permanent teeth, vital pulp therapy in the immature dentition is associated with favorable outcomes.

For necrotic immature teeth, treatment options include apexification and regenerative endodontic treatment. Apexification involves the development of a barrier at the apex of an immature necrotic tooth using long-term calcium hydroxide treatment or bioceramic materials. While both methodologies offer predictable outcomes (77% success for calcium hydroxide, 95% for bioceramics),[22] the marked reduction in treatment time associated with bioceramic barrier development makes this a more desirable treatment modality in most cases. The long-term risk associated with apexification treatment is cervical root fracture because apexification does not facilitate continued root development.[23,24] As an alternative to this procedure, regenerative endodontic therapy can be considered. This procedure uses stem cells from the apical papilla to promote hard tissue development, overcoming the fracture risk related to apexification procedures. Regenerative endodontic procedures are associated with positive outcomes,[22] but if regenerative failures are noted, apexification may be performed as a secondary procedure.

Informed Consent

Clinicians must pull from the breadth and depth of their knowledge to offer patients the appropriate treatment options. A thorough conversation with the patient about the treatment plan in terms that they understand is imperative for obtaining proper informed consent. This conversation should include a discussion of the risks and benefits of various treatment options, including their prognosis and financial and time costs, as well as the need for adjunctive treatments like restorative or surgical care. Irrespective of the diagnosis, not performing treatment or deciding to delay treatment are valid options, albeit with obvious risks involving continued or progressive signs and symptoms of pain and infection and/or a worsened prognosis should treatment eventually be pursued. Components of informed consent are listed in Fig 3-4.

Informed consent isn't simply a signature on a document. It represents a process in which the clinician and patient review the diagnosis, proposed treatment, alternatives, and associated risks. It provides patients the opportunity to ask questions

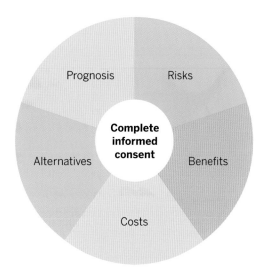

FIG 3-4 Components of complete informed consent. Informed consent involves a discussion about the recommended procedure as well as any adjunctive treatment needs. These items should be reviewed verbally and documented in the patient's chart.

about their proposed treatment and ensures that they fully comprehend their options for care. Ensuring that patients hear and understand all components of the treatment is crucial for consent, and visual, auditory, and written formats can be used to enhance patients' comprehension and recollection.[25]

While informed consent isn't simply a signature, details surrounding these conversations must be carefully documented in patient records. The use of a formal consent form allowing clinicians to lay out all the components of the discussion is recommended by most attorneys. Because an executed informed consent form is a legal document, the particulars of its components and wording should be formulated to adhere to local guidelines in consultation with a liability insurance agent and attorney. The document should be signed and dated by both patient and clinician. A sample informed consent document for NSRCT is available in Fig 3-5.

INFORMED CONSENT: NONSURGICAL ROOT CANAL THERAPY

It is our belief that you should be informed about the benefits, risks, and expenses involved in endodontic therapy and that you provide your written consent prior to treatment. You should also be informed of alternatives to our recommended treatment.

Root canal therapy involves the removal of the pulp tissues (nerves, blood vessels, and cells) or their remnants from inside the tooth, followed by sealing of the space with a filling material. Although root canal therapy has a high rate of success, the success of any medical treatment cannot be guaranteed. Occasionally, a root canal–treated tooth may require additional treatment, such as root canal retreatment, periapical surgery, or even extraction, that is not covered by the original fee. Furthermore, root canal therapy can be successful only if your tooth is restored by your general dentist following treatment in our office.

Risks specific to root canal therapy: Treatment is performed to minimize the risks. These risks include (but are not limited to) separation of an instrument fragment inside the tooth, perforation of the tooth structure when gaining access to the canals, and tooth or crown fracture. Complications of treatment and local anesthesia may include swelling, pain, restricted jaw opening, infection, bleeding, and sinus involvement. Due to the proximity of some nerves, especially in the lower teeth, it is possible that a nerve will be bruised or damaged while operations are being performed near the root tips. As a result, the lip, chin, and/or tongue may feel numb, tingle, or have a burning sensation. This sensation could continue for days or weeks or, very rarely, permanently.

During treatment, complications may be discovered that make treatment impossible. If this occurs, you will be advised, the treatment will be discontinued, and the fee will be adjusted. These complications may include deep decay (caries), splits or fractures of the tooth, inaccessible canals, etc.

Other treatment choices include: no treatment, delayed treatment, and tooth extraction. Risks involved with these options may include pain, swelling, infection, cyst formation, periodontal disease, chronic pain and discomfort, the spread of infection to other areas, loss of the tooth, or the premature loss of adjacent teeth. Delaying treatment increases the possibility that root canal therapy will not be able to be performed.

Charges are for services rendered. A successful outcome is our goal but cannot be guaranteed.

I, the undersigned, have read this form. The procedures, alternatives, risks, and fees were explained to my satisfaction by the doctor, and I consent to treatment.

Date: _____

_____
Doctor signature

_____
Patient name printed

_____
Patient/Guardian signature

FIG 3-5 A sample informed consent document for NSRCT. This document should only be adopted in consultation with an insurance agent and attorney to ensure compliance with local laws.

Part of the conversation surrounding informed consent should include considering referral of the patient to specialists when appropriate. The principle of nonmaleficence (do no harm) obliges clinicians to not only strive for optimal care but also to understand their own limitations. Because specialty care exists in endodontics, it is important for clinicians to assess the complexity level of a case when deciding whether to offer treatment or refer. A helpful standardized assessment tool like the American Association of Endodontists Case Difficulty Assessment Form, which can be found online with the link provided in the bibliography, can aid in decision-making.[26] This form delineates criteria to aid clinicians in assessing the difficulty of a case, including patient factors and diagnosis and treatment considerations. Patient factors, including medical compromise, anesthetic challenges, and issues with limited mouth opening or a gag reflex, may warrant specialty care to enhance treatment efficiency. Individual tooth factors, such as the positioning of the tooth in the arch or complex root canal anatomy, may warrant the skills and armamentarium of a specialist with extra training. Individual considerations, including the clinician's level of comfort and training or the patient's preference, may also warrant referral.

References

1. Sorensen JA, Martinoff JT. Intracoronal reinforcement and coronal coverage: A study of endodontically treated teeth. J Prosthet Dent 1984;51:780–784.
2. Salehrabi R, Rotstein I. Endodontic treatment outcomes in a large patient population in the USA: An epidemiological study. J Endod 2004;30:846–850.
3. Brännström M. Etiology of dentin hypersensitivity. Proc Finn Dent Soc 1992;88(Suppl 1):7–13.
4. AAE Position Statement on Vital Pulp Therapy. American Association of Endodontists, 2021. https://www.aae.org/wp-content/uploads/2021/05/VitalPulpTherapyPositionStatement_v2.pdf. Accessed 28 March 2023.
5. Asgary S, Hassanizadeh R, Torabzadeh H, Eghbal MJ. Treatment outcomes of 4 vital pulp therapies in mature molars. J Endod 2018;44:529–535.
6. Kundzina R, Stangvaltaite L, Eriksen HM, Kerosuo E. Capping carious exposures in adults: A randomized controlled trial investigating mineral trioxide aggregate versus calcium hydroxide. Int Endod J 2017;50:924–932.
7. de Chevigny C, Dao TT, Basrani BR, et al. Treatment outcome in endodontics: The Toronto study—Phase 4: Initial treatment. J Endod 2008;34:258–263.
8. Ng YL, Mann V, Rahbaran S, Lewsey J, Gulabivala K. Outcome of primary root canal treatment: Systematic review of the literature—Part 2. Influence of clinical factors. Int Endod J 2008;41:6–31.
9. Setzer FC, Boyer KR, Jeppson JR, Karabucak B, Kim S. Long-term prognosis of endodontically treated teeth: A retrospective analysis of preoperative factors in molars. J Endod 2011;37:21–25.
10. Krell KV, Caplan DJ. 12-month success of cracked teeth treated with orthograde root canal treatment. J Endod 2018;44:543–548.
11. Lin PY, Huang SH, Chang HJ, Chi LY. The effect of rubber dam usage on the survival rate of teeth receiving initial root canal treatment: A nationwide population-based study. J Endod 2014;40:1733–1737.
12. Baruwa AO, Martins JNR, Meirinhos J, et al. The influence of missed canals on the prevalence of periapical lesions in endodontically treated teeth: A cross sectional study. J Endod 2020;46:34–39.
13. Pratt I, Aminoshariae A, Montagnese TA, Williams KA, Khalighinejad N, Mickel A. Eight-year retrospective study of the critical time lapse between root canal completion and crown placement: Its influence on the survival of endodontically treated teeth. J Endod 2016;42:1598–1603.
14. Ray HA, Trope M. Periapical status of endodontically treated teeth in relation to the technical quality of the root filling and the coronal restoration. Int Endod J 1995;28:12–18.
15. Roda R. Nonsurgical Retreatment: Clinical Decision Making. American Association of Endodontists: Colleagues for Excellence, Spring 2017.
16. Iqbal MK, Kratchman SI, Guess GM, Karabucak B, Kim S. Microscopic periradicular surgery: Perioperative predictors for postoperative clinical outcomes and quality of life assessment. J Endod 2007;33:239–244.

17. de Chevigny C, Dao TT, Basrani BR, et al. Treatment outcome in endodontics: The Toronto study—Phases 3 and 4: Orthograde retreatment. J Endod 2008;34:131–137.

18. He J, White RK, White CA, Schweitzer JL, Woodmansey KF. Clinical and patient-centered outcomes of non-surgical root canal retreatment in first molars using contemporary techniques. J Endod 2017;43:231–237.

19. Ng YL, Mann V, Gulabivala K. Outcome of secondary root canal treatment: A systematic review of the literature. Int Endod J 2008;41:1026–1046.

20. Rubinstein RA, Kim S. Long-term follow-up of cases considered healed one year after apical microsurgery. J Endod 2002;28:378–383

21. Huang S, Chen NN, Yu VSH, Lim HA, Liu JN. Long-term success and survival of endodontic microsurgery. J Endod 2020;46:149–157.e4.

22. Jeeruphan T, Jantarat J, Yanpiset K, Suwannapan L, Khewsawai P, Hargreaves KM. Mahidol study 1: Comparison of radiographic and survival outcomes of immature teeth treated with either regenerative endodontic or apexification methods: A retrospective study. J Endod 2012;38:1330–1336.

23. Kahler SL, Shetty S, Andreasen FM, Kahler B. The effect of long-term dressing with calcium hydroxide on the fracture susceptibility of teeth. J Endod 2018;44:464–469.

24. Cvek M. Prognosis of luxated non-vital maxillary incisors treated with calcium hydroxide and filled with gutta percha. Endod Dent Traumatol 1992;8:45–55.

25. Moreira NCF, Pachêco-Pereira C, Keenan L, Cummings G, Flores-Mir C. Informed consent comprehension and recollection in adult dental patients: A systematic review. J Am Dent Assoc 2016;147:605–619.

26. American Association of Endodontists. Case Assessment Tools. https://www.aae.org/specialty/clinical-resources/treatment-planning/case-assessment-tools/. Accessed 21 March 2023.

Pharmacology

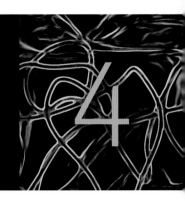

All clinicians must be aware of the breadth of prescriptions and over-the-counter medications their patients consume. That said, the scope of pharmacology in endodontic care is relatively narrow, including analgesics, antibiotics, anxiolytic medications, and anesthetics. This chapter reviews these medications, including their indications, contraindications, and prescribing strategies, as well as anesthetic delivery protocols.

Analgesics

The diagnoses of pulpitis, apical periodontitis, and abscess are associated with significant discomfort. Many of the patients experiencing these conditions present for care while already taking analgesic medications. The delivery of definitive treatment via endodontic therapy or extraction should result in immediate symptom improvement and tapering of analgesic use in the days following treatment.[1] That said, most patients undergoing endodontic therapy experience mild to moderate postoperative discomfort.[2] Therefore, clinicians must maintain an up-to-date understanding of the best pharmacologic agents to help patients manage pain.

The use of pharmacologic pain relievers in endodontics centers around oral analgesic agents. Numerous high-quality studies have established that combination therapy using nonsteroidal anti-inflammatory drugs (NSAIDs) and acetaminophen is the gold standard for managing both pre- and postoperative endodontic pain.[3] These drugs show the greatest effectiveness in pain relief along with low side-effect profiles and are readily available at low cost without the risk of dependency found with opioid family drugs.[3]

Both NSAIDs and acetaminophen exhibit a ceiling effect. This means that their peak analgesic effectiveness occurs at a dose below the maximum recommended dose.[4] Higher doses provide no added benefit but will increase the risk of adverse events. These events include hepatotoxicity and gastrointestinal upset for NSAIDs[5] and hepatotoxicity for acetaminophen.[6] Therefore, recommended doses must be kept below the maximum doses recommended by drug manufacturers, namely, 3,200 mg ibuprofen/day and 4,000 mg acetaminophen/day.

Ibuprofen is the preferred NSAID in endodontics due to its availability and convenient dosing schedule. For patients with mild pain, the first-line analgesic therapy is 400 mg ibuprofen every 6 hours.[7] For mild pain, 400 mg ibuprofen combined with 325 mg acetaminophen every 6 hours is advised.[3] For more intense pain, 600 to 800 mg ibuprofen combined with up to 1,000 mg acetaminophen every 6 hours may be indicated. Rather than alternating ibuprofen and acetaminophen, the two medications should be administered simultaneously because this combination has shown greater efficacy than alternating courses.[8] Furthermore, the combination of these two medications is more effective than any opioid or corticosteroid at reducing patient discomfort associated with endodontic care.[9] That said, 600 mg ibuprofen alone can provide pain relief equivical to what can be achieved when combined with 1,000 mg acetaminophen 6 hours after endodontic therapy. Therefore, ibuprofen alone might be preferred postoperatively in patients with even relative contraindications to acetaminophen usage.[3] If patients are unable to tolerate the NSAID/acetaminophen combination due to allergies or other medical contraindications, NSAIDs or acetaminophen alone should be used as first-line therapy.

For patients with more severe discomfort, opioid drugs, including complexes of ibuprofen or acetaminophen with codeine, hydrocodone, oxycodone and tramadol, can be considered for endodontic pain.[10] Their use, however, is associated with higher side effect profiles and the risk of dependence and abuse.[11] Consequently, expedient definitive management should be prioritized for these patients. Analgesic strategies are summarized in Table 4-1.

TABLE 4-1 Flexible analgesic prescription strategies for endodontics			
	Mild pain	**Moderate pain**	**Severe pain**
Healthy patient	400 mg ibuprofen plus 325 mg acetaminophen every 6 hours	600–800 mg ibuprofen plus 1,000 mg acetaminophen every 6 hours	600 mg ibuprofen every 6 hours plus acetaminophen/ opioid combination medication
NSAIDs contraindicated	325–650 mg acetaminophen every 6 hours	1,000 mg acetaminophen every 6 hours	Acetaminophen/ opioid combination medication

Antibiotics

While definitive dental care with endodontic therapy or extraction is essential for the management of endodontic infections, clinicians must be aware of the adjunctive role of oral antibiotics. Most endodontic infections do not require systemic antibiotic therapy. However, for severe infections exceeding the patient's immune responses, antibiotic therapy can be lifesaving. Furthermore, other clinical situations may arise in which antibiotic premedication is advisable prior to the delivery of care. This section reviews both the therapeutic uses of antibiotics and their use as a premedication.

Therapeutic usage

Systemic antibiotics are indicated for a well-defined subset of endodontic infections.[12,13] Patients with swelling, namely, a diagnosis of acute apical abscess, accompanied by systemic signs and symptoms should be prescribed oral antibiotics.[12,13] Signs of systemic spread include a fever greater than 100.4°F, unexplained trismus, lymphadenopathy, malaise, and/or tachycardia. Furthermore, immunocompromised patients presenting with a diagnosis of acute apical abscess should be prescribed antibiotics. Conditions associated with immune system compromise include uncontrolled or poorly controlled diabetes, a history of immunosuppressive medication use, chemotherapy or radiation exposure, and other poorly controlled systemic diseases. Medical consultation for these patients may be advisable. Additionally, antibiotics should be used for patients with rapidly spreading infections, those with signs of cellulitis or osteomyelitis, and those with persistent infections that are initially unresponsive to pulpal debridement.[12,13] Antibiotics may also be used for certain traumatic dental injuries, particularly soft tissue lacerations that require suturing and in the replantation of avulsed teeth.[14]

Several contraindications exist for the prescription of antibiotics. Patients presenting with localized swelling without systemic involvement and patients without immune system compromise do not require antibiotic prescriptions as long as immediate, definitive dental care can be delivered.[12,13,15] If care must be delayed, however, antibiotic therapy may be considered. Furthermore, patients with pulp necrosis and symptomatic apical periodontitis generally do not need antibiotic therapy, though a "delayed prescription" may be considered when definitive treatment is not immediately available.[15] Additionally, antibiotics are contraindicated in patients with chronic infections when the host defenses are intact, namely in the presence of a chronic apical abscess characterized by drainage or asymptomatic apical periodontitis found incidentally upon radiographic examination. Antibiotics are absolutely contraindicated in cases of symptomatic irreversible pulpitis because pulpitis is an inflammatory and not an infectious condition.[16–18] Antibiotics are also not expected to improve treatment outcomes,[19] and their use should always follow the best evidence-based guidelines. Indications and contraindications for antibiotic therapy in endodontic infections are summarized in Fig 4-1, and a breakdown of when antibiotics are and are not indicated in endodontics based on the ability to complete definitive treatment is available in Table 4-2.

Indications	Contraindications
• Acute apical abscess with systemic involvement or in a medically compromised patient • Rapidly progressive infections with cellulitis or osteomyelitis • Persistent infections • Following certain traumatic dental injuries	• Cases of irreversible pulpitis • Infection under host control, including chronic apical abscesses and acute apical abscesses without systemic involvement • Asymptomatic periapical pathology detected on radiograph • To improve outcomes • Treatment for preoperative or postoperative pain

FIG 4-1 Indications and contraindications for the use of systemic antibiotic therapy in endodontic infections.

TABLE 4-2 When antibiotics are indicated based on ability to provide immediate definitive treatment

	Definitive treatment CAN be provided	Definitive treatment CANNOT be provided
Symptomatic irreversible pulpitis with any periapical diagnosis	No antibiotics	No antibiotics
Pulpal necrosis with chronic apical abscess	No antibiotics	No antibiotics
Pulpal necrosis with symptomatic apical periodontitis	No antibiotics	Delayed antibiotics
Pulpal necrosis with acute apical abscess, no systemic symptoms	No antibiotics	Antibiotics
Pulpal necrosis with acute apical abscess, systemic symptoms or immunocompromised patient	Antibiotics	Antibiotics

When systemic antibiotic therapy is indicated, clear guidance exists regarding the best drugs and dosages to reach therapeutic levels for the treatment of endodontic infections. Antibiotics are only needed until host defenses regain control of an infection. Therefore, short duration courses are recommended to minimize toxicity and allergy.[20,21] Loading doses two times greater than the maintenance dose are advised to expedite achievement of therapeutic serum concentrations, and appropriate dosing regimens must be followed to ensure therapeutic levels of drugs are maintained throughout the course.[20] In general, 2- to 3-day antibiotic courses are recommended, along with close patient monitoring, with extensions necessary only if symptoms fail to improve. When courses are extended, close monitoring must continue, and patients should be advised to continue taking the medication for no more than 2 to 3 days beyond symptom improvement to minimize the risk of developing antibiotic resistance or other adverse events. In most cases, no more than 7 days of antibiotic therapy is warranted.[22,23] Patients should always be counseled that if their infection remains refractory to oral therapeutics or if it spreads into deeper fascial spaces, referral to medical providers for intravenous antibiotic therapy may be warranted.

The first-line drug for treating endodontic infections is penicillin VK. In an average-sized adult patient, it should be dosed at 500 mg every 6 hours.[13] In medically compromised patients where drug resistance is more likely, the slightly broader spectrum amoxicillin can be considered as the first-line antibiotic. It is dosed at 500 mg every 8 hours. If infections are unresponsive to these first-line drugs after 48 to 72 hours, clinicians should either add metronidazole to the existing prescription, dosed at 500 mg every 8 hours for 5 to 7 days, or switch to a combination of amoxicillin with clavulanic acid (Augmentin, USAntibiotics), dosed at 500/125 mg every 8 hours or 875/125 mg every 12 hours.[13] Patients who have been prescribed metronidazole must be counseled on its disulfiram-like effects when mixed with alcohol, which include nausea, vomiting, and chest pain. If the infection remains unresponsive for an additional 48 to 72 hours despite the addition of metronidazole or switching to amoxicillin plus clavulanic acid, clindamycin 300 mg every 8 hours should be considered. An antibiotic prescription strategy for patients not allergic to penicillin is provided in Fig 4-2.

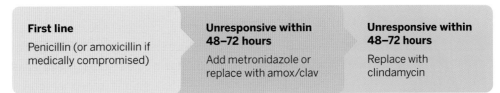

First line

Penicillin (or amoxicillin if medically compromised)

Unresponsive within 48–72 hours

Add metronidazole or replace with amox/clav

Unresponsive within 48–72 hours

Replace with clindamycin

FIG 4-2 Antibiotic prescription strategy for the penicillin-tolerant patient (amox/clav = amoxicillin/ clavulanic acid combination).

For penicillin-allergic patients, the first-line medication is cephalexin 500 mg every 6 hours. However, due to issues with cross-allergenicity, this drug should be avoided in patients with severe penicillin allergies involving anaphylaxis, angioedema, or hives.[13,24] In severely penicillin-allergic patients, azithromycin is the recommended first-line drug, with 500 mg as a loading dosage and 250 mg once per day for a total of 5 days.[13] If infections are unresponsive to these first-line medications after 48 to 72 hours, replacement with clindamycin 300 mg administered every 8 hours is advised. Although clindamycin was historically the first-line drug for penicillin-allergic patients, current guidelines suggest other drugs because of black box warnings associating clindamycin with *clostridium difficile* superinfections.[13] An antibiotic prescription strategy for penicillin-allergic patients is available in Fig 4-3, and a dosage summary for the most common antibiotics used in endodontics is presented in Table 4-3.

First line

Cephalexin OR azithromycin

Unresponsive within 48–72 hours

Replace with clindamycin

FIG 4-3 Antibiotic prescription strategy for the penicillin-allergic patient.

TABLE 4-3 Dosing strategies for the most commonly used antibiotics in endodontics

Drug	Loading dose	Adult maintenance dose
Penicillin VK	1,000 mg	500 mg four times per day for 3–7 days
Amoxicillin	1,000 mg	500 mg three times per day for 3–7 days
Metronidazole (with penicillin or amoxicillin)	NA	500 mg three times per day for 5–7 days
Amoxicillin/clavulanic acid	NA	500/125 mg three times per day or 875/125 mg twice per day for 7 days
Clindamycin	600 mg	300 mg three times per day for 3–7 days
Cephalexin	1,000 mg	500 mg four times per day for 3–7 days
Azithromycin	500 mg	250 mg once per day for 5 days

Antibiotic premedication

Premedication refers to dispensing antibiotics prior to treatment to certain at-risk patients to prevent poor outcomes related to infections secondary to treatment. Premedication is meant to address transient bacteremia (bacteria in the bloodstream), which can occur due to penetration of the mucous membranes and theoretically may result in distant infections. Endodontics falls among the procedures for which premedication is indicated, based on the presumption that bacteremia may occur following instrumentation. That said, examinations and routine imaging during consultations may not necessitate premedication if gingival tissues are not manipulated. The dental procedures for which premedication is advised, as well as those procedures for which it may not be indicated, are listed in Fig 4-4. It should be noted that transient bacteremia also develop while eating and during oral hygiene procedures, and these activities do not require antibiotic premedication.

Procedures for which antibiotic prophylaxis is recommended	**Procedures for which antibiotic prophylaxis is not required**
• All dental procedures involving manipulation of gingival tissues, the periapical region of teeth, or perforation of the oral mucosa • Surgical and nonsurgical periodontal procedures • Surgical and nonsurgical endodontic procedures • Oral surgery, including extraction	• Injection of local anesthetic through noninfected tissue • Dental radiographs • Placement of removable prosthetics • Placement or adjustment of orthodontic appliances or brackets • Exfoliation of primary teeth • Bleeding due to trauma of oral mucosa or lips

FIG 4-4 Dental procedures for which antibiotic premedication is recommended by the American Heart Association (AHA).[25]

Premedication has historically been employed for patients with certain cardiac conditions and following joint replacement surgery, as well as for patients with other medical conditions involving immune system compromise. The American Heart Association (AHA) recommends premedication for patients with certain cardiac conditions to prevent bacterial endocarditis and its associated morbidity and mortality.[25,26] Patients for whom premedication is recommended include those with prosthetic heart valves, a history of previous infective endocarditis, a history of certain congenital heart diseases, and patients who develop valvulopathy following cardiac transplants (Fig 4-5).

Cardiac conditions for which antibiotic prophylaxis is recommended	• Prosthetic heart valve • Previous infective endocarditis • Congenital heart disease – Unrepaired cyanotic CHD, which includes palliative shunts and conduits – Repaired CHD within the first 6 months following the procedure – Repaired CHD with residual defects • Cardiac transplant recipients who develop valvulopathy

FIG 4-5 Cardiac conditions for which antibiotic prophylaxis is recommended by the AHA[25] (CHD = congenital heart defects).

Recommended antibiotic regimens for premedication are presented in Table 4-4. Of note, cephalexin is not advised for patients with a history of allergy to penicillin with symptoms that include urticaria, angioedema, or anaphylaxis. Cephalosporins are also not recommended in patients already taking penicillin family drugs because of cross-resistance in the viridans group streptococci. If patients are already on a course of antibiotics related to a dental abscess or other systemic medical condition, they should be premedicated with a different class of drugs. In cases of elective dentistry, the recommendation is to space treatment to allow 10 days between antibiotic dosages or courses.

TABLE 4-4 Premedication regimens advised by the AHA[25]

Clinical scenario	Medication	Regimen: Single dose 30–60 minutes before procedure	
		Adults	*Children*
Oral	Amoxicillin	2 g	50 mg/kg
Unable to take oral medication	Ampicillin OR cefazolin or ceftriaxone	2g IM or IV 1g IM or IV	50 mg/kg IM or IV 50 mg/kg IM or IV
Allergic to penicillin (oral)	Cephalexin OR azithromycin OR doxycycline	2 g 500 mg 100 mg	50 mg/kg 15 mg/kg 2.2 mg/kg
Allergic to penicillin (unable to take oral medication)	Cefazolin or ceftriaxone	1 g IM or IV	50 mg/kg IM or IV

IM: intramuscular injection; IV: intravenous injection.

Though antibiotic premedication has historically been advised for patients with prosthetic joints, guidelines updated in 2015 no longer advise its routine use due to insufficient evidence supporting a relationship between dental procedures and joint infections.[27] That said, orthopedic surgeons may advise antibiotic premedication in certain high-risk patients and should be responsible for prescribing in these unique situations.

Antibiotic prophylaxis may also be advised by physicians for a myriad of other medical conditions outside of routine guidelines. Consequently, concerns noted during review of a patient's medical history warrant consultation with their treating physician. This medical consult not only alerts the physician to a potential risk but gives them an opportunity to make recommendations accordingly. This may include antibiotic prophylaxis or other modifications to care to minimize the chance of very specific adverse outcomes in these patients. Physicians may consider antibiotic premedication for at-risk patients scheduled for invasive dental procedures that carry the risk of postoperative infection. These may be patients with HIV, AIDS, or neutropenia; solid organ transplant patients taking antirejection drugs; or patients undergoing chemotherapy or dialysis. Furthermore, physicians may advise antibiotic premedication for patients with uncontrolled diabetes, often defined by glycosylated hemoglobin (HbA1c) levels greater than 10%.

Anxiolytics

For many patients, the delivery of dental care, particularly endodontic therapy, is associated with significant anxiety. While excellent communication, reassurance, and the provision of adequate local anesthesia is sufficient to mitigate anxiety for some, other patients may benefit from pharmacologic anxiolysis. In an endodontic setting, this may include oral anxiolytics, nitrous oxide, or deeper sedation. It should be noted that patients using anxiolytic medications cannot provide adequate informed consent, and therefore, consent should be obtained from the patient prior to the treatment date or from a healthcare proxy on the day of treatment. Furthermore, patients given pharmacologic anxiolytics should be escorted to and from their appointments and should not be permitted to drive.

Oral anxiolytics

Benzodiazepines are the oral medication of choice for patients experiencing procedure-related anxiety or who suffer from claustrophobia with the dental dam and associated dental armamentarium necessary for treatment. This class of medications does not potentiate local anesthetic agents. Consequently, its use is not advised for reasons related to inadequate local anesthesia.[28] That said, anxious patients are more likely to experience intraoperative pain.[29] Therefore, anxiolysis is warranted for the especially fearful patient. Because patients may sleep poorly the night before a procedure due to their anxiety, medications may be prescribed to be taken the evening prior to treatment and again 30 to 90 minutes prior to the procedure itself. Commonly used medications for adult patients include diazepam (Valium, Genentech) 5 to 20 mg, lorazepam (Ativan, Pfizer) 1 to 10 mg, alprazolam (Xanax, Pfizer) 0.25 to 2 mg, and triazolam (Halcion, Pfizer) 0.125 to 0.5 mg.

Nitrous oxide

Nitrous oxide is a safe and effective tool for the management of dental anxiety. It possesses a wide therapeutic margin and has the advantage over oral medication of a controlled duration. Inhaled nitrous oxide uniquely provides not only anxiolysis but also analgesia.[30] It has been shown to improve the success rates of inferior alveolar nerve block anesthesia in patients with symptomatic irreversible pulpitis.[31] Although safe and effective on its own, nitrous oxide should not be mixed with oral anxiolytics due to the risk of compounded respiratory depression.[32]

Deeper sedation

Whether due to anxiety or a strong gag reflex, or in young patients or those with disabilities, deeper sedation by way of intravenous sedation or inhalational general anesthesia is sometimes required to provide endodontic care. Specialized training in the drugs utilized is required, along with patient monitoring and emergency protocols for safe practice.[32] Clinicians may consider partnering with a dental or medical anesthesiologist or delivering care in a hospital setting in these scenarios.

Anesthetics

Endodontic pathology is often associated with significant discomfort. Furthermore, certain endodontic diagnoses can complicate the provision of profound anesthesia. For instance, the inflammation associated with symptomatic irreversible pulpitis has been shown to negatively influence the success rates of local anesthesia.[33] Even patients presenting with pulpal necrosis may experience pain due to dental dam isolation impinging on gingival tissues, subclinical vital tissue remaining within the canal, or the pressure or heat associated with endodontic procedures. Thus, all endodontic procedures require profound anesthesia so that both patient and clinician can be assured of comfort, allowing delivery of high-quality care. To that end, evidence-based protocols have been developed for achieving profound pulpal and periapical anesthesia in endodontics.[33] Anesthetic pharmacology and techniques are presented in the following discussion.

Pharmacology

Local anesthetics work by blocking sodium channels involved in the propagation of a stimulus along a neuron, thus preventing its perception within the cerebral cortex.[34] In selecting appropriate anesthetics, practitioners must consider the drug, its dose, and its onset and duration of efficacy (Fig 4-6). Though there are no major differences in the success rates of pulpal anesthesia for the commonly available anesthetic agents 2% lidocaine, 4% articaine, and 3% mepivacaine,[35–37] articaine has shown greater effectiveness for buccal local infiltration in mandibular molars.[37,38] Given its high lipid solubility, it may also spread further within maxillary bone to anesthetize palatal mucosa when administered via a buccal infiltration route.[39] Articaine and other 4% solutions, however, should not be used for block anesthesia due to the associated increased incidence of paresthesias.[40]

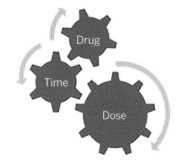

FIG 4-6 When providing local anesthesia for endodontic treatments, clinicians must select the appropriate drug at the appropriate dose and provide enough time for pulpal anesthesia to develop.

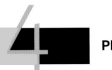

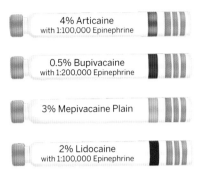

4% Articaine
with 1:100,000 Epinephrine

0.5% Bupivacaine
with 1:200,000 Epinephrine

3% Mepivacaine Plain

2% Lidocaine
with 1:100,000 Epinephrine

FIG 4-7 Common local anesthetics for endodontics.

Particularly in the mandible, bupivacaine has been shown to provide longer durations of pulpal and soft tissue anesthesia. Its use is also recommended when significant postoperative pain is expected because it can reduce this pain for up to several days following injection.[41,42] Many local anesthetic preparations contain epinephrine, which may be contraindicated for certain patients. For these patients, plain mepivacaine or prilocaine may be the drug of choice. Commonly used anesthetics for endodontics are depicted in Fig 4-7.

In addition to drug selection, the appropriate dose or volume must be administered. This is particularly important when anesthetizing inflamed teeth. For these teeth, 3.6 mL of anesthetic solution (equivalent to two carpules) is more effective than 1.8 mL (one carpule) for an inferior alveolar nerve block.[43] Therefore, in general for endodontic therapies, at least 3.6 mL total volume of anesthetic is recommended. Even if the appropriate drug and dose are selected, practitioners may still find that anesthesia is inadequate if they try to work too quickly. Adequate pulpal anesthesia, particularly for very inflamed teeth, can take anywhere from 5 to 30 minutes to develop.[33] Therefore, clinicians must be sure to allow adequate time for anesthesia to take effect.

Beyond traditional means of injectable local anesthesia, other pharmacologic agents can enhance intraoperative pain control. In patients with a history of difficulty obtaining profound pulpal anesthesia and/or severely painful symptomatic irreversible pulpitis wherein difficulties might be expected, premedication with NSAIDs, dexamethasone, and tramadol may improve anesthetic efficacy.[44] Inhaled nitrous oxide can be similarly utilized due to its analgesic effects beyond anxiolysis.[31]

Techniques

Topical anesthesia

Topical application of 20% benzocaine is recommended for 2 full minutes prior to intraoral injection of anesthetic agents to reduce the pain of needle insertion.[45] The topical preparation should be applied to dry mucosa for maximum efficacy (Fig 4-8). For more comfortable anesthetic administration following topical anesthesia, depositing a small amount of anesthetic while walking the needle slowly deeper into the tissues can allow for anesthesia to take effect as injection occurs. Careful technique can make for truly painless injections, increasing patient confidence and comfort.

Topical
Anesthesia

FIG 4-8 Topical anesthetics should be applied prior to the delivery of local anesthetics for endodontics.

Maxillary anesthesia

Pulpal anesthesia of maxillary teeth is achievable with the use of local infiltration on the buccal or facial aspects of the tooth (Fig 4-9). Administration of 4% articaine solution via buccal infiltration may often achieve sufficient palatal anesthesia without the need for additional palatal injections.[39] While palatal infiltration injections are not needed for pulpal anesthesia according to the literature, some clinicians find that additional palatal infiltration anes-

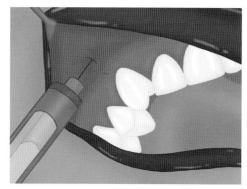

FIG 4-9 Local anesthesia for maxillary teeth undergoing endodontic treatment can be achieved via buccal infiltration.

thesia provides better pulpal anesthesia for maxillary molar teeth with a diagnosis of symptomatic irreversible pulpitis.[46,47] Additionally, palatal anesthesia may be required for dental dam isolation due to gingival hyperplasia or structural breakdown of the tooth or root anatomy that forces the clamp to impinge on the gingiva.

Mandibular anesthesia

Complete pulpal anesthesia of mandibular teeth is often more challenging to achieve than in the maxilla due to the greater complexity of innervation and alveolar bone thickness. Mandibular anterior teeth may be anesthetized by infiltrations on the buccal and lingual or by mental nerve blocks[48] but may require an inferior alveolar nerve block (Fig 4-10). Mandibular premolars may be anesthetized with a combination of mental and inferior alveolar nerve blocks.[49] Mandibular molars require inferior alveolar nerve blocks as well as local infiltration on the buccal aspect, which has been shown to provide the greatest success rates even in inflamed teeth.[38] As mentioned, although articaine solutions are not advised for use in inferior alveolar nerve blocks, they are superior agents for local infiltration in this region. A summary of location-specific local anesthesia techniques and medications is available in Table 4-5. If epinephrine is contraindicated, 3% mepivacaine without epinephrine should be substituted. In cases involving an increased risk of postoperative pain (eg, significant preoperative pain or chronic pain comorbidities), 0.5% bupivacaine with 1:200,000 epinephrine may be additionally administered to potentially reduce postoperative pain and the need for postoperative analgesia.

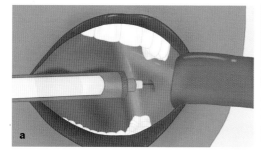
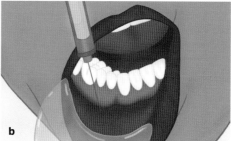

FIG 4-10 Both anterior and posterior mandibular teeth may require inferior alveolar nerve block techniques to achieve complete pulpal anesthesia (a), though premolar and anterior teeth may also be readily anesthetized by mental nerve blocks or infiltration anesthesia (b).

TABLE 4-5 Local anesthesia strategy by location

Arch	Tooth	Drug	Route
Maxilla	Anterior, premolar, and molar	1.7 mL 2% lidocaine with 1:100,000 epinephrine PLUS 1.7 mL 4% articaine	Local infiltration on buccal or facial aspect
Mandible	Anterior	1.7 mL 2% lidocaine with 1:100,000 epinephrine PLUS 1.7 mL 4% articaine with 1:100,000 epinephrine	Local infiltration on buccal aspect OR Mental nerve block and local infiltration on buccal aspect
	Premolar	3.4 mL 2% lidocaine with 1:100,000 epinephrine	Inferior alveolar nerve block and mental nerve block
	Molar	3.4 mL 2% lidocaine with 1:100,000 epinephrine PLUS 1.7 mL 4% articaine with 1:100,000 epinephrine	Inferior alveolar nerve block with lidocaine solution PLUS Local infiltration on the buccal aspect with articaine solution

Confirmation of anesthesia

Prior to proceeding with endodontic treatment, achievement of pulpal anesthesia should be confirmed. Soft tissue anesthesia can easily be confirmed by the absence of sensation as measured by light palpation of gingival tissues with the sharp end of a double-ended endodontic explorer. Pulpal anesthesia is best confirmed by cold testing on a tooth that was previously responsive.[50] If the tooth in question was not cold responsive preoperatively, cold testing of a neighboring tooth is the next best option to confirm true pulpal anesthesia (Fig 4-11).

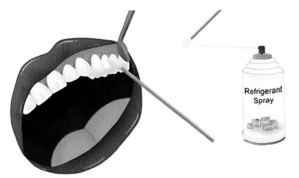

FIG 4-11 Pulpal anesthesia should always be confirmed prior to initiating care. The most predictable means of confirming pulpal anesthesia is by reapplication of the cold test utilized for diagnosis. A lack of cold response is indicative of profound pulpal anesthesia.

Adjunctive anesthetic techniques

While the aforementioned techniques are associated with a high degree of predictability, success rates for pulpal anesthesia are not 100%. Thus, clinicians providing endodontic care must have adjunctive anesthetic techniques in their skillset. These adjunctive techniques include intraligamentary, intraosseous, and intrapulpal injections.[38]

The intraligamentary injection, also called the periodontal ligament (PDL) injection, should be considered if first-line techniques for anesthesia are insufficient.[38] The technique involves injection of anesthetic solution under pressure through the gingival sulcus into the periodontal attachment tissues and cancellous bone surrounding the alveolar socket[51] (Fig 4-12). In theory, this procedure anesthetizes an individual tooth immediately via vasoconstriction of the vasculature surrounding the tooth. However, the intraligamentary injection may also anesthetize neighboring teeth and therefore cannot be reliably used for selective anesthesia in diagnosis.[52] Epinephrine-free anesthetic solutions should be used because intraligamentary injections are considered to be intravascular injections.[53]

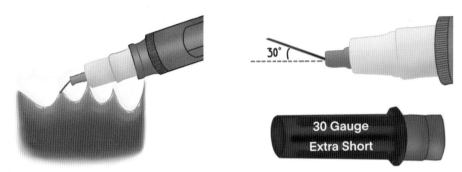

FIG 4-12 Intraligamentary injections involve the deposition of anesthetic under pressure through the gingival sulcus. This represents the first-line adjunctive anesthetic technique when block and infiltration techniques are insufficient to obtain pulpal anesthesia.

The technique is performed with a syringe loaded with mepivacaine plain and an ultrashort 30-gauge needle bent at 30 degrees to the long axis of the tooth, with the bevel facing the root surface.[54] The needle should be inserted into the sulcus at one line angle of the tooth until a hard stop is reached and a tight fit is felt. Injection should proceed to deposit 0.2 mL of anesthetic solution with significant backpressure until the adjacent tissue blanches. This typically takes at least 20 to 30 seconds. If a tight fit and backpressure is not felt, a different spot should be located for injection. Leakage of anesthetic solution into the oral cavity should not occur if this technique is performed properly; however, given the risk of bitter-tasting anesthetic solutions leading to patient discomfort, a surgical suction may be placed adjacent to the needle tip. Commercially available devices such as the LigaJect (Micro-Mega) or the Ligmaject (HenkeSassWolf) may be used to overcome the challenge of injecting under pressure. That said, they have not shown greater efficacy over the manual technique using a conventional dental syringe.[55]

Intraligamentary injections can produce vasoconstriction and damage the pulp circulation, so their use should be reserved for endodontic procedures or extractions wherein the pulp will be removed.[54] Furthermore, they should be avoided in cases of severe infection like cellulitis or osteomyelitis due to concerns about spreading infection. Patients given intraligamentary injections should be counseled on the expectation of postoperative discomfort relating to the soft tissue trauma and swelling of the apical tissues. While occlusal reduction may minimize these symptoms, preemptive use of postoperative analgesics is recommended.[51]

An intraosseous injection can be utilized if the above techniques are insufficient to provide pulpal anesthesia.[38] This method involves the use of a commercially available system such as the X-tip dental anesthesia system (Dentsply Maillefer) (Fig 4-13) to create a small opening in the cancellous bone for direct deposition of anesthesia. Following soft tissue anesthesia of the overlying tissues and identification of a safe space just apical and interproximal to the root tips, and avoiding anatomical structures like the mental foramen, a proprietary "perforator" drill tip is advanced through the cancellous bone with a slow-speed handpiece (Fig 4-14). Following this, mepivacaine can be introduced with a short, 30-gauge needle directly into the opening. Epinephrine-free anesthetic solutions are advised for intraosseous anesthesia due to the high vascularity of cancellous bone, which may lead to tachycardia secondary to epinephrine.[56] The intraosseous injection is also contraindicated in cases of active infection and when root or neural anatomy cannot be easily avoided. Care must be taken with these injections due to the risks of perforator separation, thermal injuries, and postoperative infections.[57]

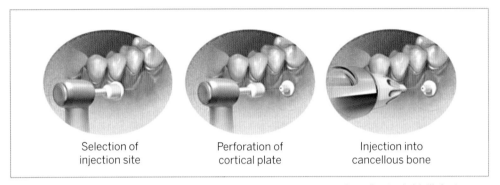

| Selection of injection site | Perforation of cortical plate | Injection into cancellous bone |

FIG 4-13 The commercially available X-tip intraosseous injection system from Dentsply Maillefer is one means of providing intraosseous anesthesia.

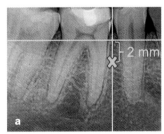 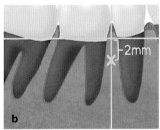

FIG 4-14 (*a and b*) Intraosseous anesthetic systems require identification of a safe space for insertion of the perforator to avoid damage to the root structure or other vital anatomical structures.

Intrapulpal injections should be used only when all other methods fail to provide complete pulpal anesthesia. In certain cases, small amounts of incompletely anesthetized tissue will remain inside the canals or chamber or pulpal anesthesia will wear off during the course of treatment, and intrapulpal anesthesia will then be indicated. In cases where pain is felt prior to accessing pulpal tissues, other adjunctive methodologies should instead be employed. Intrapulpal injections involve direct deposition of anesthetic solution into the sensitive tissues (Fig 4-15). Resultantly, the injection can be quite painful for a few seconds until anesthesia is complete, and patients should be duly warned. The effectiveness of intrapulpal anesthesia is directly related to the clinician's ability to administer the medication under pressure.[58] This is most easily done with a short, 30-gauge needle inserted into a minimally unroofed pulp chamber or all the way into the canal space when accessible until resistance is encountered. Epinephrine-free anesthetic solutions are advised because intrapulpal anesthesia uses an intravascular injection.

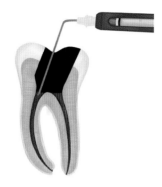

FIG 4-15 Intrapulpal anesthesia should be delivered under pressure for maximum efficacy.

References

1. Elzaki WM, Abubakr NH, Ziada HM, Ibrahim YE. Double-blind randomized placebo-controlled clinical trial of efficiency of nonsteroidal anti-inflammatory drugs in the control of post-endodontic pain. J Endod 2016;42:835–842.
2. Sathorn C, Parashos P, Messer H. The prevalence of postoperative pain and flare-up in single- and multiple-visit endodontic treatment: A systematic review. Int Endod J 2008;41:91–99.
3. Smith EA, Marshall JG, Selph SS, Barker DR, Sedgley CM. Nonsteroidal anti-inflammatory drugs for managing postoperative endodontic pain in patients who present with preoperative pain: A systematic review and meta-analysis. J Endod 2017;43:7–15.
4. Hargreaves KM, Keiser K. Development of new pain management strategies. J Dent Educ 2002;66:113–121.
5. Risser A, Donovan D, Heintzman J, Page T. NSAID prescribing precautions. Am Fam Physician 2009;80:1371–1378.
6. American Dental Association. ADA Dental Drug Handbook: A Quick Reference. Chicago: American Dental Association, 2019.
7. Aminoshariae A, Kulild JC, Donaldson M. Short-term use of nonsteroidal anti-inflammatory drugs and adverse effects: An updated systematic review. J Am Dent Assoc 2016;147:98–110.
8. Derry CJ, Derry S, Moore RA. Single dose oral ibuprofen plus paracetamol (acetaminophen) for acute postoperative pain. Cochrane Database Syst Rev 2013;2013:CD010210.
9. Zanjir M, Sgro A, Lighvan NL, et al. Efficacy and safety of postoperative medications in reducing pain after nonsurgical endodontic treatment: A systematic review and network meta-analysis. J Endod 2020;46:1387–1402.e4.
10. Richards D. The Oxford Pain Group League table of analgesic efficacy. Evid Based Dent 2004;5:22–23.
11. Miech R, Johnston L, O'Malley PM, Keyes KM, Heard K. Prescription opioids in adolescence and future opioid misuse. Pediatrics 2015;136:e1169–e1177.
12. American Association of Endodontists. AAE position statement: AAE guidance on the use of systemic antibiotics in endodontics. J Endod 2017;43:1409–1413.
13. Johnson M. Antibiotics and the treatment of dental infections. American Association of Endodontists: Colleagues for Excellence, Fall 2019.
14. American Association of Endodontists. The Recommended Guidelines of the American Association of Endodontists for the Treatment of Traumatic Dental Injuries. 2013. http://www.aae.org/clinical-resources/trauma-resources.aspx. Accessed 22 March 2023.
15. Lockhart PB, Tampi MP, Abt E, et al. Evidence-based clinical practice guideline on antibiotic use for the urgent management of pulpal- and periapical-related dental pain and intraoral swelling: A report from the American Dental Association. J Am Dent Assoc 2019;150:906.e12–921.e12.
16. Nagle, D, Reader A, Beck M, Weaver J. Effect of systemic penicillin on pain in untreated irreversible pulpitis. Oral Surg Oral Med Oral Pathol Oral Radiol Endod 2000;90:636–640.
17. Walton RE, Chiappinelli J. Prophylactic penicillin: Effect on posttreatment symptoms following root canal treatment of asymptomatic periapical pathosis. J Endod 1993;19:466–470.
18. Fouad AF, Rivera EM, Walton RE. Penicillin as a supplement in resolving the localized acute apical abscess. Oral Surg Oral Med Oral Pathol Oral Radiol Endod 1996;81:590–595.
19. Ng YL, Mann V, Gulabivala K. A prospective study of the factors affecting outcomes of nonsurgical root canal treatment: Part 1: Periapical health. Int Endod J 2011;44:583-609.
20. Pallasch TJ. Pharmacokinetic principles of antimicrobial therapy. Periodontol 2000;10:5–11.

21. Llewelyn MJ, Fitzpatrick JM, Darwin E, et al. The antibiotic course has had its day. BMJ 2017;358:j3418.
22. Martin MV, Longman LP, Hill JB, Hardy P. Acute dentoalveolar infections: An investigation of the duration of antibiotic therapy. Br Dent J 1997;183:135–137.
23. Segura-Egea JJ, Gould K, Şen BH, et al. European Society of Endodontology position statement: The use of antibiotics in endodontics. Int Endod J 2018;51:20–25.
24. Macy E. Penicillin and beta-lactam allergy: Epidemiology and diagnosis. Curr Allergy Asthma Rep 2014;14:476.
25. Wilson W, Taubert KA, Gewitz M, et al. Prevention of infective endocarditis: Guidelines from the American Heart Association: A guideline from the American Heart Association Rheumatic Fever, Endocarditis and Kawasaki Disease Committee, Council on Cardiovascular Disease in the Young, and the Council on Clinical Cardiology, Council on Cardiovascular Surgery and Anesthesia, and the Quality of Care and Outcomes Research Interdisciplinary Working Group. Circulation 2007;116:1736–1754.
26. Wilson WR, Gewitz M, Lockhart PB, et al. Prevention of Viridans group streptococcal infective endocarditis: A scientific statement from the American Heart Association. Circulation 2021;143:e963–e978 [erratum 2021;144:e192].
27. Sollecito TP, Abt E, Lockhart PB, et al. The use of prophylactic antibiotics prior to dental procedures in patients with prosthetic joints. J Am Dent Assoc 2015;146:11–16.e8.
28. Lindemann M, Reader A, Nusstein J, Drum M, Beck M. Effect of sublingual triazolam on the success of inferior alveolar nerve block in patients with irreversible pulpitis. J Endod 2008;34:1167–1170.
29. Murillo-Benítez M, Martín-González J, Jimenez-Sánchez MC, Cabanillas-Balsera D, Velasco-Ortega E, Segura-Egea JJ. Association between dental anxiety and intraoperative pain during root canal treatment: A cross sectional study. Int Endod J 2020;53:447–454.
30. Becker DE, Rosenberg M. Nitrous oxide and the inhalation anesthetics. Anesth Prog 2008;55:124–130.
31. Stanley W, Drum M, Nusstein J, Reader A, Beck M. Effect of nitrous oxide on the efficacy of the inferior alveolar nerve block in patients with symptomatic irreversible pulpitis. J Endod 2012;38:565–569.
32. Goodchild JH, Donaldson M. New sedation and general anesthesia guidelines: Why the changes? J Am Dent Assoc 2017;148:138–142.
33. Drum M, Reader A, Nusstein J, Fowler S. Successful pulpal anesthesia for symptomatic irreversible pulpitis. J Am Dent Assoc 2017;148:267–271.
34. Malamed SF. Handbook of Local Anesthesia, ed 7. St Louis: Mosby, 2019.
35. McLean C, Reader A, Beck M, Meryers WJ. An evaluation of 4% prilocaine and 3% mepivacaine compared with 2% lidocaine (1:100,000 epinephrine) for inferior alveolar nerve block. J Endod 1993;19:146–150.
36. Kanaa MD, Whitworth JM, Meechan JG. A comparison of the efficacy of 4% articaine with 1:100,000 epinephrine and 2% lidocaine with 1:80,000 epinephrine in achieving pulpal anesthesia in maxillary teeth with irreversible pulpitis. J Endod 2012;38:279–282.
37. Kung J, McDonagh M, Sedgley CM. Does articaine provide an advantage over lidocaine in patients with symptomatic irreversible pulpitis? A systematic review and meta-analysis. J Endod 2015;41:1784–1794.
38. Kanaa MD, Whitworth JM, Meechan JG. A prospective randomized trial of different supplementary local anesthetic techniques after failure of inferior alveolar nerve block in patients with irreversible pulpitis in mandibular teeth. J Endod 2012;38:421–425.
39. Gholami M, Banihashemrad A, Mohammadzadeh A, Ahrari F. The efficacy of 4% articaine versus 2% lidocaine in inducing palatal anesthesia for tooth extraction in different maxillary regions. J Oral Maxillofac Surg 2021;79:1643–1649.
40. Garisto GA, Gaffen AS, Lawrence HP, Tenenbaum HC, Haas DA. Occurrence of paresthesia after dental local anesthetic administration in the United States. J Am Dent Assoc 2010;141:836–844.
41. Gordon SM, Dionne RA, Brahim J, Jabir F, Dubner R. Blockade of peripheral neuronal barrage reduces postoperative pain. Pain 1997;70:209–215.
42. Jebeles JA, Reilly JS, Gutierrez JF, Bradley EL Jr, Kissin I. Tonsillectomy and adenoidectomy pain reduction by local bupivacaine infiltration in children. Int J Pediatr Otorhinolaryngol 1993;25:149–154.
43. Aggarwal V, Singla M, Miglani S, Kohli S, Singh S. Comparative evaluation of 1.8 mL and 3.6 mL of 2% lidocaine with 1:200,000 epinephrine for inferior alveolar nerve block in patients with irreversible pulpitis: A prospective, randomized single-blind study. J Endod 2012;38:753–756.
44. Pulikkotil SJ, Nagendrababu V, Veettil SK, Jinatongthai P, Setzer FC. Effect of oral premedication on the anaesthetic efficacy of inferior alveolar nerve block in patients with irreversible pulpitis—A systematic review and network meta-analysis of randomized controlled trials. Int Endod J 2018;51:989–1004.
45. Bhalla J, Meechan JG, Lawrence HP, Grad HA, Haas DA. Effect of time on clinical efficacy of topical anesthesia. Anesth Prog 2009;56:36–41.
46. Guglielmo A, Drum M, Reader A, Nusstein J. Anesthetic efficacy of a combination palatal and buccal infiltration of the maxillary first molar. J Endod 2011;37:460–462.
47. Aggarwal V, Singla M, Miglani S, Ansari I, Kohli S. A prospective, randomized, single-blind comparative evaluation of anesthetic efficacy of posterior superior alveolar nerve blocks, buccal infiltrations, and buccal plus palatal infiltrations in patients with irreversible pulpitis. J Endod 2011;37:1491–1494.

48. Kumar U, Aggarwal V, Singh S, Singh SP, Gauba K. Is mental incisive nerve block better than unilateral mental incisive nerve block during the endodontic management of mandibular incisors with symptomatic irreversible pulpitis? A prospective single-blind randomized clinical trial. J Endod 2020;46:471–474.

49. Aggarwal V, Singla M, Miglani S, Kohli S. Comparative evaluation of mental incisal nerve block, inferior alveolar nerve block, and their combination on the anesthetic success rate in symptomatic mandibular premolars: A randomized double-blind clinical trial. J Endod 2016;42:843–845.

50. Hsiao-Wu GW, Susarla SM, White RR. Use of the cold test as a measure of pulpal anesthesia during endodontic therapy: A randomized, blinded, placebo-controlled clinical trial. J Endod 2007;33:406–410.

51. Smith GN, Walton RE. Periodontal ligament injection: Distribution of injected solutions. Oral Surg Oral Med Oral Pathol 1983;55:232–238.

52. White JJ, Reader A, Beck M, Meyers WJ. The periodontal ligament injection: A comparison of the efficacy in human maxillary and mandibular teeth. J Endod 1988;14:508–514.

53. Brkovic BMB, Savic M, Andric M, Jurisic M, Todorovic L. Intraseptal vs. periodontal ligament anaesthesia for maxillary tooth extraction: Quality of local anaesthesia and haemodynamic response. Clin Oral Investig 2010;14:675–681.

54. Malamed SF. Handbook of Local Anesthesia, ed 6. St Louis: Mosby, 2013.

55. Ryan RM. Ligmaject system for local anaesthesia in otology. J Laryngol Otol 1990;104:606–607.

56. Wood M, Reader A, Nusstein J, Beck M, Padgett D, Weaver J. Comparison of intraosseous and infiltration injections for venous lidocaine blood concentrations and heart rate changes after injection of 2% lidocaine with 1:100,000 epinephrine. J Endod 2005;31:435–438.

57. Woodmansey KF, White RK, He J. Osteonecrosis related to intraosseous anesthesia: Report of a case. J Endod 2009;35:288–291.

58. VanGheluwe J, Walton R. Intrapulpal injection: Factors related to effectiveness. Oral Surg Oral Med Oral Pathol Oral Radiol Endod 1997;83:38–40.

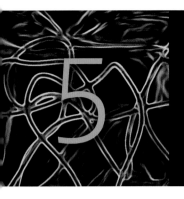

Nonsurgical Endodontics

Nonsurgical endodontics includes nonsurgical root canal therapy (NSRCT) and nonsurgical retreatment, as well as vital pulp therapy, apexification, and regenerative endodontics. The foundation of nonsurgical endodontics is the disinfection and prevention of re-infection of the root canal spaces. This chapter covers, in detail, all the procedures and materials related to NSRCT, some of which may apply broadly to other nonsurgical endodontic procedures. The protocols and materials pertinent to the remaining procedures are reviewed in separate chapters.

Armamentarium

Armamentarium for NSRCT should include anesthetic syringes, a mouth mirror, cotton pliers, an explorer, a periodontal probe, Schilder pluggers or similar gutta-percha pluggers, scissors, irrigation needles, paper points, gutta-percha points, and file storage (Fig 5-1). Armamentarium for simple dental dam isolation includes dental dam clamps, dental dam frames, dental dams (both latex and nonlatex in case of patient allergy), and dental floss (Fig 5-2).

Dental Dam Isolation

Dental dam isolation is the standard of care for safety and surgical isolation in the delivery of nonsurgical endodontic care.[1,2] Endodontic procedures performed without the use of the dental dam fall outside of legally sound care.[2] Not only does dental dam isolation eliminate the reintroduction of microbial salivary contaminants into the root canal space, but it also minimizes the aspiration risk associated with small endodontic instruments and irrigants. No alternative means of isolation have proven as effective as the dental dam, and no other device or protocol can take its place.[2,3] Furthermore, the dental dam can serve to minimize the transmission of patient respiratory droplets.[4]

For most nonsurgical endodontic procedures, single tooth isolation is appropriate. Clamps should be selected based on tooth size and clinician preference. Most anterior and premolar teeth can easily be isolated with a butterfly-style clamp (9A). Larger premolars may require the use of a size 0 or 2 clamp. Intact molars in the first (ie, maxillary right) and third (ie, mandibular left) quadrants

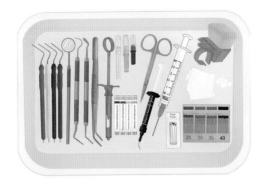

FIG 5-1 The armamentarium for root canal therapy should include the local anesthetic armamentarium (syringes, needles, drugs), a mouth mirror, cotton pliers, an explorer, a periodontal probe, Schilder pluggers or similar gutta-percha pluggers, scissors, irrigation needles, paper points, gutta-percha points, file storage, plastic instruments, and temporary restorative materials.

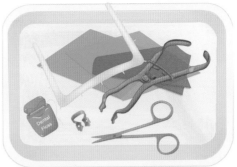

FIG 5-2 The armamentarium for dental dam isolation should include dental dam clamps, dental dam frames, dental dam (both latex and nonlatex in case of patient allergy), and dental floss.

are best isolated with 13A clamps, whereas those in quadrants two (ie, maxillary left) and four (ie, mandibular right) are best isolated with 12A clamps (Fig 5-3). That said, clinicians should be prepared for clamp placement on unusually shaped teeth outside these standard recommendations.

Winged clamps are advantageous for dental dam isolation in endodontics because the dam, clamp, and frame can be delivered as a single unit into the patient's mouth. Floss should be tied around the clamp to facilitate retrieval and prevent swallowing or aspiration if it is accidentally dislodged. After placement, the dam should be passed over the clamp wings, flossed between contacts, and

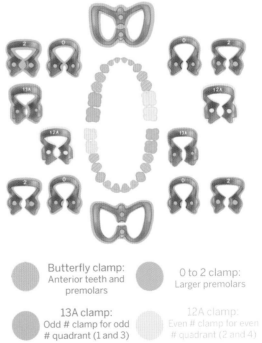

Butterfly clamp: Anterior teeth and premolars

0 to 2 clamp: Larger premolars

13A clamp: Odd # clamp for odd # quadrant (1 and 3)

12A clamp: Even # clamp for even # quadrant (2 and 4)

FIG 5-3 Dental dam clamp selection for endodontic procedures by tooth.

inverted around the tooth or teeth (Fig 5-4). If there are concerns about leakage surrounding the tooth, isolation adjuncts, such as OpalDam (Ultradent), can be placed around the tooth to create a leak-proof seal.

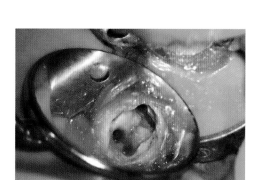

FIG 5-4 Single tooth isolation is appropriate for most endodontic procedures. (Photo courtesy of Dr Yen-jung Chen.)

Certain teeth require creative modifications for isolation. For teeth with extensive fractures or caries, restoration of the defect prior to isolation may be indicated to facilitate clamp placement. Bonded materials, including resin-modified glass ionomers and composite restorative materials, or other appropriate temporary restorative materials may be used to restore the tooth to facilitate isolation and maintenance of a coronal seal during the delivery of endodontic care. Neighboring teeth may also be utilized as the anchor for a dental dam clamp when the tooth being treated has insufficient structure.

Dental dam isolation can provoke fear and claustrophobia in certain patients. Talking patients through the practicalities of how the dental dam will be placed, as well as trimming the dam, may aid in patient acceptance. The use of bite blocks, usually in pediatric sizes, can be helpful for certain patients, though may be intolerable for others. Placing a saliva ejector behind the dam may relieve patient fears of saliva buildup or of being unable to swallow with the bite block or dam in place. Anxiolysis with oral medications or nitrous oxide may allow certain patients to better tolerate the dental dam, though deeper sedation may be necessary for patients with severe anxiety, claustrophobia, or gag reflexes.

Preoperative Rinses

The use of preoperative oral rinses has been advised for disinfecting the operative field prior to invasive dental procedures.[5–7] Rinses may be used throughout the oral cavity or applied via syringe to the surface of the tooth following dental dam isolation. Chlorhexidine gluconate, hydrogen peroxide, cetylpyridinium chloride, and iodopovidone, among others, represent available and realistic options for oral and irrigation-based preoperative rinsing solutions[7,8] and have been shown to be effective to reduce viral loads in saliva for up to 45 minutes following use.[8] The use of these mouth rinses poses little additional cost or time and carries potential benefits to reduce cross-contamination of the operative or surgical space.

Magnification

One cannot treat what one cannot see. The necessity of magnification in endodontics cannot be overemphasized. Magnification aids clinicians in locating normal anatomical structures during nonsurgical and surgical endodontic therapy,[9] detecting cracks and fractures,[10] removing obstructions, and managing complications.[11] At a minimum, magnification loupes with a headlight or, ideally, a surgical operating microscope should be employed to ensure adequate visualization of the miniscule structures germane to endodontics (Fig 5-5).[12] The surgical operating microscope has the added benefit of integrated illumination. Even in conservative access cavities, the surgical operating microscope enhances one's ability to detect canal anatomy.[13] Of course, in cases of pulp canal obliteration or calcification of the pulp chamber, normal anatomical clues may be absent, and extra care is needed to locate canals safely and conservatively. Magnification is but one means to provide such extra care.

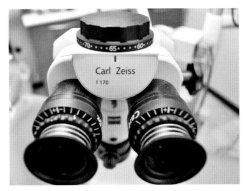

FIG 5-5 Loupes or a surgical operating microscope are necessary to provide adequate visualization during endodontic care.

Access

The purpose of an endodontic access is to expose the full extent of the pulp chamber and canal network to facilitate cleaning, shaping, and obturation. While all canals must be visualized, endodontic access should be performed with care to conserve dental hard tissues to the greatest extent possible. Overzealous endodontic access openings can predispose teeth to future fractures or result in inadequately retained restorations and, in cases where the access extends too deep, lead to immediate perforations. Conversely, an undersized access risks leaving tissue remnants and infection behind.[14] Therefore, the size of an access should balance complete removal of pulpal soft tissues and infectious debris with the absolute need to conserve tooth structure to reduce risks related to fracture and perforation.[15]

Armamentarium for access includes a high-speed handpiece and appropriate burs. Adjunctive armamentarium should include spoon excavators and slow-speed handpieces and burs for caries removal, as well as ultrasonic instruments when microscopes are available (Fig 5-6). Access openings through natural tooth structure should be made using a high-speed handpiece. In operative dentistry, water coolant is necessary to minimize pulpal damage.[16] While this isn't a concern in endodontics, water coolant may still be needed when accessing through porcelain, zirconia, or metal restorations to prevent heat-related damage to these restorative materials. Water coolants may also aid in flushing away debris.

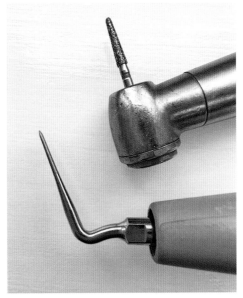

FIG 5-6 The access armamentarium should include a high-speed handpiece and appropriate burs, as well as ultrasonic instruments when microscopes are available.

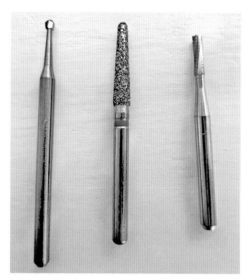

FIG 5-7 Clinicians should have a selection of burs at their disposal for access, including surgical-length round burs, tapered diamond burs, metal-cutting burs, and zirconia-cutting burs.

A wide variety of burs are available, including products with non-cutting tips designed specifically for endodontic access, and the choice of what to use ultimately lies with the clinician. New dentists often feel most comfortable with a no. 2 or no. 4 round bur for initial entry to the chamber, switching to a safe-end bur to unroof the remainder of the chamber. More experienced clinicians may work entirely with a tapered diamond bur, which is also indicated when drilling through porcelain to minimize fractures. Metal cutting or zirconia-specific burs are often needed in the presence of full-coverage restorations comprised of these materials, not only for improved efficacy but to minimize material fracture (Fig 5-7).

Generally, intracoronal restorations should be removed in their entirety during endodontic access, with the notable exception being in those cases where restorations have been placed recently and have excellent marginal integrity. This process of coronal disassembly facilitates inspection of the remaining tooth structure for fractures or other compromise. Temporary crowns can be removed for access but may also be left in place if securely cemented, with access performed through their occlusal surface as with the natural tooth. In some cases, removal of temporary crowns facilitates access of the pulp by minimizing the materials that must be drilled through; in others, it can complicate dental dam isolation due to inadequate retention without the crown in place. Permanent crowns need not be removed. Access should be performed through the occlusal surface of the existing crown, and patients should be informed of the risks of intraoperative complications, including loss of retention or recurrent caries, necessitating crown removal and postendodontic replacement.

The shape of the access preparation is determined by the anatomy of the individual tooth. Knowledge of both clinical and radiographic dental anatomy should facilitate access shape development. Access openings should mirror the size and shape of the pulp chamber and permit clinicians to locate all the canals contained within the tooth. The shape of the pulp chamber reflects the external tooth anatomy at the level of the cementoenamel junction (CEJ) and is concentric with the external tooth surface. Exposure of the entirety of the pulpal floor will reveal a change in coloration at the wall-floor junction. These anatomical rules are referred to as Krasner and Rankow's laws for pulp chamber location (Fig 5-8).

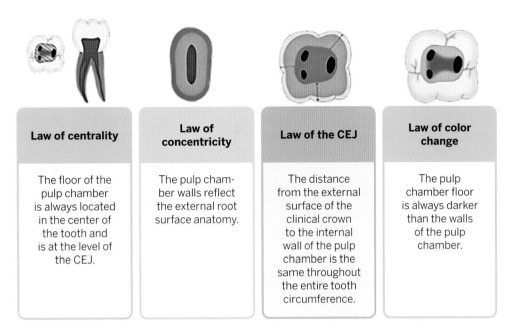

Law of centrality	Law of concentricity	Law of the CEJ	Law of color change
The floor of the pulp chamber is always located in the center of the tooth and is at the level of the CEJ.	The pulp chamber walls reflect the external root surface anatomy.	The distance from the external surface of the clinical crown to the internal wall of the pulp chamber is the same throughout the entire tooth circumference.	The pulp chamber floor is always darker than the walls of the pulp chamber.

FIG 5-8 Krasner and Rankow's laws for pulp chamber location.

Radiographic anatomy, like clinical anatomy, is essential for access development. In addition to their utility in diagnosis, bitewing radiographs are especially useful for planning the endodontic access because they accurately depict the mesiodistal and coronal-apical dimensions of the pulp chamber.[17] When available, CBCT imaging accurately demonstrates the faciolingual position of the pulp chamber and can therefore be of particular use for access planning. In the future, novel methods involving 3D-guided access will no doubt revolutionize endodontics.[18,19] Access shapes produced by these anatomical guides often follow trends, and the common shapes are depicted in Fig 5-9.

Access shape should facilitate straight-line access into the canal spaces. Straight-line access, wherein tooth structure is removed so that canal spaces can be entered longitudinally, allows for reduced stress on instruments entering curved spaces and ensures complete

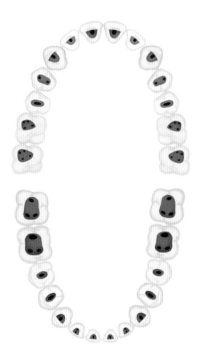

FIG 5-9 Common access shapes are depicted.

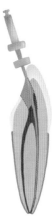

FIG 5-10 Straight-line access, wherein tooth structure is removed so that canal spaces can be entered longitudinally, allows for reduced stress on instruments entering curved spaces and ensures complete removal of tissue within the pulp chamber.

removal of tissue within the chamber (Fig 5-10). In teeth that will receive full-coverage restorations following treatment, the occlusal reduction can be performed prior to access to provide a flat, reproducible reference point and to reduce the risk of fracture or postoperative pain.[20]

With the external anatomy and radiographs to guide initial access shape, access depth must be determined. The average distance between the cusp tip to the roof of the chamber is 6 to 7 mm, and the average pulp chamber height is 2 to 3 mm.[21] That said, measurements for individual teeth should be assessed via careful radiographic study. A rubber stopper placed on a DG16 double-ended endodontic explorer provides an easy means of measuring the depth of access opening as one proceeds, and intraoperative bitewing angle radiographs or even CBCT images may be used to ensure an appropriate access angle if the chamber is not located as expected (Fig 5-11).

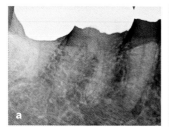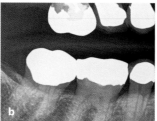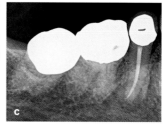

FIG 5-11 Bitewing radiographs and CBCT images can be used during access to ensure that the access remains in line with the pulp chamber and canal spaces. This mandibular second premolar (a) required an access bitewing (b) because the coronal chamber was quite calcified and the access was difficult. The completed root canal is seen in the final radiograph (c).

Anterior access

Anterior teeth generally follow a triangular or ovoid pattern of access once the full extent of the pulp horns is unroofed. Because anterior teeth lack a flat occlusal surface, small amounts of additional tooth structure must often be removed on both the facial and lingual or palatal surfaces of the chamber to fully clean the space and obtain direct access into the canal (Fig 5-12). The access should be directed along the long axis of the tooth, as opposed to perpendicular to the lingual or palatal surface, to provide straight-line access into the canal space (Fig 5-13). In the case of two-canaled mandibular incisors, additional removal of lingual dentin may be required to access the additional anatomy. Care must be taken to stop drilling within the pulp chamber to avoid perforation through the facial wall.

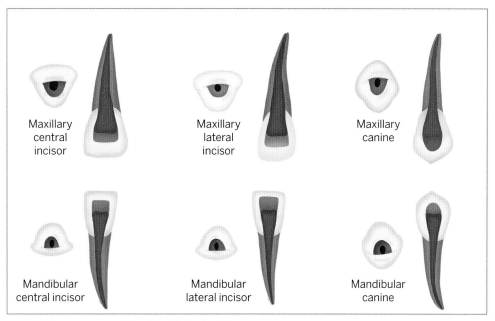

FIG 5-12 Access preparations for anterior teeth.

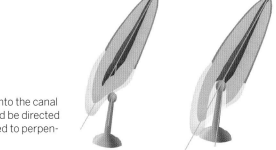

FIG 5-13 To achieve straight-line access into the canal spaces of anterior teeth, the access should be directed along the long axis of the tooth, as opposed to perpendicular to the tooth surface.

Premolar access

Access of premolars requires extreme care because of their narrow mesiodistal dimensions. Attention must be paid to the orientation of canal anatomy within the tooth, especially when the tooth is rotated or when a full-coverage restoration is present, because the restoration anatomy may change the perceived crown-to-root orientation. Furthermore, mandibular premolars have lingually inclined occlusal tables, whereas maxillary premolars may have proximal root concavities. Cervical perforations can easily occur if the unique anatomy is not respected.

The premolar access shape follows that of the pulp chamber anatomy and canal configuration, ranging from a circular shape in the case of a single-canaled tooth, an oval in the case of two canals, and triangular in the rare three-canaled premolar (Fig 5-14). Mandibular premolars require access toward the buccal cusp to achieve straight-line access given their lingually inclined occlusal table (Fig 5-15).

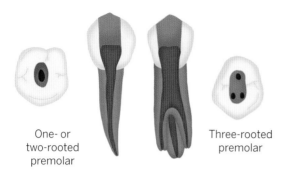

One- or
two-rooted
premolar

Three-rooted
premolar

FIG 5-14 Access preparations for premolar teeth.

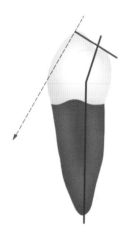

FIG 5-15 Mandibular premolars have lingually inclined occlusal tables, necessitating an access directed more closely toward the buccal cusps. If access is directed only perpendicular to the occlusal table, buccal perforation may occur.

Molar access

Molars possess complex occlusal features, making access challenging. Care should be taken because of discrepancies in the mesiodistal width of the occlusal table and the cervical portions of teeth. If the occlusal width is used as a landmark for access, clinicians risk cervical perforation. For maxillary molars, the access should be placed mesial to the oblique ridge. For mandibular molars, access should begin in the central fossa (Fig 5-16). Some clinicians first aim toward the largest canal, usually the distal canal in mandibular molars and the palatal canal in maxillary molars. Others aim for the highest pulp horn seen on the bitewing radiograph, where the chamber space is largest, which is often toward the mesiobuccal aspect in maxillary and mandibular molars.

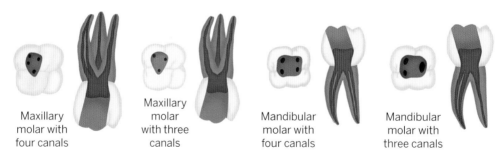

Maxillary
molar with
four canals

Maxillary
molar
with three
canals

Mandibular
molar with
four canals

Mandibular
molar with
three canals

FIG 5-16 Access preparations for molar teeth.

Access challenges

Excessive bleeding may make visualization difficult when accessing inflamed teeth. Small spoon excavators can be useful to remove large pieces of pulp tissue within the chamber to lessen bleeding. As long as perforation is not suspected, gentle irrigation with sodium hypochlorite or hydrogen peroxide can also be used to remove inflamed pulp tissue in order to slow bleeding and enhance visualization. Accessed canals may be a source of bleeding, and in some cases, it makes sense to complete a pulpectomy in the accessible canals before locating further canals to complete the access.

If orientation loss occurs during access due to rotations in the tooth, fractures, or prior restorations, the dental dam may be removed to better visualize the CEJ of the root, as this outlines the canal shape most accurately. The tooth should be temporized prior to dam removal. Of course, the dental dam should be replaced prior to cleaning and shaping of the canal space. In some cases, an intraoperative bitewing radiograph or CBCT image might showcase the orientation of the access opening relative to canal orifices.

Canal Location

Ultimately, completion of an endodontic access requires identification and initial instrumentation of all canals so that straight-line access is confirmed. This requires knowledge of root canal morphology, both in general and specific to the tooth being treated. Canal morphology has been well documented in the endodontic literature, and clinicians should be familiar with the average canal numbers per tooth as a starting place for their anatomical search (Table 5-1).[22–28]

TABLE 5-1 Summary of root canal morphology[22–28]

Tooth	No. of canals/roots
Maxillary central incisors	1 canal (100%)
Maxillary lateral incisors	1 canal (100%)
Maxillary canines	1 canal (100%)
Maxillary first premolars	2 canals (69%) 1 canal (26%) 3 canals (5%)
Maxillary second premolars	1 canal (75%) 2 canals (24%) 3 canals (1%)
Maxillary first molars	4 canals (96%) 3 canals (4%)
Maxillary second molars	4 canals (94%) 3 canals (6%)
Mandibular central incisors	1 canal/1 foramen (70%) 2 canals/1 foramen (27%) 2 canals/2 foramina (3%)
Mandibular lateral incisors	1 canal/1 foramen (75%) 2 canals/1 foramen (23%) 2 canals/2 foramina (2%)
Mandibular canines	1 canal (94%) 2 canals (6%)
Mandibular first premolars	1 canal/1 foramen (70%) 2 canals/2 foramina (25.5%) 2 canals/1 foramen (4%) 3 canals (0.5%)
Mandibular second premolars	1 canal (97.5%) 2 canals (2.5%)
Mandibular first molars	3 canals (64.8%) 4 canals (35.1%) 2 canals (0.1%) *Middle mesial canals present in 4–32% of patients*
Mandibular second molars	3 canals (89.4%) 4 canals (5.5%) 2 canals (4.1%) 1 canal (1%)

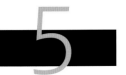

Nonsurgical Endodontics

First law of symmetry	**Second law of symmetry**	**First law of orifice location**	**Third law of orifice location**
In teeth with multiple canal orifices, the orifices are separated equidistant from a line drawn in a mesiodistal direction through the center of the pulp chamber floor. Maxillary molars are the exception.	Canal orifices are perpendicular to a line drawn in a buccolingual direction across the center of the pulp chamber floor. Maxillary molars are the exception.	Root canal orifices are always located at the junction of the walls and the floor.	Root canal orifices are always located at the terminus of the developmental fusion lines of the roots.
		Second law of orifice location	
		Root canal orifices are always located at the angles in the floor-wall junction.	

FIG 5-17 Krasner and Rankow's laws for canal location.

Locating canals, however, requires anatomical knowledge beyond knowing the average presentations. Just as Krasner and Rankow described anatomical laws for pulp chamber location, so too did they delineate laws for canal location.[10] Canals are located at the junction of the pulp chamber walls and the floor, at the angles in the floor-wall junctions, and at the terminus of the developmental fusion lines. Furthermore, except for maxillary molars, in teeth with multiple canal orifices, canals are separated equidistant from a line drawn in a mesiodistal direction through the center of the pulp chamber floor and are perpendicular to a line drawn in a buccolingual direction across the center of the pulp chamber floor (Fig 5-17). CBCT imaging is the next best alternative outside of visualizing anatomy within the tooth itself. However, clinicians must be aware of the myriad variations in pulp chamber and canal anatomy that fall outside the norm, including but not limited to C-shaped molar or premolar anatomy and the radix entomolaris (Fig 5-18).[29,30] When normal anatomical markers are present, such as chamber floor staining, Krasner and Rankow's laws generally do apply.

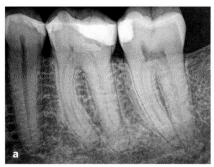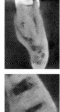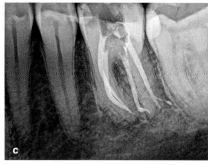

FIG 5-18 *(a to c)* Exceptions to Krasner and Rankow's laws for root canal morphology and symmetry, including the radix entomolaris anatomical anomaly shown here, warrant consideration of CBCT imaging to identify canals. In this case in particular, pulp chamber calcifications masked the clinical presence of this distolingual canal, whereas preoperative CBCT imaging made its presence clear, allowing for canal cleaning and obturation.

Endodontic access and canal location are interrelated procedures. Canals must be located to make the endodontic access. However, initial drilling is done before canals are found. Most clinicians aim for the easiest point of access into the pulp chamber. From there, one can "take what the tooth gives them," meaning locating, and sometimes instrumenting, the first canal space accessible and extending the access opening from there. In sum, endodontic access and initial canal location often occur simultaneously.

Canals can be scouted with a sharp, double-ended endodontic (DG16) explorer, or a small-diameter stainless steel hand instrument (eg, 0.06-mm-diameter, 25-mm-length K file or Hedstrom file) bent at 90 degrees when searching for calcified spaces (Fig 5-19). Great care must be taken with the DG16 as its sharp tip combined with pressure on dentin can create false stickiness suggestive of a canal orifice where one is not present. Because these instruments are usually too large, calcified canals are best scouted by alternative means. Stiffened stainless steel instruments, such as C files, can be especially useful for scouting calcified spaces that might catch a more flexible instrument and force it to kink or bend. Once the coronal portion of the canal is patent, a file of corresponding diameter can be introduced into the length of the canal and working length determination can begin.

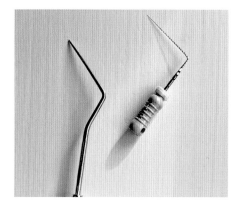

FIG 5-19 Canals can be scouted with a sharp, double-ended endodontic (DG16) explorer or a stainless steel hand file bent at 90 degrees, which is especially useful when searching for calcified root anatomy.

Often, canals can be located by tactile sensation alone. However, if chamber calcifications exist, visualization via magnification is crucial for locating the full extent of canal anatomy. When searching for hard-to-find canals, many clinicians switch from the initial access bur to smaller cutting burs, such as a no. 0.5 round bur, or ultrasonic drills with appropriately sized cutting tips (eg, Endo 3 or Endo 4 ProUltra Ultrasonic Tip, Dentsply Sirona). This shift should come with appropriate magnification because the risk of perforation is high when drilling on the chamber floor. Burs and ultrasonic drills with small diameter cutting tips require the use of a surgical operating microscope, as the divot that they create can easily be mistaken for a canal orifice.

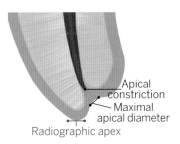

FIG 5-20 The cementodentinal junction, also known as the apical constriction, is the anatomical point at which instrumentation should terminate.

Working Length Determination

The aim of endodontics is the disinfection of the entire root canal system. Doing so requires the establishment of an accurate working length, defined as the measurement from a reference point to the apical terminus, or, more specifically, to the cementodentinal junction, or apical constriction (Fig 5-20).[31] Accurate working length determination is crucial for successful root canal therapy given the need to clean the entirety of the root canal space and to avoid undertreatment, overinstrumentation, or overfilling and their resultant negative effects on the periapical tissues.[31,32]

In practice, to maintain an apical stop against which to pack obturation materials, instrumentation and obturation should terminate at the apical constriction.[1] It should be noted, however, that this constriction may be absent in an incompletely formed tooth[33] or may be lost due to apical external inflammatory root resorption, which often occurs secondary to apical pathology. The apical constriction is usually proximal to the radiographic apex,[34] though it may not correspond directly in canals with a lateral portal of exit, and it often resides 0.5 mm short of the external tooth surface.[35]

Determination of working length requires the establishment of an occlusal reference point and the location of the apical termination of the root canal space. Commercial rulers with clearly legible markers and space for file stoppers, such as the EndoRing line of products (Jordco) that also allows for file storage on disposable sponges, are convenient for this purpose. Establishing a reproducible reference point is crucial and

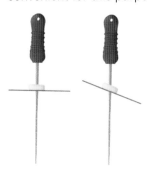

FIG 5-21 A reproducible reference point is best achieved when measured against a flat surface on the occlusal table. This may require occlusal adjustment.

is best achieved using a flat surface, with the rubber file stopper placed perpendicular to the length of the file (Fig 5-21). As previously mentioned, occlusal reduction should be performed prior to working length establishment, and this will also aid in creating the necessary flat surface.

Apical termination can be measured either radiographically or by electronic apex locators (EALs). Some clinicians may gain a tactile sense of instrumentation around the apical terminus. However, this methodology is grossly inaccurate compared to the described techniques and risks apical over-enlargement and traumatizing the periapical tissues. Similarly, methodologies incorporating a fluid line as seen on paper points taken beyond the apical terminus may risk the introduction of foreign bodies or mechanical trauma to the periapical tissues and are not advised.

Working lengths should be estimated preoperatively via radiograph. Digital software facilitates reasonable measurement estimates even with periapical images, though the dimensional accuracy of CBCT images provides even more reliable estimates.[36] When using radiographs alone to determine working length or when the measurements seem unreliable, estimated working lengths should

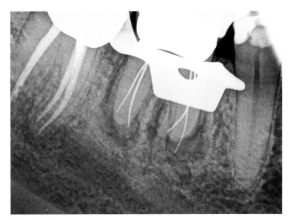

FIG 5-22 Working length radiographs, or file shots, in which no. 10 or no. 15 K files are introduced into the root canal spaces to the estimated working length and then a radiograph taken, are a useful tool in working length determination.

be confirmed via a working length radiograph prior to canal enlargement. Images may be taken with any file that is a no. 10 diameter or larger, as smaller files are generally not visualizable (Fig 5-22).[37] Not only do file shots confirm estimated working lengths, but they also show canal curvatures that may not be visible in the initial radiograph.

That said, determining the curvatures in roots and variability in the apical portal of exit require greater accuracy in working length determination than radiographs alone provide. EALs are now ubiquitous in endodontics, offering a reliable and noninvasive means for working length confirmation.[36,38] The EAL is a small, computerized device that measures impedance to accurately determine the change in resistance as the canal terminates within the apical periodontal ligament (PDL). EALs capitalize on the constant level of resistance that exists between the PDL and the oral cavity.[39,40] A circuit is created between the two via a metallic clip placed on the opposing lip commissure and an attachment to a file placed within the canal space. Measuring working length with the EAL is completed by the introduction of a file into the canal space while attached to the unit, typically the first scouting file. As the file approaches the periapex, a computer output depicts the approach. It is important to note that the point measured as "zero" on most EALs corresponds to the maximal apical diameter rather than the diameter of the apical constriction.[41] Because the apical constriction is typically located 0.5 to 1 mm short of the maximal diameter, the working length measured is usually at the "0.5" reading on the EAL monitor (Fig 5-23). When working with files smaller than a no. 10, the file should be passed through the apex to confirm patency because the

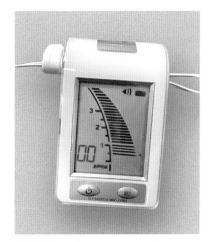

FIG 5-23 As the minimal apical constriction is typically located 0.5 to 1 mm short of the maximal diameter, the working length measured is usually at the "0.5" reading on the EAL monitor.

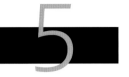

EAL measurement is most accurate when backing into the canal from patency. The EAL should be clipped on each hand instrument inserted into the tooth up to the master apical file (MAF). EAL technology has been adapted to integrate directly into slow-speed handpieces with the objective of continually measuring the working length throughout rotary instrumentation.[42] Beyond these generalizations, EAL function is manufacturer specific, and product manuals should be consulted.

EAL readings are accurate under a variety of conditions. They can accurately locate the apical foramen 96% of the time[38] but may be more useful for determining the major diameter than the minor diameter.[41] Their accuracy is not impacted by the pulpal diagnosis[43] or by the presence of apical root resorption[44] or apical periodontitis.[45] The EAL is also unaffected by neighboring electronic devices, including cellphones, and current evidence indicates that they do not interfere with the functionality of cardiac pacemaker devices.[46] Though EAL accuracy is unaffected by irrigation solutions in general,[47] the presence of fluid may matter in certain circumstances because EAL accuracy can be negatively impacted by metal restorations, particularly when fluid, including tissue fluid and irrigation solutions, is present in the canal space. Care must therefore be taken to keep the file away from metal surfaces while taking a reading.

The most common clinical issue with EAL use is the lack of a reading. Clinicians should first determine whether the lack of reading arises from a problem with the EAL unit or an issue within the tooth. Instrument function can be tested by attaching the lead clip to the ground. A lack of reading when doing so indicates malfunction of one of the EAL components, most often the lead, due to wear and tear, and each lead can be swapped out individually to discern where the issue is. If the unit immediately registers a reading when the lead is attached to the ground, the lack of read is likely due to a lack of patency within the canal, either caused by an abrupt anatomical curvature or the creation of a ledge within the canal space.

Though EALs may serve as reliable guides for initial instrumentation, radiographs remain the gold standard for working length determination,[1] and radiographic imaging must be used to confirm working lengths at some point during nonsurgical endodontics. At least one radiograph should be taken during root canal therapy to confirm the accuracy of EAL measurements. However, additional imaging may be performed at the clinician's discretion. Working length images can include a file shot, as discussed previously, an MAF film, or a cone fit radiograph, taken with gutta-percha in place

Working lengths should be reconfirmed during treatment because they can change slightly over the course of treatment. Rechecking lengths at several points during instrumentation accounts for changes due to canal widening and straightening of curvatures. Working lengths should similarly be reconfirmed during each visit of multistage therapy to account for calibration variability in rulers as well as aberrations in reference points. Confirmation of working lengths with small files, such as no. 08 or 10, can also serve to recapitulate and ensure patency of the canal from chamber to apex. If inconsistencies are noted at any point in working length determination, be it with EAL or radiographic confirmation, care should be taken to revisit and confirm the accuracy of working length measurements before proceeding.

Instrumentation

Following access and discovery of the canal systems and working length determination, cleaning and shaping of the root canal system is necessary to debride and prepare the space for obturation.[48] In endodontics, this is referred to as *chemomechanical preparation* because it combines mechanical instrumentation with disinfecting irrigants and medicaments. Although instrumentation and irrigation are used together to render the root canal system free of bacteria and tissue debris, they are discussed separately in this text.

Armamentarium

Armamentarium for instrumentation includes both hand and rotary files. Sizing for both is universal and follows the International Organization for Standardization (ISO) sizing guide. Each size is associated with a standardized color, which should be consistent across brands and instrument types (Fig 5-24). No matter the protocol followed, multiple hand and rotary instruments are required for every nonsurgical endodontic procedure. Because these tiny and sharp instruments pose a safety risk when left loose on a bracket table or tray, sponge storage is recommended. Additionally, instead of passing instruments directly between clinicians, files should be pushed into the sponge by one clinician and retrieved by another. Convenient holding devices, such as the previously mentioned EndoRing line of products, allow for ergonomic and safe access to instruments (Fig 5-25).

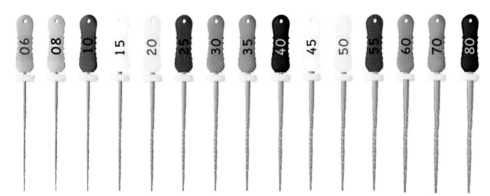

FIG 5-24 Sizing for both hand and rotary files is universal and follows the ISO sizing guide. Size is indicated by a standardized color, consistent across brands and instrument types.

Hand files

Hand files are single-use items composed of stainless steel. They are used for canal scouting during access until rotary instruments can be introduced into the root canal space. They follow the canal space from the chamber to the apex to aid in working length determination and to create a smooth glide path at the established working length. In theory, hand instruments can be used alone to fully instrument the canal spaces, but this is not often practiced due to the superior efficiency of nickel-titanium (NiTi) rotary instruments.

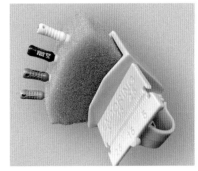

FIG 5-25 Convenient holding devices allow for ergonomic and safe access to both hand and rotary instruments. (EndoRing, Jordco).

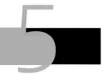

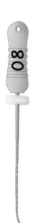

Hand files all follow a similar design with a rubber handle and fluted end. Generally, they are available in lengths of 21, 25, and 31 mm, all of which have a 16-mm cutting surface. The tip of the file (D0) corresponds to the number on the file. For example, a no. 10 file has a 0.1-mm diameter at D0. Each diameter is color coded according to ISO standards. Hand files have a standard taper of 0.02 mm (or 02 taper)—meaning that for every 1 mm of distance from D0, the diameter of the file increases by 0.02 mm. Thus, the diameter of a no. 10 0.02 taper file at D16 is 0.42 mm (0.10 + 16 × 0.02).

Smaller hand instruments, up to size no. 20, should be gently pre-curved prior to introduction into the canal space (Fig 5-26). This can be done by making a gentle pass over the file with a thumb and forefinger or with the tip of a pair of cotton pliers. Files larger than no. 20 prove difficult for gentle curvatures and can risk ledging. For this reason, curved canals are generally instrumented with the more flexible NiTi rotary instruments once an adequate glide path is created with no. 15 or 20 files.

FIG 5-26 Small hand instruments up to no. 20 should be gently pre-curved prior to introduction into the canal space.

K FILES

K files are the mainstay stainless steel hand instruments and are available in 0.02-mm taper and ISO diameters beginning with nos. 06 (0.06-mm apical diameter), 08, and 10, and increasing in denominations of 0.05 mm from there. Cross sections of square or rhomboid wire are twisted to create flutes that can engage the walls of the canal for a cutting motion (Fig 5-27). These files are marked by a square surrounding the number label on the handle. In smaller diameters, K files are relatively flexible and conducive to pre-curving. They are a versatile file, ideal for scouting and creating a glide path, as well as for the step-back hand instrumentation method described later in this chapter.

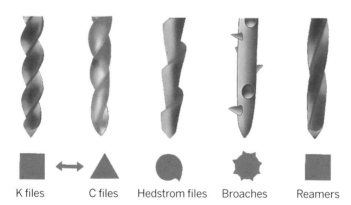

| K files | C files | Hedstrom files | Broaches | Reamers |

FIG 5-27 Hand file instrument types, including their cross-sectional shapes.

Endodontic instrumentation requires the use of several small-diameter K files, at minimum, usually up to at least no. 10 or 15 in apical diameter, to create a glide path of sufficient size and shape prior to introduction of NiTi rotary instruments. Small and calcified canals may require starting instrumentation with a no. 06 file, whereas wider canals can be initially instrumented with a no. 10 file.

C FILES

C files are similar in design to K files, but with greater stiffness This improves their ability to navigate teeth with calcifications, where more flexible files are prone to bend or kink. They are only available in sizes ranging from nos. 06 to 10, for use as stiffer alternatives to the more flexible K files in this size range.

HEDSTROM FILES

Hedstrom files are an alternative stainless steel hand file. Their cutting edges are inclined so that the instruments cut only on withdrawal from the canal. They are fabricated from a circular cross-section of wire with machined flutes. These files are marked with a circle surrounding their number label on the handle. They should be used in a longitudinal filing motion and can rapidly enlarge canals. Therefore, care should be taken to avoid ledging or transportation with these aggressive instruments. That said, the aggressive nature of Hedstrom files embodies them with qualities similar to a broach, making them useful for removing loose debris, such as tissue fragments, cotton pellets, and remnants of gutta-percha during retreatment procedures.

REAMERS

Reamers are fabricated from a cross-section of square or triangular wire twisted to create more cutting edges than a K file to engage with more walls of the tooth for more aggressive cutting. For that reason, use of these instruments risks overinstrumentation or transportation of canals, and they have been largely replaced by NiTi rotary instruments.

BROACHES

Broaches have machined barbs on a circular wire and are useful for pulp tissue removal and retrieval of cotton pellets, remnants of gutta-percha, and other debris.

Rotary files

Prior to the advent of NiTi rotary instruments, stainless steel coronal-flaring instruments were developed. These include both Gates Glidden Drills, Peeso reamers, and proprietary post drills (Fig 5-28). All may be used with an air-driven slow-speed drill, or electric slow-speed motor at high rotation.

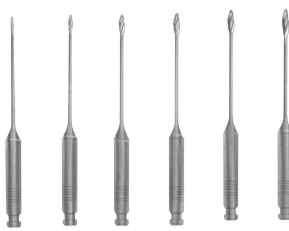

FIG 5-28 Stainless steel rotary instruments include Gates Glidden Drills (shown here), Peeso reamers, and post drills. They may be used with either torque-controlled or air-driven handpieces. Caution should be used with these instruments due to the aggressive dentin removal that results from their use.

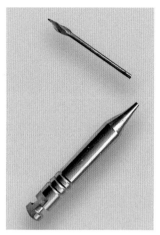

FIG 5-29 Gates Glidden drills are designed to fracture at the hub under stress, making them easily retrievable upon breakage.

Gates Glidden instruments possess limited cutting areas and are used solely for coronal flaring. They have a flame-shaped cutting tip and widening diameters with increasing size, indicated by the number of notches on their handle and sometimes by color. Gates Glidden instruments are considered the safest of the stainless steel flaring instruments given their limited area of cutting and their weak point at the hub, which allows the instrument to break in a manner allowing for easy retrieval from the chamber or canal space (Fig 5-29). That said, these instruments are aggressive, and care should be exercised if they are used. Improper use of Gates Glidden drills, particularly along furcal walls of canals, in roots with external grooves, or in curved canals, can result in excessive thinning or perforation. They have a propensity to create their own path if pushed apically, resulting in canal transportation or ledging.

Peeso drills and proprietary post drills have a similar design, with a longer and generally parallel cutting tip. These drills can only be used in extremely straight and wide canals, such as in the palatal roots of maxillary molars and the distal roots of mandibular molars. Great care must be taken to avoid pushing the instruments apically, resulting in canal ledging or perforation. Now that more flexible and conservative NiTi rotary instruments are available, application of these instruments is generally in the creation of post spaces, made even more rare as posts have been largely obviated by adhesive dentistry.

NiTi rotary instruments represent the gold standard in rotary instrument technology to date. Both early adaptations of NiTi as well as newer heat-treated instruments are available to practitioners. As a material, NiTi is utilized for power-driven rotary instrumentation due to its greater flexibility as compared to stainless steel, allowing it to maintain natural root curvatures without transportation. However, compared to stainless steel instruments, NiTi instruments have a greater risk of fracture due to torsional strain.[49] For this reason, most manufacturers advise that these instruments are single use.

It is important to recognize generalities existing in most of the rotary instrument systems on the market. Most systems include some form of coronal-flaring instrument, with other rotary instruments that can be taken to the full working length. The length of instruments varies by manufacturer, though they generally coordinate with 21-, 25-, and 31-mm hand instruments. Files may have constant taper (0.02, 0.04, or 0.06 mm) or variable taper, depending on design. Though manufacturers market rotary instruments as a "system" wherein the manufacturer prescribes the use of every instrument in a particular order, most experienced endodontists adopt different instruments from different systems to create their own protocols (Fig 5-30). Certain canal types, sizes, and shapes may warrant the use of different instruments depending on the situation, and understanding the strengths, weaknesses, and applications of many different instrument types allows for creation of efficiently tailored protocols unique to the individual patient and tooth.

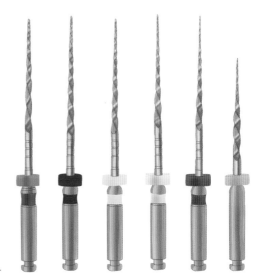

FIG 5-30 Manufacturers of rotary files often market systems containing multiple instruments.

NiTi rotary instruments require careful control of speed and torque according to manufacturer instructions to minimize stress on the file, which risks instrument separation. Resultantly, torque control electrically powered motors are essential for rotary instrumentation, and air-driven handpieces that lack speed and torque control should not be used with these files (Fig 5-31). Most file systems have preprogrammed settings on the torque control motor for practitioner convenience.

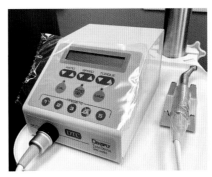

FIG 5-31 Careful control of both torque and speed are essential when using NiTi rotary instruments. Consequently, torque control motors are required. Shown here is the discontinued Dentsply DTC Motor.

Instrumentation methods

While rotary and hand instrumentation techniques differ in many respects, both necessitate the development of a glide path as well as coronal flaring. Depending on the clinical scenario, it may be advantageous to perform one or the other first. Glide path refers to the ability to reproducibly insert small hand files to the working length without resistance or stoppage. To develop a glide path, pre-curved nos. 06, 08, and 10 files are inserted to the working length and used in a gentle filing motion. The working length should be confirmed with an EAL with each incremental increase in file size. A smooth path must be created to ensure that larger instruments, whether rotary or hand instruments, can be inserted to the working length. Maintaining the glide path is essential to prevent ledging and transportation of the canal. Coronal flaring refers to the enlargement of the coronal portion of the canal, typically with rotary instruments. Instruments used for this purpose can include the more aggressive stainless steel instruments like Gates Glidden burs or more conservative NiTi coronal-flaring instruments. Following coronal flaring, recapitulation of small instruments to the working length is advisable.

The step-back technique

The step-back technique is performed with stainless steel hand instruments. Its major disadvantages include its inefficiency and the risk of debris compaction and ledging. That said, it is a useful technique when rotary instruments are unavailable. Following working length determination, glide path development, and coronal flaring, the canal should be sequentially enlarged to the MAF, as described next. Irrigation should occur between every instrument, as well as recapitulation to the working length with a small no. 10 K file to confirm patency. Working length should also be repeatedly confirmed with an EAL.

No hard and fast rules exist for establishing MAF size. While some authors suggest that a minimum of a no. 30 K file is necessary,[50] most agree that it should be at least three ISO sizes larger than the file that first binds apically.[51] For example, if a no. 10 file binds tightly, such as in a narrow root, the MAF may be a no. 25 file, whereas in a wide incisor where a no. 30 file is the first to bind apically, the MAF may be larger than no. 45.

The term *step-back* refers to the development of the apical taper preparation. This involves an increase in file size while stepping back in 1-mm increments. Five step-backs are usually indicated to allow for an increase of 0.25 mm in diameter moving from the apex to the coronal root. For example, if the MAF is a no. 30, the next file should be the no. 35 stepped back 1 mm short of the working length, then a no. 40 at 2 mm back, a no. 45 at 3 mm back, a no. 50 at 4 mm back, and a no. 55 at 5 mm back. Between each instrument, recapitulation with a no. 10 file to the working length is necessary (Fig 5-32). The final step should involve the MAF, used to smooth the walls.

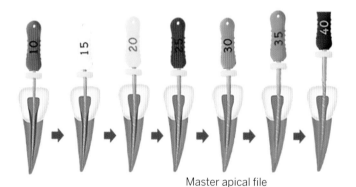

FIG 5-32 Sequential files for the step-back technique.

Master apical file

The crown-down technique

The crown-down technique is typically performed with NiTi rotary instruments. Its advantages include its efficiency over hand instrumentation and the decreased risk of packing debris into the apical canal. As opposed to the step-back technique, where instrument size is incrementally increased from the apex, the crown-down technique involves an incremental decrease in instrument size. Following working length determination, glide path development, and coronal flaring, larger rotary files are introduced into the canal space short of the working length. Rotary file size is then decreased, and the next instrument is inserted farther into the canal. This is repeated until the rotary file reaches the working length, with recapitulation performed between files (Fig 5-33).

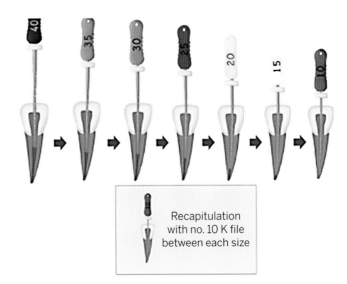

FIG 5-33 Sequential files for the crown-down technique.

Recapitulation with no. 10 K file between each size

The size of the final instrument used to create the glide path ultimately depends on the rotary system being used. Many rotary instrument system manufacturers recommend specific sequencing and techniques that differ from the basic crown-down technique. Any time rotary systems are incorporated into clinical practice, clinicians must synthesize their clinical judgment with manufacturer recommendations to ensure that appropriate instrumentation is completed. Some NiTi rotary systems use variably tapered instruments to engage different areas of the dentin walls moving from crown to apex. Others use uniformly tapered files beginning with larger diameters to shape the crown, moving through a series of smaller diameters to the apex. Some systems, and some clinicians, favor a mixture of variable and uniform tapers. Familiarity with many systems allows for flexibility to deliver care that is appropriately tailored to the individual tooth.

Irrigation

Whereas endodontic instrumentation shapes the canal space, irrigation represents the most essential means of cleaning and disinfecting.[48,52] Irrigation not only eradicates intracanal microbes but also lubricates instruments within the canal spaces and physically removes debris created during instrumentation.

Armamentarium

A multitude of options exists for irrigation solutions, and each option has its own benefits and drawbacks. Clinicians must consider the needs of the individual case when selecting irrigation solutions (Fig 5-34).

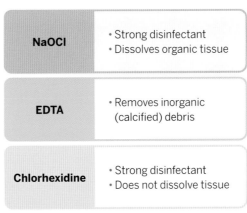

NaOCl	• Strong disinfectant • Dissolves organic tissue
EDTA	• Removes inorganic (calcified) debris
Chlorhexidine	• Strong disinfectant • Does not dissolve tissue

FIG 5-34 The three most common endodontic irrigants are sodium hypochlorite (NaOCl), ethylenediaminetetraacetic acid (EDTA), and chlorhexidine.

Sodium hypochlorite

Sodium hypochlorite (NaOCl) is considered the gold standard endodontic irrigant.[1] It is not only a strong disinfectant that is able to effectively target endodontic pathogens,[52,53] but it also dissolves organic tissue debris.[54,55] Notably, a 5-minute soak in sodium hypochlorite inactivates prions on stainless steel instruments,[56] showcasing its efficacy in neutralizing these neurologic pathogens known to withstand even autoclave disinfection.[57]

Sodium hypochlorite is an inexpensive and readily procured irrigant. As long as contact times are adequate, it is most effective in full-strength concentrations between 5% and 6%.[58,59] Sodium hypochlorite requires at least 10 minutes of contact time with necrotic tissues for complete debridement, which can easily be achieved during hand and rotary instrumentation with consistent irrigation.[60] The tissue should be rinsed and the solution replenished frequently during this time due to expiration of the chlorine ion and the need to continuously remove debris during instrumentation.[61] When referring to this solution during endodontic procedures, be careful to refer to it as "sodium hypochlorite" or "hypochlorite" for short rather than the colloquial "bleach" to make patients feel comfortable with the care they are receiving.

Although tissue dissolution is considered a favorable property in the debridement of canal spaces, this property does pose a risk if sodium hypochlorite is extruded beyond the confines of the tooth. This could lead to the sodium hypochlorite accident, an injury characterized by immediate, severe pain and swelling, with potentially dangerous sequelae.[62,63] More details on this intraoperative complication can be found in chapter 10. Special care must be taken in the presence of perforations or in teeth with open apices. Sodium hypochlorite also has an especially foul taste and will immediately and irreversibly bleach fabric if splashed. Dental dam isolation and the practice of four-handed dentistry with careful surgical suctioning during irrigation is crucial to avoid leakage of the solution outside the working field.[1] Finally, sodium hypochlorite is also subject to several chemical interactions. When combined with chlorhexidine, it forms a brown precipitate consisting at least partially of para-chloroaniline, a potentially toxic substance that may additionally occlude dentinal tubules.[64,65] When mixed with ethylenediaminetetraacetic acid (EDTA) solutions, the chlorine ion is inactivated, rendering sodium hypochlorite ineffective,[66,67] so care should be taken to rinse with saline or water between these solutions or to use them in the appropriate order (ie, sodium hypochlorite first, EDTA second) to ensure their efficacy (Fig 5-35).

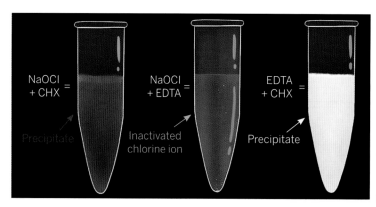

FIG 5-35 Care must be taken when using different irrigation solutions during endodontic treatment because interactions are known to occur between the most common irrigants (CHX=chlorhexidine gluconate).

EDTA

Commercially available EDTA in a 17% solution is routinely used as a secondary irrigation solution. It is a calcium chelator that dissolves inorganic debris, including the inorganic portion of the smear layer lining the canal space following cleaning and shaping.[68] EDTA also exposes the dentinal tubules that create the scaffold loaded with growth factors for regenerative endodontic procedures. In NSRCT and retreatment, EDTA is often used as a final irrigation solution prior to obturation. Based on the interaction between EDTA and sodium hypochlorite and the precipitates that are known to form when EDTA is mixed with chlorhexidine,[69] care should be taken to rinse with saline or water between solutions. For similar reasons, although NiTi instruments should never be used in a dry environment, EDTA-based lubricants should not be used.

Chlorhexidine gluconate

Chlorhexidine gluconate (CHX) in a 2% solution is an alternative disinfectant solution that can be used when sodium hypochlorite is contraindicated, such as when a perforation has occurred or the apex of the tooth being treated is significantly open.[70] Although CHX is effective against endodontic microbes and possesses substantivity (an extended duration of activity),[71] it lacks the tissue dissolution properties of sodium hypochlorite.[72] Additionally, it produces precipitates when mixed with other common irrigation solutions, including sodium hypochlorite and EDTA.[64,69] Consequently, care should be taken to rinse with saline or sterile water between the use of CHX and other solutions.

Alternative irrigation solutions

Using stand-alone alternative irrigants, including commercially available preparations of some of the above agents and others like hydrogen peroxide, is not generally advisable for endodontic irrigation. That said, they may be beneficial as adjunctive irrigants, and novel solutions may offer improved results. Clinicians must do their research before modifying irrigation protocols.

Delivery devices

Syringes equipped with side-vented safety needles are the instrument of choice for the delivery of endodontic irrigants[1] (Fig 5-36). The syringe barrels are conveniently available in 1-, 3-, 5-, and 10-mL volumes. The needle should be bent to improve accessibility, as shown in Fig 5-36, and inserted into only the coronal half of the canal space, without any engagement.

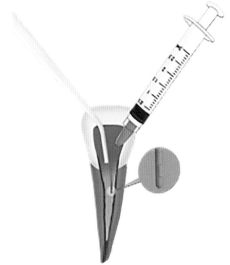

FIG 5-36 Side-vented needles should be used for the delivery of irrigation solutions.

Methods

To balance the most favorable properties of irrigation solutions, an irrigation protocol for NSRCT that combines full-strength sodium hypochlorite with 17% EDTA, delivered via syringe with a side-vented needle, should be used.[1] The irrigant should be injected slowly and without pressure to ensure that none of the solution is spread to extraradicular spaces. High-volume surgical suction should be placed upon the access opening to prevent overflow of the irrigation solution onto the dental dam. To maximize irrigant contact time with the tooth, the sodium hypochlorite solution is introduced to fill the pulp space immediately after access, with the solution changed between every instrument to remove loose debris. Instruments, particularly NiTi rotary instruments, should never be used in a dry environment. Therefore, irrigant solutions should be maintained as a bath within the canal spaces. The use of sodium hypochlorite irrigation should continue until the final stages of instrumentation, just prior to obturation. The suggested protocol calls for active irrigation (described in the following section) with the sodium hypochlorite solution, followed by a final rinse with EDTA. This protocol combines the removal of organic debris during instrumentation with a final rinse that allows for removal of the smear layer, which is thought to interfere with the adhesion of sealers[73–75] (Fig 5-37).

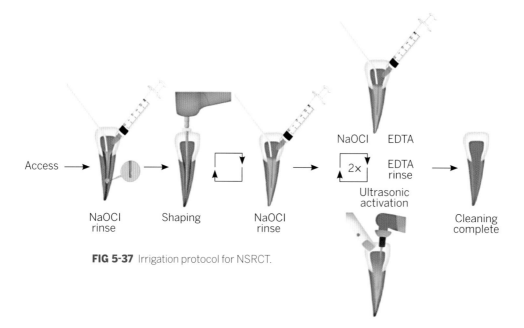

FIG 5-37 Irrigation protocol for NSRCT.

Active irrigation

The endodontic literature supports the performance of enhanced cleaning by activation of irrigant solutions. This can be accomplished using either sonic or ultrasonic instruments.[76,77] As both methods produce similar results, the choice of system lies with the clinician.[78] Ultrasonic activation of an irrigation solution is most easily performed with a specialized tip applied to an ultrasonic motor (eg, piezostyle). Sonic activation can be easily performed using a commercially available handle with corresponding plastic tips, such as the EndoActivator (Dentsply Sirona) (Fig 5-38). Activation of irrigation solutions should be performed as the final step in cleaning following complete instrumentation of thc canal spaces. Most protocols recommend activation of a sodium hypochlorite solution in each canal space for at least 45 seconds, but specific manufacturer recommendations should be followed. Other proprietary systems, marketed as enhancements of irrigation-based cleaning, have been introduced to the marketplace in recent years and may serve

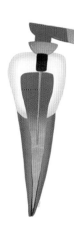

FIG 5-38 Active irrigation involves the insertion of a device into the canal spaces to agitate the irrigation solution. Commercially available devices for this purpose include the EndoActivator, as well as specialized ultrasonic tips and other proprietary irrigation devices.

similar purposes.[79] Alternatively, lasers have been proposed to enhance the antimicrobial efficacy of irrigant solutions in a similarly activated manner.[80]

Intracanal Medicaments

The discussion of intracanal medication ultimately begins with the decision of whether treatment is to be performed in a single visit or over multiple visits. Single-visit therapy refers to treatment where cleaning, shaping, and obturation are completed in one visit. Multiple-visit therapy refers to treatment where cleaning and shaping are performed and an intracanal medicament is placed for a period of time. Obturation is then usually performed at a second visit. Performing NSRCT in a single visit offers clear benefits of convenience for both patients and clinicians[81] and minimizes loss to follow-up that may result. High-quality evidence has failed to show the superiority of either single-visit therapy or multivisit therapy in terms of postoperative pain, risk of flare-up, and long-term success.[82-89]

Single-visit therapy is appropriate for patients with a diagnosis of irreversible pulpitis or pulpal necrosis or a periapical diagnosis of symptomatic or asymptomatic apical periodontitis. Certain situations, however, may require multivisit therapy, including when swelling or sinus tracts are present. In addition to the antimicrobial effects on the evolved microbial communities present in chronically draining infections, exhibited as sinus tracts or periodontal-endodontic drainage, the ability to monitor healing of these pathologies in real time warrants consideration for multivisit therapy. The second visit allows for direct visualization of a healed sinus tract or periodontal defect, and if a refractory lesion is observed, an opportunity remains for re-medication with an alternative drug, such as triple antibiotic paste, after the first-line use of calcium hydroxide.[90] Similarly, when preoperative swelling is present, the opportunity to assess clinical healing prior to obturation necessitates multivisit therapy.

Multivisit therapy may also be indicated when patients present with significant preoperative pain. Single-visit endodontics makes for longer appointments, and greater jaw soreness is expected to follow. Though data is inconclusive regarding the levels of postoperative pain following single- versus multiple-visit treatment,[82,83,87,88] patients with significant preoperative pain are more likely to suffer from greater postoperative pain.[91-93] Multivisit therapy not only reduces the appointment time for the first visit but also gives clinicians the chance to confirm symptom resolution at the follow-up appointment. The decision to plan multivisit therapy may simply be a matter of scheduling. The delivery of definitive endodontic treatment is the best means of relieving the symptoms of painful pulpitis and apical periodontitis. Sometimes, emergency appointments may only permit the delivery of palliative care including pulpotomy or pulpectomy. Rather than rushing through a procedure or risking breakthrough pain as anesthesia wears off (not to mention the stress of running late for the next scheduled patient), the placement of an interappointment medication allows for the delivery of safe and effective care that accommodates the unique challenges of performing clinical endodontics (Fig 5-39). Finally, in certain circumstances when multivisit therapy may traditionally be considered, clinicians may elect to provide single-visit treatment with good reason. For example, if patients will be undergoing medical care or pursuing travel that would make them unable to come in for an expedient second visit or if sedation is required for treatment, the benefits of single-visit therapy may outweigh the risks.

Potential contraindications to single-visit therapy	Contraindications to single-visit therapy
• Severe preoperative pain • Delivery of emergency treatment • Retreatments	• Sinus tracts • Swelling • Time constraints

FIG 5-39 Caution should be exercised when determining whether to provide single-visit therapy.

Whenever NSRCT cannot be completed in a single visit, interappointment, intracanal medications should be used to maintain and enhance disinfection of the root canal space.[94,95] Calcium hydroxide is the first-line medication.[1] It both disinfects canal spaces and dissolves necrotic tissue remnants.[96–98] In cases where calcium hydroxide is ineffective, as in when a second visit reveals refractory signs of infection presenting as persistent sinus tracts, periodontal-endodontic lesions, or intracanal drainage from the apex, a second round of intracanal medication can be considered. Clinicians can elect to use additional calcium hydroxide or alternative medicaments. Alternative medicaments, including 2% chlorhexidine gel[99–101] and antibiotic pastes, offer coverage of different endodontic microbes, and their topical application avoids the use of systemic drugs with these persistent infections[90,102] (Fig 5-40).

First line	Unresponsive infection
Calcium hydroxide	Calcium hydroxide OR antibiotic pastes OR 2% chlorhexidine gel

FIG 5-40 Whenever multivisit therapy is performed, intracanal medicaments should be used.

Antibiotic pastes rely on topical activity and may therefore be utilized in patients whose gastrointestinal tracts cannot tolerate oral antibiotic therapy or who may present with an undue risk of superinfections with oral antibiotic use (eg, patients with a history of *Clostridium difficile* superinfection). Typically compounded in a propylene glycol medium,[103] a triple antibiotic paste is classically composed of minocycline, metronidazole, and ciprofloxacin for broad-spectrum activity.[90,104] Double antibiotic pastes may not include minocycline due to its potential to cause tooth discoloration.[105–107]

Prior to placement of intracanal medicaments, canal spaces should be dried with absorbent paper points, with care taken to avoid extrusion of the points into extraradicular spaces. If apical drainage occurs, efforts should be made to dry the canals as completely as possible. Flexible plastic capillary tips (UltraCal, Ultradent) may be attached to the end of a surgical suction tip to evacuate canals exhibiting copious drainage. Hyperemic drainage may be controlled with calcium hydroxide either in powder or gel formulation due to its hemostatic properties. Calcium hydroxide, along with the alternative medications, can be easily placed using commercially available dispensing systems such as the syringe and flexible plastic capillary tips (UltraCal), or it may be mixed from raw materials and placed with a Lentulo spiral.[108] Care should be taken to avoid apical extrusion of calcium hydroxide because foreign body or neurotoxic reactions can occur if it contacts extraradicular tissues.[109] Therefore, the medicament should be introduced into the canal without any pressure and into the apical portion of the canal using a measured Lentulo spiral (Fig 5-41). Intracanal medicaments can be removed at a second visit with irrigants, including sodium hypochlorite, saline, and EDTA. Light instrumentation or active irrigation can enhance removal of the medicament. All medicament should be removed prior to obturation so as not to interfere with the setting of endodontic sealers.

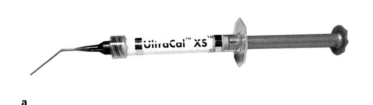

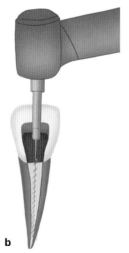

FIG 5-41 *(a)* Calcium hydroxide, as well as alternative medications, can easily be placed with commercially available dispensing systems, such as a syringe with a flexible plastic tip. *(b)* Medicaments must not be expressed into the periapical tissues. Lentulo spirals used to place mixed raw materials can serve the double purpose of ensuring length control.

Obturation

The cleaned and shaped canal space must be filled to prevent ingress of tissue fluid and reinfection of the root canal spaces. The filling material must adapt three dimensionally to the root canal space and create a complete apical seal.[110] The ideal obturation material is flexible, dimensionally stable, biocompatible, and bacteriostatic. Additionally, it must be retrievable from the root canal spaces in case retreatment is required[111] (Fig 5-42). The chosen obturation material should extend exactly to the working length, wherein the minimal apical constriction confines it within the tooth. Tugback, the sensation that

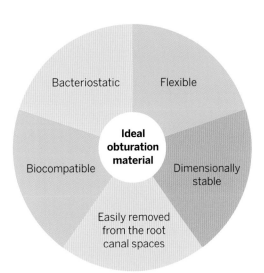

FIG 5-42 Properties of an ideal obturation material.

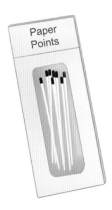

FIG 5-43 Prior to placing any root filling material, canals should be completely dried with absorbent paper points. Paper points should be sterile and are available in various sizes to match individual canal preparations.

the master cone is resistant to displacement in the canal when seated to length and tugged coronally, is essential to ensure that gutta-percha is sealing the apical extent of the root canal space and not likely to be pushed apically during compaction. Underextending filling materials can create a harbor for infection, whereas overextension is associated with foreign body reactions.[32,110,112]

Prior to placement of any obturation material, canals should be completely dried with absorbent paper points.[1] Most of the drying can be done with coarse or extra coarse paper points, with medium or fine points used for the apical portion of canal spaces (Fig 5-43). The paper points should be carefully premeasured to ensure that they do not extend into the extraradicular space, which could cause bleeding into the apical spaces. If needed, hemostasis of apical bleeding can be obtained by inserting a small amount of calcium hydroxide powder on a paper point into the canal space. However, excessive bleeding of apical drainage is an indication for placement of intracanal calcium hydroxide, with obturation at a second visit.

Armamentarium

Though many materials have been used historically, and future commercial interests will no doubt continue to bring more products to market, gutta-percha combined with sealer remains the gold standard obturation material in endodontic practice (Fig 5-44). Historic obturation materials, including formaldehyde-containing pastes (ie, Sargenti pastes), silver points, and Resilon, are associated with unfavorable outcomes and should no longer be used.[113–115] Gutta-percha is not only safe and effective but also fulfills many criteria of the ideal obturation material when paired with appropriate sealers.[111] Most notably, gutta-percha can easily be removed from canal spaces in cases when treatment failure or coronal leakage necessitates nonsurgical or surgical retreatment.[116] Carrier-based materials are less easily removed and are associated with more leakage compared to other materials and should therefore be used with caution.[117] Gutta-percha cones should be sterilized by soaking them in a sodium hypochlorite solution prior to placement within the canal.[1,118] Because sodium hypochlorite can create crystals with unkown consequences on the exterior surface of gutta-percha cones, some clinicians propose removing the crystals with an isopropyl alcohol wipe before insertion.[119]

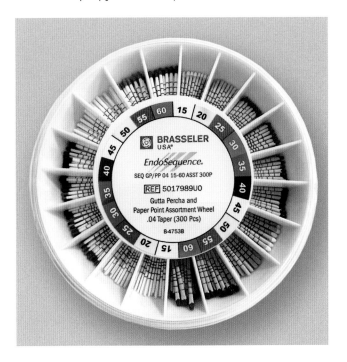

FIG 5-44 Gutta-percha remains the gold standard obturation material. For clinical efficiency, gutta-percha cones and paper points can be organized in wheel devices like this one from Brasseler USA.

To complete the 3D obturation, sealer is used to fill the complex root canal spaces not reached by gutta-percha.[120] Many products are available from commercial sources, including those composed of resin materials, zinc-oxide and eugenol, tricalcium silicate cements (also known as bioceramics), and calcium hydroxide,[121] all of which show similar efficacy and toxicity effects when confined to the root canal spaces and periradicular tissues.[122–124] The materials do, however, exhibit different effects when exposed to structures beyond the periapex, including the periapical bone, maxillary sinuses,[125] and inferior alveolar nerve bundles,[126] necessitating extra care when choosing a sealer for the individual tooth.

Sealers are an essential component to fill the voids between the gutta-percha and the dentinal wall.[120] Many safe and effective endodontic sealers exist for the clinician to choose from. Generally, most clinicians choose eugenol, resin, or tricalcium silicate cement sealers, but others, including glass ionomer, silicone, epoxy, and calcium hydroxide-based products, are useful for those rare cases of documented patient sensitivity. It is most convenient to choose one sealer for everyday practice, but familiarity with others is important for situations where another may be more appropriate. The most biocompatible sealer possible should be used in case of unintentional sealer extrusion into the extradicular spaces and associated anatomy. Sealers should be mixed to a consistency that is thick enough to minimize unnecessary extrusion because all sealers possess some degree of toxicity for periapical tissues.[127] That said, sealers should remain flowable enough to fill the unique root canal anatomy.

Sealer may be inserted on paper points, K files, Lentulo spirals, and even gutta-percha cones.[128] Each gutta-percha cone introduced into the canal space can be rolled in sealer to thoroughly coat its surface prior to introduction into the canal space. Care must be taken to ensure that the cone is not excessively coated, which could cause apical extrusion of the sealer that can contribute to chronic inflammation.[32] Excess sealer on the master cone placed to the apex should be removed prior to placement of the cone. Some clinicians coat the tip of their thermoplastic backfill device with sealer to ensure sufficient placement during the backfill process.

Resin-based sealers (eg, AH Plus, Dentsply Sirona) offer versatility in endodontic obturation. They mix readily, sometimes in commercially available premixing syringes; create an even radiopaque density[129]; exhibit minimal toxicity in the extraradicular spaces[130,131]; and have antibacterial properties similar to other sealers.[132] These sealers are readily available and popular among clinicians. Notably, early iterations of these materials (eg, AH 26, Dentsply Sirona) were found to release formaldehyde upon setting and should not be used.[133,134]

Zinc-oxide eugenol (ZOE) sealers (eg, Master-Dent Roth Root Canal Sealer from Dentonics, and Pulp Canal Sealer EWT from Kerr) are a mainstay in endodontics due to their many advantageous properties.[135] They handle easily, create an even radiopaque density,[129] and are antibacterial.[132] Additionally, their eugenol component may have palliative properties.[136] The use of ZOE sealers raises several clinical concerns, however. Extrusion of eugenol-containing materials into the inferior alveolar nerve (IAN) canal that sometimes runs proximal to mandibular molar root apices can cause neurotoxicity and permanent paresthesia,[126,137] so care must be taken when using these materials in the vicinity of the IAN. Additionally, case reports have shown that zinc-containing substances can support maxillary sinus fungal infections,[138–140] so extrusion into the maxillary sinus must be absolutely avoided.

Calcium hydroxide–based sealers (eg, Sealapex, Kerr) are an alternative and clinically acceptable option,[138] especially when patients have documented or suspected allergies to other sealers. These sealers are considered safe enough for use. However, cytotoxicity is reported in periapical tissues exposed to calcium hydroxide sealer overfills, so extra care should be taken to avoid apical extrusion of this sealer.[138–140] That said, most endodontic sealers exhibit some degree of cytotoxicity to the periapical tissues,[130,131,141,142] and most clinicians elect not to use calcium hydroxide–based sealers simply because of differences in handling and radiographic appearance.

Tricalcium silicate cement sealers (eg, EndoSequence BC Sealer, Brasseler USA), also termed bioceramics, are newer materials that have gained favor among clinicians due to certain ideal properties. They are flowable and radiopaque, and they have good sealing abilities.[143–145] Notably, tricalcium silicate cements are hydrophilic, and their setting is enhanced in a moist environment. They are also highly alkaline, creating an antibacterial microenvironment.[146–148] Tricalcium silicate cement sealers, however, may be difficult to retrieve.[123] The manufacturer of Endosequence BC Sealer advises its use with their proprietary gutta-percha points that contain bioceramics to which the sealer can chemically bond. Placement of the material is also unique and should follow a hydraulic condensation methodology using a single cone.[149] That said, this high-flow sealer is meant to be used with the warm vertical condensation technique described in the next section and used by many endodontists (Fig 5-45).

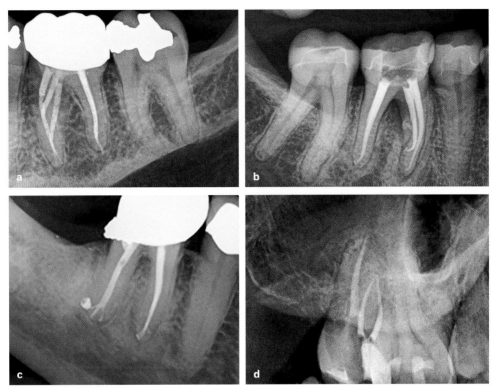

FIG 5-45 Several options exist for endodontic sealers, with similar clinical and radiographic results and prognoses. These include resin-based sealer (AH Plus) *(a)*, calcium hydroxide–based sealer (Sealapex) *(b)*, zinc-oxide eugenol sealer (Pulp Canal Sealer EWT) *(c)*, and bioceramic sealer (EndoSequence BC Sealer) *(d)*.

Methods

There are several methods for obturation. Clinicians should master several techniques to best adapt to individual teeth and unique situations. With all obturation techniques, cone fit radiographs are advisable to reconfirm working length and ensure an appropriate fit prior to compaction (Fig 5-46).

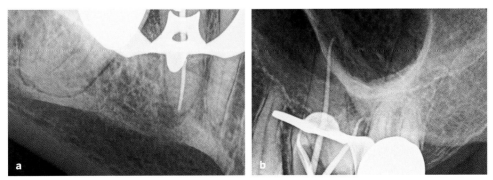

FIG 5-46 *(a and b)* With all obturation techniques, cone fit films are advisable to reconfirm the working length and ensure an appropriate fit.

Cold lateral compaction

Also called lateral condensation, cold lateral compaction involves placing tightly fitted narrow cones of gutta-percha laterally against a master cone within the canal space without introducing heat into the canal space. This method is appropriate for filling canals of varying shapes, including oval canals and those with fins or isthmuses. It is a useful technique for novice clinicians because errors can easily be corrected prior to making the definitive seal and it involves a low risk of apical extrusion. Moreover, a hybrid of this technique is often useful for canals with a wider diameter than a single cone, even when warm vertical techniques are used.

To perform cold lateral compaction, a standardized master gutta-percha cone (available in 0.02-, 0.04-, and 0.06-mm taper) with an apical diameter equal to that of the MAF is lightly coated with sealer and placed to the working length with tugback. Many clinicians will also use a dry paper point coated in sealer to first coat the canal walls prior to cone insertion. A spreader is then inserted to within 2 mm of the working length to create space for accessory cones, and the process is repeated, with the spreader reaching shorter depths each time until there is no more room for spreader and accessory canal insertion (Fig 5-47). Finger spreaders are preferred for greater access and flexibility, whereas fully handled spreaders should be used with caution to avoid excess force within the root (Fig 5-48).

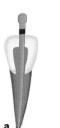 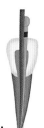 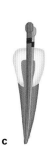 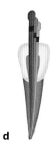

a   b   c   d

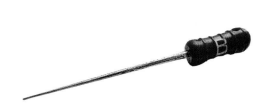

FIG 5-47 *(a)* In the lateral condensation technique, a standardized master gutta-percha cone is coated with sealer and placed to the working length with tugback. *(b)* A spreader is then inserted to within 2 mm of the working length to create space for accessory cones. *(c and d)* The process is repeated with the spreader reaching shorter depths each time until there is no room for spreader and accessory canal insertion.

FIG 5-48 Finger spreaders are preferred for their greater flexibility and access, whereas fully handled spreaders should be used with care to avoid excess force within the root.

Accessory cones, most useful in nonstandard sizes ranging from fine to medium, are added until the spreader can no longer fit within the coronal one-third of the canal space. Traditionally, a radiograph is exposed with this "bouquet" in place, allowing confirmation of adequate length control and density of the filling material. Excess gutta-percha is removed with a heated implement (Fig 5-49) (eg, Touch 'n Heat or System B, Kerr) and compacted with a plugger to just below the canal orifice. Pluggers are available in a variety of sizes and designs, and most cases can be treated using equivalents to Schilder pluggers in sizes 8.5 (0.5 mm) and 9 (0.6 mm), as the smaller plugger tips can compact even the narrowest canal orifices (Fig 5-50).

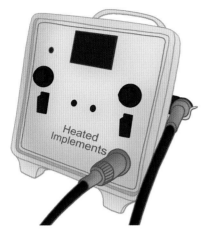

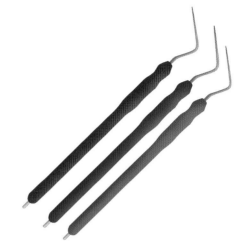

FIG 5-49 Heated implements with careful temperature and power controls should be used to remove gutta-percha from the canal orifice in lateral condensation techniques and within the apical third in warm vertical techniques.

FIG 5-50 Pluggers are available in a variety of sizes and designs. Most cases may be treated using equivalents to Schilder pluggers.

Warm vertical condensation

Warm vertical condensation, or compaction, is the recommended method for obturation whenever possible given its 3D seal and association with improved outcomes.[150] The most common method currently used was proposed by Dr Steven Buchanan, who coined the term *continuous wave of condensation*.[151] This involves the use of a heated element to condense obturation material into the apical portion of a canal space, followed by backfill with warm gutta-percha. As with the lateral condensation technique, a dry paper point coated in sealer may be used to apply sealer directly to the canal walls. A standardized master cone is lightly coated in sealer and placed to working length with tugback. A controlled heat source (eg, System B, Kerr) set between 200 and 250° F is advanced in the canal to the apical third of the root, as premeasured by a stopper on the instrument. Careful monitoring of temperature is crucial to avoid overheating and periodontal ligament damage.[152] The heated element should remain on while the instrument is introduced and advanced, then turned off once it reaches length. With the heat off, the element is left in place for 5 seconds to cool, then the heat is applied in a burst as the element is removed, to separate the excess coronal gutta-percha (Fig 5-51). If a post space is needed, the fill is complete. If not, backfilling can be completed with a cartridge-based commercial obturation unit (eg, Obtura III Max, Young Specialties) to the level of the canal orifice

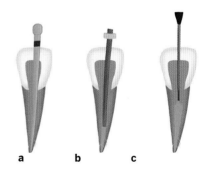

a   b   c

FIG 5-51 *(a)* In the vertical condensation technique, a standardized master cone seated with sealer is used according to manufacturer instructions. *(b)* A controlled heat source set between 200 and 250 degrees Fahrenheit is advanced in the canal to the apical third of the root, as premeasured by a stopper on the instrument. The heat should remain on while the instrument is introduced and advanced, then turned off once it reaches length. *(c)* With the heat off, the implement is left in place for 5 seconds to cool, then the heat is applied in a burst as the element is removed to separate the excess coronal gutta-percha.

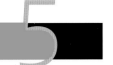

(Fig 5-52). For canals with a wide diameter, a modification of the cold lateral compaction technique can be used, wherein spreaders are used to insert accessory gutta-percha cones to the appropriate level to create a dense apical filling. From there, the downpack and backfill procedures can be completed.

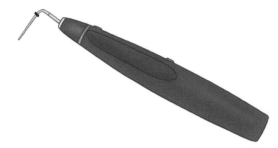

FIG 5-52 Commercially available devices are used to backfill gutta-percha into the coronal canal spaces during warm vertical condensation.

Alternative techniques

Alternative techniques, including thermoplastic injection methods where backfill devices are used to fill the entirety of the canal space, are extremely technique sensitive and useful only in very experienced hands.[153] As mentioned, carrier-based gutta-percha techniques require the use of materials that are not sized to fit every canal accurately and completely and are therefore associated with leakage.[117] As a result, as well as due to challenges in retrieval when root canal retreatment becomes necessary, carrier-based obturation methods are not advised.

In canals without intact apical constrictions, bioceramic materials, including mineral trioxide aggregate (MTA) and EndoSequence BC Root Repair Material Fast Set Putty (Brasseler USA), may be utilized to create an apical barrier.[154] These materials are biocompatible, antibacterial, compactible, and radiopaque,[155,156] making them ideal for open or overprepared apices where gutta-percha and sealer would not be able to produce a seal. Bioceramic materials are non-irritating and promote periodontal ligament and bony healing, so even a slight overextension of the material is inconsequential.[156] Materials may be introduced using the same methods as for MTA-based apexification procedures, discussed in chapter 9. Following instrumentation to working length, a small bolus of bioceramic material can be inserted with a plugger into a dried canal without the use of sealer and compacted to the estimated working length with a plugger with a premeasured stopper. Radiographic confirmation of the filling is advised prior to placing more bioceramic material to fill the entirety of the canal space. Alternatively, sealer and gutta-percha backfill can be used in the coronal portion of the canal in lieu of additional bioceramic materials.

Restorative Care

Appropriate restorative care is crucial to the success of endodontic treatment. Restorative care in endodontics can be divided into temporary and definitive restorative phases. Both are of equal importance and act to prevent coronal leakage and the leakage of saliva, salivary bacteria, and other contaminants into the canal space, which are all associated with near immediate failures of endodontic treatment.[157–159] Ultimately, definitive restorative care should be completed as soon as possible, not only to reduce the risk of failing temporary restorations but also to provide cuspal protection from fracture when indicated.[160,161]

Temporary restorative care

If endodontic therapy is completed over multiple visits or if definitive restorative care is to be completed at an appointment other than that scheduled for endodontic treatment, temporary restorations must be used. Temporary restorations must seal well and be easily removable. Clinicians often place spacers under temporary restorations to facilitate their removal (Fig 5-53). These spacers can include sterile cotton pellets or cut pieces of sterile sponge. Nonsterilizable materials should not be used. The spacer should be large enough to prevent restorative clinicians from having to drill deeply into the tooth before reaching the spacer but not so large that they impinge upon the appropriate thickness of temporary materials. When post spaces are present, care should be taken to not push the spacer into the post space.

Temporary restorations should also provide an excellent seal that can be maintained for a reasonable amount of time until they are replaced. Because unforeseen delays in placing the definitive restoration occur often, materials known to leak within weeks, including Cavit (3M) and IRM (Dentsply Sirona), are not advised.[162,163] Resin-modified glass-ionomer materials balance a long-lasting seal with ease of placement and removal[163] (Fig 5-54).

In addition to temporary restorative materials, intraorifice barriers can be placed on the chamber floor to minimize the risk of coronal leakage until the tooth is restored. Their use assures maintenance of the coronal seal even in the absence of dental dam isolation during placement of the definitive restoration.[164,165] Intraorifice barriers are also thought to reinforce fractured teeth until a full-coverage restoration can be placed.[166,167] Materials like EndoSequence BC Liner (Brasseler USA) combine ease of use with excellent sealing properties and can be considered for this purpose (Fig 5-55).

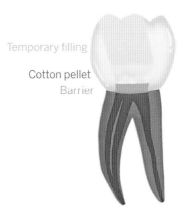

FIG 5-53 Temporary restorative materials should be placed over a spacer.

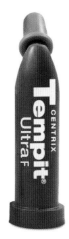

FIG 5-54 Resin-modified glass-ionomer temporary restorations (eg, Tempit Ultra-F, Centrix) balance a long-lasting seal with ease of placement and removal.

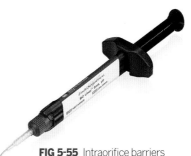

FIG 5-55 Intraorifice barriers can be placed across the pulpal floor to prevent coronal leakage.

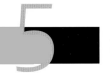

Nonsurgical Endodontics

Definitive restorative care

In an ideal and efficient world, the definitive restoration would be placed immediately after endodontic therapy, and some clinicians place the core buildup at the time of obturation (Fig 5-56). The quality of the restoration is the most important factor for success following endodontic and restorative care.[168] No matter the restoration, clinicians must carefully monitor biologic width[169] and maintain an adequate ferrule.[170–172] The type of restoration selected depends both on the location of the tooth in the arch and the amount of missing tooth structure. For anterior teeth with sufficient remaining tooth structure, direct restorations are appropriate. However, anterior teeth with extensive prior restorations or traumatic fractures may require indirect, full-coverage restorations. Posterior teeth, on the other hand, should always receive indirect, cuspal-coverage restorations such as onlays or crowns.[173] Numerous studies point to the risk of catastrophic fractures in posterior teeth lacking cuspal coverage following root canal therapy[174–176] (Fig 5-57). Whether in the anterior or posterior region, restorative care should be completed with dental dam isolation to prevent coronal leakage.[177]

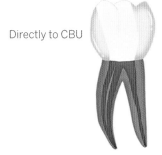

Directly to CBU

FIG 5-56 Ideally, the definitive restoration, or at a minimum the core buildup, would be placed immediately following endodontic therapy.

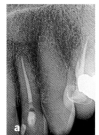
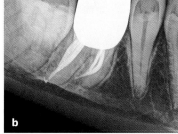

FIG 5-57 (a) Following nonsurgical endodontic therapy, anterior teeth may be restored with a direct composite restoration or full-coverage restorative care, depending on the coronal tooth structure loss. (b) Cuspal coverage is necessary to restore posterior teeth.

Posts

Posts are indicated only when insufficient tooth structure remains for adequate core retention. Either prefabricated or custom posts can be used. Prefabricated posts are made of metal or fiberglass. Posts do not strengthen the root and may increase the risk of fracture if the root requires greater preparation for post placement or suffers from deeper force concentration by way of the post itself[175,178,179] (Fig 5-58). Even fiber posts placed with bonded cements may not provide the root strengthening some authors suggest.[180–182] Clinicians must take care to justify the use of a post. When posts are placed, they should be passively inserted within a straight canal to prevent uneven force distribution. Furthermore, they should be limited to the prepared canal spaces to avoid unnecessary loss of tooth structure.[183]

FIG 5-58 *(a and b)* Poor post design is associated with fracture and perforation.

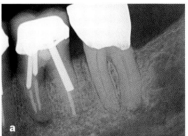
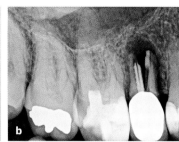

Parallel, nonthreaded posts are preferred over tapered and threaded posts due to risk of fracture. Whenever a post is placed, it is important to ensure that at least 5 mm of apical gutta-percha remains to maintain the canal seal[184] because insufficient gutta-percha can predispose the tooth to leakage.[185] Additionally, the length of the post should be equal to the height of the clinical crown or two-thirds of the length of the root, whichever is greater.[186] When selecting a post diameter, the size and shape of the root must be considered to minimize excessive dentinal thinning. In general, preparations should not exceed a size 3 Gates Glidden drill, or a diameter of 0.9 mm[183] (Fig 5-59).

Post spaces can be created using a variety of methods. The simplest way is to skip the backfill stage of the warm vertical condensation method of obturation. Post spaces may also be created mechanically with Gates Glidden drills or proprietary post drills (Fig 5-60). These mechanical means for gutta-percha removal are considered safe,[184] but care is necessary to minimize root dentin removal. If post drills are used, manufacturer instructions should be followed. Post drills should not be used to enlarge the canal space to fit a larger post than what passively fits the canal space created by NSRCT. Care must always be taken to ensure a passive fit of the post itself before drill preparation to create the parallel footing for the post terminus.

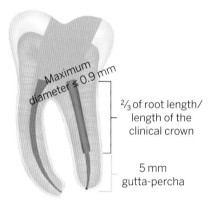

Maximum diameter ≤ 0.9 mm

⅔ of root length/length of the clinical crown

5 mm gutta-percha

FIG 5-59 The ideal post space should leave a minimum of 5 mm of gutta-percha apically. The length of the space should equal the height of the clinical crown or two-thirds the length of the root, whichever is greater. To minimize thinning, the diameter of the post space should not exceed the size of the root shape, with a safe maximal diameter no greater than 0.9 mm, equivalent to a size 3 Gates Glidden drill.

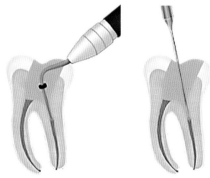

FIG 5-60 Post spaces can be left during warm vertical condensation or prepared manually with Gates Glidden drills or proprietary post drills.

Postoperative Care

Endodontics represents an unknown for many patients, both during and after the procedure. Consequently, they must be counseled regarding both what to expect and what to do postoperatively. Postoperative instructions should be delivered orally, and written instructions should be given to reinforce patient understanding (Fig 5-61). Patients should be advised if they should delay eating or drinking while materials set, as well as on the expected duration of local anesthesia. Patients often require a reminder not to eat on the anesthetized side due to risks of soft tissue injury. Although discussions about the need for definitive restorative care should have occurred during the informed consent process, patients should again be advised of the necessity and timing of required restorative care following endodontic treatment. Patients often ask how soon they should seek restorative care, and they should be advised that a 7-day delay is typically appropriate to allow time for recovery from normal postoperative symptoms.[187] That said, especially in the case of posterior teeth requiring full-coverage restorative care, the longer the wait to receive a definitive restoration, the greater the risk of fracture or leakage.[160,161] In the interim, the patient should avoid chewing hard foods to reduce the risk of fracture.

Dentist's Information

(123) 456-7890

Analgesic regimen advised:
Generally 400 mg ibuprofen + 325 mg acetaminophen every 6 hours

Postoperative Instructions: Root Canal Therapy and Retreatment

1. Please refrain from eating or drinking for 30 minutes after your appointment to allow for filling materials to set. After that time, please be cautious not to bite your lip, cheek, or tongue until the local anesthetic wears off.
2. Please refrain from biting on your treated tooth while the temporary restoration is in place.
3. Postoperative discomfort is normal and to be expected following treatment, and often lasts between 2 to 7 days. Your doctor will review appropriate pain management strategies. If you begin to notice worsening discomfort that isn't relieved by over-the-counter medication, or if swelling develops, please call your doctor immediately.
4. It is essential that you have your root canal–treated tooth definitively restored following treatment. Please be sure to schedule restorative care after your root canal is completed.
5. Please contact the office with any questions. Emergency numbers for the doctors are available if issues arise after hours.

FIG 5-61 Postoperative instructions should be given orally and in written form to enhance patient comprehension.

A discussion should occur about which symptoms are normal postoperatively and which are not. Patients must be advised that mild to moderate postoperative discomfort is normal and to be expected, but symptoms should be manageable with the use of oral analgesics. Chewing discomfort is expected on the treated tooth for at least a few days, and the surrounding soft tissues and muscles may feel bruised from the trauma of the procedure, including the use of local anesthesia. Most patients will experience mild to moderate discomfort that peaks approximately 24 hours after NSRCT, with some experiencing symptoms for up to 7 days.[91,187] Patients can be advised to prepare softer foods to ease chewing-associated discomfort. Furthermore, preemptive analgesic use is advisable. As previously discussed, combination therapy with ibuprofen and acetaminophen is considered most effective, and the dosage profile advised following routine NSRCT is 400 mg ibuprofen with 325 mg acetaminophen dosed every 6 hours.[188,189]

Due to unique qualities related to the patient and procedure, some patients may experience greater levels of postoperative discomfort, and setting these expectations is of the utmost importance for at-risk individuals. For instance, patients with severe preoperative pain, female patients, and those with a history of chronic pain conditions are more prone to experiencing severe postoperative symptoms[190] (Fig 5-62). Consequently, clinicians may consider administration of long-acting anesthesia via bupivacaine, as well as advising these patients to use slightly higher doses of analgesics, such as 600 to 800 mg ibuprofen and up to 1,000 mg acetaminophen.

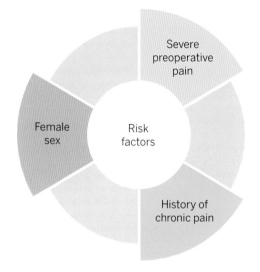

FIG 5-62 Risk factors for more severe postoperative discomfort following nonsurgical endodontics.

Finally, patients should be warned of the risk of a postoperative flare-up, in which pain worsens rather than subsides in the 48 hours or so following treatment[191] due to a change in the immune system's equilibrium in the extraradicular space secondary to treatment.[192] Flare-ups occur in approximately 8% of patients following initiation or continuation of endodontic treatment.[193] This risk should be communicated to all patients as part of normal postoperative discussions, which itself can serve as reassurance if a flare-up occurs. Patients should additionally be counseled that flare-up symptoms do not impact the long-term treatment prognosis.[194,195] Predisposing factors for flare-up include older age; female sex; a history of atopy, high levels of preoperative pain, or analgesic use; and patients undergoing endodontic retreatments[92,196] (Fig 5-63).

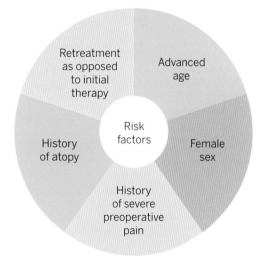

FIG 5-63 Risk factors for the development of flare-up symptoms following nonsurgical endodontics.

Patients should be counseled to contact the doctor on call if flare-up symptoms develop. Management is palliative in most cases, but patients will require counseling on how best to manage their symptoms. Simply communicating to a patient that their experiences have a documented name and etiology with an expected timeline of resolution can be reassuring. In most cases, analgesics alone are used to manage the flare-up with the higher doses of ibuprofen and acetaminophen previously mentioned. If swelling develops, however, re-accessing the tooth for cleaning and re-medication or even incision and drainage may be indicated,[88] in addition to the judicious use of systemic antibiotics.[88,192,197]

1-year follow-up for all cases

3- and/or 6-month follow-up for large lesions, sinus pathology

> 1-year follow-up for larger or slowly healing lesions

FIG 5-64 Recommended follow-up schedule after NSRCT. Follow-up schedules are case specific but incorporate certain general benchmarks.

Follow-Up Appointments

Patients having undergone root canal therapy should be seen for follow up. This allows the clinician to monitor healing and assess for other complications. Patients with more severe pathology, particularly lesions that sit close to neighboring teeth, may be recalled as soon as 3 months postoperatively for follow-up. Most patients should be seen 1 year postoperatively for a clinical and radiographic assessment.[198,199] Follow-ups may continue beyond 1 year postoperatively depending on the findings. Larger lesions may take longer to heal and should be followed until they are resolved.[200] Certain conditions, such as diabetes mellitus, may slow healing and therefore require monitoring for a longer duration.[201] Furthermore, the stability of presumed apical scars can be monitored[202] (Fig 5-64).

Generally, follow-up radiography should follow the principles of as low as reasonable achievable (ALARA). Therefore, periapical images are recommended for the vast majority of follow up exams (Fig 5-65). Limited field-of-view CBCT may be necessary to visualize early signs of healing, particularly in areas with significant anatomical noise, such as the posterior maxilla.[203] In particular, endodontic pathology that has created secondary maxillary sinus mucositis should be followed up with early CBCT imaging to ensure that the sinusitis resolves[204,205] (Fig 5-66).

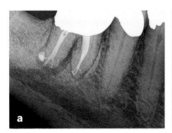 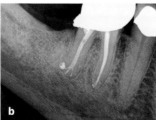

FIG 5-65 Periapical images are appropriate for follow-up radiography in the vast majority of cases. *(a)* Following endodontic treatment. *(b)* At the 1-year follow-up.

FIG 5-66 Limited field-of-view CBCT imaging is an appropriate follow-up tool to assess for early periapical healing or the resolution of endodontically derived sinus pathology. In this case, the maxillary left first molar showed evidence of apical healing and resolution of adjacent maxillary sinus mucositis 6 months after NSRCT.

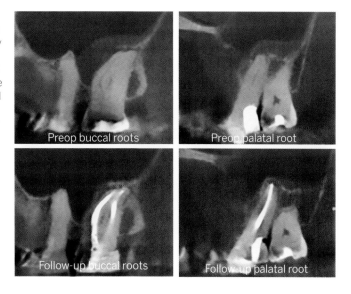

Preop buccal roots

Preop palatal root

Follow-up buccal roots

Follow-up palatal root

References

1. Treatment Standards. AAE Position Statement. American Association of Endodontists, 2019. https://www.aae.org/specialty/clinical-resources/guidelines-position-statements/. Accessed 23 March 2023.
2. Dental Dams. AAE position statement. American Association of Endodontists, 2017. https://www.aae.org/specialty/wp-content/uploads/sites/2/2017/06/dentaldamstatement.pdf. Accessed 23 March 2023.
3. Kameyama A, Asami A, Noro A, Abo H, Hirai Y, Tsunoda M. The effects of three dry-field techniques on intraoral temperature and relative humidity. J Am Dent Assoc 2011;142:274–280.
4. Cochran MA, Miller CH, Sheldrake MA. The efficacy of the rubber dam as a barrier to the spread of microorganisms during dental treatment. J Am Dent Assoc 1989;119:141–144.
5. Marui VC, Souto MLS, Rovai ES, Romito GA, Chambrone L, Pannuti CM. Efficacy of preprocedural mouthrinses in the reduction of microorganisms in aerosol: A systematic review. J Am Dent Assoc 2019;150:1015–1026.e1.
6. Samaranayake LP, Fakhruddin KS, Buranawat B, Panduwawala C. The efficacy of bio-aerosol reducing procedures used in dentistry: A systematic review. Acta Odontol Scand 2021;79:69–80.
7. Vergara-Buenaventura A, Castro-Ruiz C. Use of mouthwashes against COVID-19 in dentistry. Br J Oral Maxillofac Surg 2020;58:924–927.
8. Chaudhary P, Melkonyan A, Meethil A, et al. Estimating salivary carriage of severe acute respiratory syndrome coronavirus 2 in nonsymptomatic people and efficacy of mouthrinse in reducing viral load: A randomized controlled trial. J Am Dent Assoc 2021;152:903–912.
9. Krasner P, Rankow HJ. Anatomy of the pulp-chamber floor. J Endod 2004;30:5–16.
10. Slaton CC, Loushine RJ, Weller RN, Parker MH, Kimbrough WF, Pashley DH. Identification of resected root-end dentinal cracks: A comparative study of visual magnification. J Endod 2003;29:519–522.
11. Carr GB, Murgel CAF. The use of operating microscopes in endodontics. Dent Clin N Am 2004;54:191–214.
12. Use of Microscopes and Other Magnification Techniques. AAE Position Statement. American Association of Endodontists, 2012. https://www.aae.org/specialty/wp-content/uploads/sites/2/2017/06/microscopesstatement.pdf. Accessed 23 March 2023.
13. Rover G, Belladonna FG, Bortoluzzi EA, De-Deus G, Silva EJNL, Teixeira CS. Influence of access cavity design on root canal detection, instrumentation efficacy, and fracture resistance assessed in maxillary molars. J Endod 2017;43:1657–1662.
14. Vieira GCS, Pérez AR, Alves FRF, et al. Impact of contracted endodontic cavities on root canal disinfection and shaping. J Endod 2020;46:655–661.
15. Silva EJNL, Rover G, Belladonna F, De-Deus G, Teixeira CS, Silva Fidalgo TK. Impact of contracted endodontic cavities on fracture resistance of endodontically treated teeth: A systematic review of in vitro studies. Clin Oral Investig 2018;22:109–118.
16. Hamilton AI, Kramer IR. Cavity preparation with and without waterspray. Effects on the human dental pulp and additional effects of further dehydration of the dentine. Br Dent J 1967;123:281–285.
17. Robinson D, Goerig AC, Neaverth EJ. Endodontic access: An update, Part I. Compendium 1989;10:290–292, 294–296, 298.

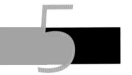

18. Connert T, Zehnder MS, Weiger R, Kühl S, Krastl G. Microguided endodontics: Accuracy of a miniaturized technique for apically extended access cavity preparation in anterior teeth. J Endod 2017;43:787–790.

19. Lara-Mendes STO, Barbosa CFM, Santa-Rosa CC, Machado VC. Guided endodontic access in maxillary molars using cone-beam computed tomography and computer-aided design/computer-aided manufacturing system: A case report. J Endod 2018;44:875–879.

20. Rosenberg PA, Babick PJ, Schertzer L, Leung A. The effect of occlusal reduction on pain after endodontic instrumentation. J Endod 1998;24:492–496.

21. Deutsch AS, Muskikant BL. Morphological measurements of anatomic landmarks in human maxillary and mandibular molar pulp chambers. J Endod 2004;30:388–390.

22. Bellizzi R, Hartwell G. Radiographic evaluation of root canal anatomy of in vivo endodontically treated maxillary premolars. J Endod 1985;11:37–39.

23. Carns EJ, Skidmore AE. Configurations and deviations of root canals of maxillary first premolars. Oral Surg Oral Med Oral Pathol 1973;36:880–886.

24. Kulild JC, Peters DD. Incidence and configuration of canal systems in the mesiobuccal root of maxillary first and second molars. J Endod 1990;16:311–317.

25. Hartwell G, Bellizzi R. Clinical investigation of in vivo endodontically treated mandibular and maxillary molars. J Endod 1982;8:555–557.

26. Nosrat A, Deschenes RJ, Tordik PA, Hicks ML, Fouad AF. Middle mesial canals in mandibular molars: Incidence and related factors. J Endod 2015;41:28–32.

27. Nosrat A, Deschenes RJ, Tordik PA, Hicks ML, Fouad AF. Middle mesial canals in mandibular molars: Incidence and related factors. J Endod 2015;41:28–32.

28. Vertucci FJ. Root canal anatomy of the human permanent teeth. Oral Surg Oral Med Oral Pathol 1984;58:589–599.

29. Calberson FL, De Moor RJ, Deroose CA. The radix entomolaris and paramolaris: Clinical approach in endodontics. J Endod 2007;33:58–63.

30. De Moor RJG, Deroose CAJG, Calberson FLG. The radix entomolaris in mandibular first molars: An endodontic challenge. Int Endod J 2004;37:789–799.

31. Ricucci D. Apical limit of root canal instrumentation and obturation, part 1. Literature review. Int Endod J 1998;31:384–393.

32. Seltzer S, Soltanoff W, Smith J. Biologic aspects of endodontics. V. Periapical tissue reactions to root canal instrumentation beyond the apex and root canal fillings short of and beyond the apex. Oral Surg Oral Med Oral Pathol 1973;36:725–737.

33. Meder-Cowherd L, Williamson AE, Johnson WT, Vasilescu D, Walton R, Qian F. Apical morphology of the palatal roots of maxillary molars by using micro-computed tomography. J Endod 2011;37:1162–1165.

34. Burch JG, Hulen S. The relationship of the apical foramen to the anatomic apex of the tooth root. Oral Surg Oral Med Oral Pathol 1972;34:262–268.

35. Kuttler Y. Microscopic investigation of root apexes. J Am Dent Assoc 1955;50:544–552.

36. Jeger FB, Janner SF, Bornstein MM, Lussi A. Endodontic working length measurement with preexisting cone-beam computed tomography scanning: A prospective, controlled clinical study. J Endod 2012;38:884–888

37. Lozano A, Forner L, Llena C. In vitro comparison of root-canal measurements with conventional and digital radiology. Int Endod J 2002;35:542–550.

38. Shabahang S, Goon WW, Gluskin AH. An in vivo evaluation of Root ZX electronic apex locator. J Endod 1996;22:616–618.

39. Sunada I. New method for measuring the length of the root canal. J Dent Res 1962;141:375–387.

40. Suzuki K. Experimental study on ionophoresis. J Jap Stomatol 1942;116:411–429.

41. Ounsi HF, Naaman A. In vitro evaluation of the reliability of the Root ZX electronic apex locator. Int Endod J 1999;32:120–123.

42. Arslan H, Güven Y, Karataş E, Doğanay E. Effect of the simultaneous working length control during root canal preparation on postoperative pain. J Endod 2017;43:1422–1427.

43. Dunlap CA, Remeikis NA, BeGole EA, Rauschenberger CR. An in vivo evaluation of an electronic apex locator that uses the ratio method in vital and necrotic canals. J Endod 1998;24:48–50.

44. Goldberg F, De Silvio AC, Manfré S, Nastri N. In vitro measurement accuracy of an electronic apex locator in teeth with simulated apical root resorption. J Endod 2002;28:461–463.

45. Saatchi M, Aminozarbian MG, Hasheminia SM, Mortaheb A. Influence of apical periodontitis on the accuracy of 3 electronic root canal length measurement devices: An in vivo study. J Endod 2014;40:355–359.

46. Wilson BL, Broberg C, Baumgartner JC, Harris C, Kron J. Safety of electronic apex locators and pulp testers in patients with implanted cardiac pacemakers or cardioverter/defibrillators. J Endod 2006;32:847–852.

47. Jenkins JA, Walker WA 3rd, Schindler WG, Flores CM. An in vitro evaluation of the accuracy of the Root ZX in the presence of various irrigants. J Endod 2001;27:209–211.

48. Schilder H. Cleaning and shaping the root canal. Dent Clin North Am 1974;18:269–296.

49. Iqbal MK, Kohli MR, Kim JS. A retrospective clinical study of incidence of root canal instrument separation in an endodontics graduate program: A PennEndo database study. J Endod 2006;32:1048–1052.

50. Salzgeber RM, Brilliant JD. An in vivo evaluation of the penetration of an irrigating solution in root canals. J Endod 1977;3:394–398.

51. Mickel AK, Chogle S, Liddle J, Huffaker K, Jones JJ. The role of apical size determination and enlargement in the reduction of intracanal bacteria. J Endod 2007;33:21–23.

52. Haapasalo M, Shen Y, Qian W, Gao Y. Irrigation in endodontics. Dent Clin North Am 2010;54:291–312.

53. Del Carpio-Perochena AE, Bramante CM, Duarte MAH, et al. Biofilm dissolution and cleaning ability of different irrigant solutions on intraorally infected dentin. J Endod 2011;37:1134–1138.

54. Baumgartner JC, Mader CL. A scanning electron microscopic evaluation of four root canal irrigation regimens. J Endod 1987;13:147–157.

55. Rosenfeld EF, James GA, Burch BS. Vital pulp tissue response to sodium hypochlorite. J Endod 1978;4:140–146.

56. Williams K, Hughson AG, Chesebro B, Race B. Inactivation of chronic wasting disease prions using sodium hypochlorite. PLoS One 2019;14:e0223659.

57. Azarpazhooh A, Fillery ED. Prion disease: The implications for dentistry. J Endod 2008;34:1158–1166.

58. Hand RE, Smith ML, Harrison JW. Analysis of the effect of dilution on the necrotic tissue dissolution property of sodium hypochlorite. J Endod 1978;4:60–64.

59. Senia ES, Marshall FJ, Rosen S. The solvent action of sodium hypochlorite on pulp tissue of extracted teeth. Oral Surg Oral Med Oral Pathol 1971;31:96–103.

60. D'Arcangelo C, Di Nardo Di Maio CF, Stracci N, Spoto G, Malagnino VA, Caputi S. Pulp-dissolving ability of several endodontic irrigants: A spectrophotometric evaluation. Int J Immunopathol Pharmacol 2007;20:381–386.

61. Estrela C, Estrela CRA, Barbin EL, Spanó JCE, Marchesan MA, Pécora JD. Mechanism of action of sodium hypochlorite. Braz Dent J 2002;13:113–117.

62. Guivarc'h M, Ordioni U, Ahmed HMA, Cohen S, Catherine JH, Bukiet F. Sodium hypochlorite accident: A systematic review. J Endod 2017;43:16–24.

63. Hülsmann M, Hahn W. Complications during root canal irrigation—Literature review and case reports. Int Endod J 2000;33:186–193.

64. Basrani BR, Manek S, Sodhi RNS, Fillery E, Manzur A. Interaction between sodium hypochlorite and chlorhexidine gluconate. J Endod 2007;33:966–969.

65. Bui TB, Baumgartner JC, Mitchell JC. Evaluation of the interaction between sodium hypochlorite and chlorhexidine gluconate and its effect on root dentin. J Endod 2008;34:181–185.

66. Clarkson RM, Podlich HM, Moule AJ. Influence of ethylenediaminetetraacetic acid on the active chlorine content of sodium hypochlorite solutions when mixed in various proportions. J Endod 2011;37:538–543.

67. Tartari T, Guimarães BM, Amoras LS, Duarte MAH, Silva e Souza PAR, Bramante CM. Etidronate causes minimal changes in the ability of sodium hypochlorite to dissolve organic matter. Int Endod J 2015;48:399–404.

68. Calt S, Serper A. Time-dependent effects of EDTA on dentin structures. J Endod 2002;28:17–19.

69. Rasimick BJ, Nekich M, Hladek MM, Musikant BL, Deutsch AS. Interaction between chlorhexidine digluconate and EDTA. J Endod 2008;34:1521–1523.

70. Jeansonne MJ, White RR. A comparison of 2.0% chlorhexidine gluconate and 5.25% sodium hypochlorite as antimicrobial endodontic irrigants. J Endod 1994;20:276–278.

71. Baca P, Junco P, Arias-Moliz MT, Castillo F, Rodríguez-Archilla A, Ferrer-Luque CM. Antimicrobial substantivity over time of chlorhexidine and cetrimide. J Endod 2012;38:927–930.

72. Okino LA, Siqueira EL, Santos M, Bombana AC, Figueiredo JAP. Dissolution of pulp tissue by aqueous solution of chlorhexidine digluconate and chlorhexidine digluconate gel. Int Endod J 2004;37:38–41.

73. Sen BH, Safavi KE, Spångberg LS. Antifungal effects of sodium hypochlorite and chlorhexidine in root canals. J Endod 1999;25:235–238.

74. Taylor JK, Jeansonne BG, Lemon RR. Coronal leakage: Effects of smear layer, obturation technique, and sealer. J Endod 1997;23:508–512.

75. Madison S, Krell KV. Comparison of ethylenediamine tetraacetic acid and sodium hypochlorite on the apical seal of endodontically treated teeth. J Endod 1984;10:499–503.

76. Gutarts R, Nusstein J, Reader A, Beck M. In vivo debridement efficacy of ultrasonic irrigation following hand-rotary instrumentation in human mandibular molars. J Endod 2005;31:166–170.

77. Malki M, Verhaagen B, Jiang LM, et al. Irrigant flow beyond the insertion depth of an ultrasonically oscillating file in straight and curved root canals: Visualization and cleaning efficacy. J Endod 2012;38:657–661.

78. Beus C, Safavi K, Stratton J, Kaufman B. Comparison of the effect of two endodontic irrigation protocols on the elimination of bacteria from root canal system: A prospective, randomized clinical trial. J Endod 2012;38:1479–1483.

79. Haapasalo M, Wang Z, Shen Y, Curtis A, Patel P, Khakpour M. Tissue dissolution by a novel multisonic ultracleaning system and sodium hypochlorite. J Endod 2014;40:1178–1181.
80. Christo JE, Zilm PS, Sullivan T, Cathro PR. Efficacy of low concentrations of sodium hypochlorite and low-powered Er,Cr: YSGG laser activated irrigation against an Enterococcus faecalis biofilm. Int Endod J 2016;49:279–286.
81. Vela KC, Walton RE, Trope M, Windschitl P, Caplan DJ. Patient preferences regarding 1-visit versus 2-visit root canal therapy. J Endod 2012;38:1322–1325.
82. Figini L, Lodi G, Gorni F, Gagliani M. Single versus multiple visits for endodontic treatment of permanent teeth: A Cochrane systematic review. J Endod 2008;34:1041–1047.
83. Manfredi M, Figini L, Gagliani M, Lodi G. Single versus multiple visits for endodontic treatment of permanent teeth. Cochrane Database Syst Rev 2016;12:CD005296.
84. Roane JB, Dryden JA, Grimes EW. Incidence of postoperative pain after single- and multiple-visit endodontic procedures. Oral Surg Oral Med Oral Pathol 1983;55:68–72.
85. Eleazer PD, Eleazer KR. Flare-up rate in pulpally necrotic molars in one-visit versus two-visit endodontic treatment. J Endod 1998;24:614–616.
86. Sathorn C, Parashos P, Messer H. The prevalence of postoperative pain and flare-up in single- and multiple-visit endodontic treatment: A systematic review. Int Endod J 2008;41:91–99.
87. Pekruhn RB. The incidence of failure following single-visit endodontic therapy. J Endod 1986;12:68–72.
88. Walton R, Fouad A. Endodontic interappointment flare-ups: A prospective study of incidence and related factors. J Endod 1992;18:172–177.
89. Penesis VA, Fitzgerald PI, Fayad MI, Wenckus CS, BeGole EA, Johnson BR. Outcome of one-visit and two-visit endodontic treatment of necrotic teeth with apical periodontitis: A randomized controlled trial with one-year evaluation. J Endod 2008;34:251–257.
90. Windley W 3rd, Teixeira F, Levin L, Sigurdsson A, Trope M. Disinfection of immature teeth with a triple antibiotic paste. J Endod 2005;31:439–443.
91. Law AS, Nixdorf DR, Rabinowitz I, et al. Root canal therapy reduces multiple dimensions of pain: A national dental practice-based research network study. J Endod 2014;40:1738–1745.
92. Torabinejad M, Kettering JD, McGraw JC, Cummings RR, Dwyer TG, Tobias TS. Factors associated with endodontic interappointment emergencies of teeth with necrotic pulps. J Endod 1988;14:261–266.
93. Polycarpou N, Ng YL, Canavan D, Moles DR, Gulabivala K. Prevalence of persistent pain after endodontic treatment and factors affecting its occurrence in cases with complete radiographic healing. Int Endod J 2005;38:169–178.
94. Byström A, Sundqvist G. Bacteriologic evaluation of the efficacy of mechanical root canal instrumentation in endodontic therapy. Scand J Dent Res 1981;89:321–328.
95. Shuping GB, Orstavik D, Sigurdsson A, Trope M. Reduction of intracanal bacteria using nickel-titanium rotary instrumentation and various medications. J Endod 2000;26:751–755.
96. Sjögren U, Figdor D, Spångberg L, Sundqvist G. The antimicrobial effect of calcium hydroxide as a short-term intracanal dressing. Int Endod J 1991;24:119–125.
97. Safavi KE, Nichols FC. Alteration of biological properties of bacterial lipopolysaccharide by calcium hydroxide treatment. J Endod 1994;20:127–129.
98. Hasselgren G, Olsson B, Cvek M. Effects of calcium hydroxide and sodium hypochlorite on the dissolution of necrotic porcine muscle tissue. J Endod 1988;14:125–127.
99. Waltimo TM, Orstavik D, Sirén EK, Haapasalo MP. In vitro susceptibility of Candida albicans to four disinfectants and their combinations. Int Endod J 1999;32:421–429.
100. Wang CS, Arnold RR, Trope M, Teixeira FB. Clinical efficiency of 2% chlorhexidine gel in reducing intracanal bacteria. J Endod 2007;33:1283–1289.
101. Leonardo MR, da Silva LA, Filho MT, Bonifácio KC, Ito IY. In vitro evaluation of the antimicrobial activity of a castor oil-based irrigant. J Endod 2001;27:717–719.
102. Arruda MEF, Neves MAS, Diogenes A, et al. Infection control in teeth with apical periodontitis using a triple antibiotic solution or calcium hydroxide with chlorhexidine: A randomized clinical trial. J Endod 2018;44:1474–1479.
103. Faria G, Rodrigues EM, Coaguila-Llerena H, et al. Influence of the vehicle and antibiotic formulation on cytotoxicity of triple antibiotic paste. J Endod 2018;44:1812–1816.
104. Hoshino E, Kurihara-Ando N, Sato I, et al. In-vitro antibacterial susceptibility of bacteria taken from infected root dentine to a mixture of ciprofloxacin, metronidazole and minocycline. Int Endod J 1996;29:125–130.
105. AlSaeed T, Nosrat A, Melo MA, et al. Antibacterial efficacy and discoloration potential of endodontic topical antibiotics. J Endod 2018;44:1110–1114.
106. Kim JH, Kim Y, Shin SJ, Park JW, Jung IY. Tooth discoloration of immature permanent incisor associated with triple antibiotic therapy: A case report. J Endod 2010;36:1086–1091.

107. Iwaya S, Ikawa M, Kubota M. Revascularization of an immature permanent tooth with periradicular abscess after luxation. Dent Traumatol 2011;27:55–58.

108. Sigurdsson A, Stancill R, Madison S. Intracanal placement of Ca(OH)2: A comparison of techniques. J Endod 1992;18:367–370.

109. Gluskin AH, Lai G, Peters CI, Peters OA. The double-edged sword of calcium hydroxide in endodontics: Precautions and preventive strategies for extrusion injuries into neurovascular anatomy. J Am Dent Assoc 2020;151:317–325.

110. Schilder H. Filling root canals in three dimensions. Dent Clin North Am 1967;11:723–744.

111. Grossman LI. Endodontic Practice. Philadelphia: Lea and Febiger, 1978.

112. Sjögren U, Sundqvist G, Nair PN. Tissue reaction to gutta-percha particles of various sizes when implanted subcutaneously in guinea pigs. Eur J Oral Sci 1995;103:313–321.

113. Use of Silver Points. AAE Position Statement. American Association of Endodontists, 2017. https://www.aae.org/specialty/wp-content/uploads/sites/2/2017/06/silverpointsstatement.pdf. Accessed 27 March 2023.

114. Paraformaldehyde-Containing Endodontic Filling Materials and Sealers. AAE Position Statement. American Association of Endodontists, 2017. https://www.aae.org/specialty/wp-content/uploads/sites/2/2017/06/paraformaldehydefillingmaterials.pdf. Accessed 27 March 2023.

115. Barborka BJ, Woodmansey KF, Glickman GN, Schneiderman E, He J. Long-term clinical outcome of teeth obturated with resilon. J Endod 2017;43:556–560.

116. Xu LL, Zhang L, Zhou XD, Wang R, Deng YH, Huang DM. Residual filling material in dentinal tubules after gutta-percha removal observed with scanning electron microscopy. J Endod 2012;38:293–296.

117. Baumgardner KR, Taylor J, Walton R. Canal adaptation and coronal leakage: Lateral condensation compared to Thermafil. J Am Dent Assoc 1995;126:351–356.

118. Gomes BP, Vianna ME, Matsumoto CU, et al. Disinfection of gutta-percha cones with chlorhexidine and sodium hypochlorite. Oral Surg Oral Med Oral Pathol Oral Radiol Endod 2005;100:512–517.

119. Short RD, Dorn SO, Kuttler S. The crystallization of sodium hypochlorite on gutta-percha cones after the rapid-sterilization technique: An SEM study. J Endod 2003;29:670–673.

120. Marshall FJ, Massler M. The sealing of pulpless teeth evaluated with radioisotopes. J Dent Med 1961;16:172–184.

121. Vitti RP, Prati C, Silva EJ, et al. Physical properties of MTA Fillapex sealer. J Endod 2013;39:915–918.

122. Lodiene G, Morisbak E, Bruzell E, Ørstavik D. Toxicity evaluation of root canal sealers in vitro. Int Endod J 2008;41:72–77.

123. Aminoshariae A, Primus C, Kulild JC. Tricalcium silicate cement sealers: Do the potential benefits of bioactivity justify the drawbacks? J Am Dent Assoc 2022;153:750–760.

124. Saleh IM, Ruyter IE, Haapasalo M, Ørstavik D. Survival of enterococcus faecalis in infected dentinal tubules after root canal filling with different root canal sealers in vitro. Int Endod J 2004;37:193–198.

125. Giardino L, Pontieri F, Savoldi E, Tallarigo F. Aspergillus mycetoma of the maxillary sinus secondary to overfilling of a root canal. J Endod 2006;32:692–694.

126. González-Martín M, Torres-Lagares D, Gutiérrez-Pérez JL, Segura-Egea JJ. Inferior alveolar nerve paresthesia after overfilling of endodontic sealer into the mandibular canal. J Endod 2010;36:1419–1421.

127. Jung S, Sielker S, Hanisch MR, Libricht V, Schäfer E, Dammaschke T. Cytotoxic effects of four different root canal sealers on human osteoblasts. PLoS One 2018;13:e0194467.

128. Wiemann AH, Wilcox LR. In vitro evaluation of four methods of sealer placement. J Endod 1991;17:444–447.

129. Tanomaru-Filho M, Jorge EG, Guerreiro Tanomaru JM, Gonçalves M. Radiopacity evaluation of new root canal filling materials by digitalization of images. J Endod 2007;33:249–251.

130. Miletić I, Jukić S, Anić I, Zeljezić D, Garaj-Vrhovac V, Osmak M. Examination of cytotoxicity and mutagenicity of AH26 and AH Plus sealers. Int Endod J 2003;36:330–335.

131. Leyhausen G, Heil J, Reifferscheid G, Waldmann P, Geurtsen W. Genotoxicity and cytotoxicity of the epoxy resin-based root canal sealer AH plus. J Endod 1999;25:109–213.

132. Siqueira JF Jr, Favieri A, Gahyva SM, Moraes SR, Lima KC, Lopes HP. Antimicrobial activity and flow rate of newer and established root canal sealers. J Endod 2000;26:274–277.

133. Spångberg LS, Barbosa SV, Lavigne GD. AH 26 releases formaldehyde. J Endod 1993;19:596–598.

134. Leonardo MR, Bezerra da Silva LA, Filho MT, Santana da Silva R. Release of formaldehyde by 4 endodontic sealers. Oral Surg Oral Med Oral Pathol Oral Radiol Endod 1999;88:221–225.

135. Grossman LI. Physical properties of root canal cements. J Endod 1976;2:166–175.

136. Kamatou GP, Vermaak I, Viljoen AM. Eugenol—From the remote Maluku Islands to the international market place: A review of a remarkable and versatile molecule. Molecules 2012;17:6953–6981.

137. Kozam G, Mantell GM. The effect of eugenol on oral mucous membranes. J Dent Res 1978;57:954–957.

138. Desai S, Chandler N. Calcium hydroxide-based root canal sealers: A review. J Endod 2009;35:475–480.

139. Miletić I, Anić I, Karlović Z, Marsan T, Pezelj-Ribarić S, Osmak M. Cytotoxic effect of four root filling materials. Endod Dent Traumatol 2000;16:287–290.

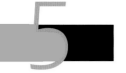

140. Leonardo MR, da Silva LA, Tanomaru Filho M, Bonifácio KC, Ito IY. In vitro evaluation of antimicrobial activity of sealers and pastes used in endodontics. J Endod 2000;26:391–394.

141. Langeland K. Root canal sealants and pastes. Dent Clin N Am 1974;18:309–327.

142. Fonseca DA, Paula AB, Marto CM, et al. Biocompatibility of root canal sealers: A systematic review of in vitro and in vivo studies. Materials (Basel) 2019;12:4113.

143. Zhou HM, Shen Y, Zheng W, Li L, Zheng YF, Haapasalo M. Physical properties of 5 root canal sealers. J Endod 2013;39:1281–1286.

144. Candeiro GTM, Correia FC, Duarte MAH, Ribeiro-Siqueira DC, Gavini G. Evaluation of radiopacity, pH, release of calcium ions, and flow of a bioceramic root canal sealer. J Endod 2012;38:842–845.

145. Ballullaya SV, Vinay V, Thumu J, Devalla S, Bollu IP, Balla S. Stereomicroscopic dye leakage measurement of six different root canal sealers. J Clin Diagn Res 2017;11:ZC65–ZC68.

146. Zhang W, Li Z, Peng B. Effects of iRoot SP on mineralization-related genes expression in MG63 cells. J Endod 2010;36:1978–1982.

147. Wang Z, Shen Y, Haapasalo M. Dentin extends the antibacterial effect of endodontic sealers against Enterococcus faecalis biofilms. J Endod 2014;40:505–508.

148. Giacomino CM, Wealleans JA, Kuhn N, Diogenes A. Comparative biocompatibility and osteogenic potential of two bioceramic sealers. J Endod 2019;45:51–56.

149. Koch KA, Brave GD, Nasseh AA. Bioceramic technology: Closing the endo-restorative circle, Part I. Dent Today 2010;29:100–105.

150. de Chevigny C, Dao TT, Basrani BR, et al. Treatment outcome in endodontics: The Toronto study—Phase 4: Initial treatment. J Endod 2008;34:258–263.

151. Buchanan LS. Continuous wave of condensation technique. Endod Prac 1998;1:7–10, 13–16.

152. Floren JW, Weller RN, Pashley DH, Kimbrough WF. Changes in root surface temperatures with in vitro use of the system B HeatSource. J Endod 1999;25:593–595.

153. Yee FS, Marlin J, Krakow AA, Gron P. Three-dimensional obturation of the root canal using injection-molded, thermoplasticized dental gutta-percha. J Endod 1977;3:168–174.

154. Torabinejad M, Parirokh M. Mineral trioxide aggregate: A comprehensive literature review—Part II: Leakage and biocompatibility investigations. J Endod 2010;36:190–202.

155. Parirokh M, Torabinejad M. Mineral trioxide aggregate: A comprehensive literature review—Part I: chemical, physical, and antibacterial properties. J Endod 2010;36:16–27.

156. Parirokh M, Torabinejad M. Mineral trioxide aggregate: A comprehensive literature review—Part III: Clinical applications, drawbacks, and mechanism of action. J Endod 2010;36:400–413.

157. Swanson K, Madison S. An evaluation of coronal microleakage in endodontically treated teeth. Part I. Time periods. J Endod 1987;13:56–59.

158. Madison S, Wilcox LR. An evaluation of coronal microleakage in endodontically treated teeth. Part III. In vivo study. J Endod 1988;14:455–458.

159. Torabinejad M, Ung B, Kettering JD. In vitro bacterial penetration of coronally unsealed endodontically treated teeth. J Endod 1990;16:566–569.

160. Yee K, Bhagavatula P, Stover S, et al. Survival rates of teeth with primary endodontic treatment after core/post and crown placement. J Endod 2018;44:220–225.

161. Chugal NM, Clive JM, Spångberg LSW. Endodontic treatment outcome: Effect of the permanent restoration. Oral Surg Oral Med Oral Pathol Oral Radiol Endod 2007;104:576–582.

162. Lamers AC, Simon M, van Mullem PJ. Microleakage of Cavit temporary filling material in endodontic access cavities in monkey teeth. Oral Surg Oral Med Oral Pathol 1980;49:541–543.

163. Barthel CR, Strobach A, Briedigkeit H, Göbel UB, Roulet JF. Leakage in roots coronally sealed with different temporary fillings. J Endod 1999;25:731–734.

164. Kumar G, Tewari S, Sangwan P, Tewari S, Duhan J, Mittal S. The effect of an intraorifice barrier and base under coronal restorations on the healing of apical periodontitis: A randomized controlled trial. Int Endod J 2020;53:298–307.

165. Schwartz RS, Fransman R. Adhesive dentistry and endodontics: Materials, clinical strategies and procedures for restoration of access cavities: A review. J Endod 2005;31:151–165.

166. Davis MC, Shariff SS. Success and survival of endodontically treated cracked teeth with radicular extensions: A 2- to 4-year prospective cohort. J Endod 2019;45:848–855.

167. Nagas E, Uyanik O, Altundasar E, et al. Effect of different intraorifice barriers on the fracture resistance of roots obturated with Resilon or gutta-percha. J Endod 2010;36:1061–1063.

168. Ray HA, Trope M. Periapical status of endodontically treated teeth in relation to the technical quality of the root filling and the coronal restoration. Int Endod J 1995;28:12–18.

169. Gargiulo A, Krajewski J, Gargiulo M. Defining biologic width in crown lengthening. CDS Rev 1995;88:20–23.

170. Juloski J, Radovic I, Goracci C, Vulicevic ZR, Ferrari M. Ferrule effect: A literature review. J Endod 2012;38:11–19.

171. Naumann M, Schmitter M, Frankenberger R, Krastl G. "Ferrule comes first. Post is second!" Fake news and alternative facts? A systematic review. J Endod 2018;44:212–219.

172. Sarkis-Onofre R, Fergusson D, Cenci MS, Moher D, Pereira-Cenci T. Performance of post-retained single crowns: A systematic review of related risk factors. J Endod 2017;43:175–183.

173. Chrepa V, Konstantinidis I, Kotsakis GA, Mitsias ME. The survival of indirect composite resin onlays for the restoration of root filled teeth: A retrospective medium-term study. Int Endod J 2014;47:967–973.

174. Reeh ES, Messer HH, Douglas WH. Reduction in tooth stiffness as a result of endodontic and restorative procedures. J Endod 1989;15:512–516.

175. Sorensen JA, Martinoff JT. Intracoronal reinforcement and coronal coverage: A study of endodontically treated teeth. J Prosthet Dent 1984;51:780–784.

176. Suksaphar W, Banomyong D, Jirathanyanatt T, Ngoenwiwatkul Y. Survival rates from fracture of end-odontically treated premolars restored with full-coverage crowns or direct resin composite restorations: A retrospective study. J Endod 2018;44:233–238.

177. Goldfein J, Speirs C, Finkelman M, Amato R. Rubber dam use during post placement influences the success of root canal-treated teeth. J Endod 2013;39:1481–1484.

178. Figueiredo FED, Martins-Filho PRS, Faria-E-Silva AL. Do metal post-retained restorations result in more root fractures than fiber post-retained restorations? A systematic review and meta-analysis. J Endod 2015;41:309–316.

179. Doyle SL, Hodges JS, Pesun IJ, Baisden MK, Bowles WR. Factors affecting outcomes for single-tooth implants and endodontic restorations. J Endod 2007;33:399–402.

180. Sagsen B, Zortuk M, Ertas H, Er O, Demirbuga S, Arslan H. In vitro fracture resistance of endodontically treated roots filled with a bonded filling material or different types of posts. J Endod 2013;39:1435–1437.

181. Maroulakos G, He J, Nagy WW. The post-endodontic adhesive interface: Theoretical perspectives and potential flaws. J Endod 2018;44:363–371.

182. Guldener KA, Lanzrein CL, Siegrist Guldener BE, Lang NP, Ramseier CA, Salvi GE. Long-term clinical outcomes of endodontically treated teeth restored with or without fiber post-retained single-unit restorations. J Endod 2017;43:188–193.

183. Kuttler S, McLean A, Dorn S, Fischzang A. The impact of post space preparation with Gates-Glidden drills on residual dentin thickness in distal roots of mandibular molars. J Am Dent Assoc 2004;135:903–909.

184. Mattison GD, Delivanis PD, Thacker RW Jr, Hassell KJ. Effect of post preparation on the apical seal. J Prosthet Dent 1984;51:785–789.

185. Abramovitz L, Lev R, Fuss Z, Metzger Z. The unpredictability of seal after post space preparation: A fluid transport study. J Endod 2001;27:292–295.

186. Shillingburg HT. Fundamentals of Fixed Prosthodontics, ed 3. Chicago: Quintessence, 1997.

187. Pak JG, White SN. Pain prevalence and severity before, during, and after root canal treatment: A systematic review. J Endod 2011;37:429–438.

188. Richards D. The Oxford Pain Group League table of analgesic efficacy. Evid Based Dent 2004;5:22–23.

189. Menhinick KA, Gutmann J, Regan JD, Taylor SE, Buschang PH. The efficacy of pain control following non-surgical root canal treatment using ibuprofen or a combination of ibuprofen and acetaminophen in a randomized, double-blind, placebo-controlled study. Int Endod J 2004;37:531–541.

190. Polycarpou N, Ng YL, Canavan D, Moles DR, Gulabivala K. Prevalence of persistent pain after endodontic treatment and factors affecting its occurrence in cases with complete radiographic healing. Int Endod J 2005;38:169–178.

191. American Association of Endodontists. Glossary of Endodontic Terms. 2020. https://www.aae.org/specialty/clinical-resources/glossary-endodontic-terms/. Accessed 29 March 2023.

192. Walton R. Interappointment flare-ups: Incidence, related factors, prevention, and management. Endod Topics 2002;3:67–76.

193. Tsesis I, Faivishevsky V, Fuss Z, Zukerman O. Flare-ups after endodontic treatment: A meta-analysis of literature. J Endod 2008;34:1177–1181.

194. Sjögren U, Hagglund B, Sundqvist G, Wing K. Factors affecting the long-term results of endodontic treatment. J Endod 1990;16:498–504.

195. Friedman S, Abitbol S, Lawrence HP. Treatment outcome in endodontics: The Toronto Study. Phase 1: Initial treatment. J Endod 2003;29:787–793.

196. Siqueira JF Jr. Microbial causes of endodontic flare-ups. Int Endod J 2003;36:453–463.

197. Johnson M. Antibiotics and the treatment of dental infections. American Association of Endodontists: Colleagues for Excellence Fall 2019.

198. Friedman S, Mor C. The success of endodontic therapy—Healing and functionality. J Calif Dent Assoc 2004;32:493–503.

199. Orstavik D. Time-course and risk analyses of the development and healing of chronic apical periodontitis in man. Int Endod J 1996;29:150–155.

200. Molven O, Halse A, Fristad I, MacDonald-Jankowski D. Periapical changes following root-canal treatment observed 20-27 years postoperatively. Int Endod J 2002;35:784–790.
201. Fouad AF, Burleson J. The effect of diabetes mellitus on endodontic treatment outcome: Data from an electronic patient record. J Am Dent Assoc 2003;134:43–51.
202. Murphy WK, Kaugars GE, Collett WK, Dodds RN. Healing of periapical radiolucencies after nonsurgical endodontic therapy. Oral Surg Oral Med Oral Pathol 1991;71:620–624.
203. Low KMT, Dula K, Bürgin W, von Arx T. Comparison of periapical radiography and limited cone-beam tomography in posterior maxillary teeth referred for apical surgery. J Endod 2008;34:557–562.
204. Langella J, Blicher B, Lucier Pryles R. Clinical update: Maxillary sinusitis of endodontic origin (MSEO). J Mass Dental Soc 2020;69:14–17.
205. Maxillary Sinusitis of Endodontic Origin. AAE Position Statement. American Association of Endodontists, 2018. https://www.aae.org/specialty/wp-content/uploads/sites/2/2018/04/AAE_PositionStatement_MaxillarySinusitis.pdf. Accessed 29 March 2023.

Nonsurgical Retreatment

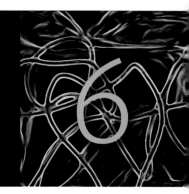

6

Nonsurgical retreatment refers to the treatment of recurrent or persistent endodontic pathology, otherwise known as posttreatment pathology, via an occlusal endodontic access. The incidence of recurrent and persistent pathology can be estimated by examining the prognosis literature. Success rates following nonsurgical root canal therapy (NSRCT) are exceptionally favorable, ranging between 86% and 97%.[1,2] This means that 3% to 14% of patients with a history of NSRCT may experience posttreatment disease that requires further care.

The etiology of posttreatment pathology relates to the quality of the initial NSRCT,[3,4] extraradicular infections,[5] problems related to restorative care,[6] and fracture[4] (Fig 6-1). Because NSRCT involves the complete debridement, disinfection, and obturation of the canal space, leaving canal spaces undertreated or untreated means bacteria and debris are left behind, resulting in posttreatment disease. In cases with excellent restorative care and untreated anatomy that present with pathology in only one root (confirmed by CBCT imaging), selective root retreatment may be appropriate.[7] Extraradicular infections may also cause posttreatment disease, evading host defenses via protective mechanisms within the multispecies infection. Leakage of salivary bacteria is another common cause of posttreatment disease. Excellent posttreatment restorative care is essential for positive outcomes after NSRCT. Conversely, failure to provide a definitive restoration or providing an inadequate restoration is known to result in coronal leakage. Finally, root fractures are a known cause of posttreatment pathology.

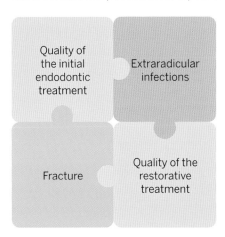

FIG 6-1
Causes of posttreatment disease following NSRCT.

Nonsurgical Retreatment

The myriad etiologies of posttreatment pathology underscore the importance of both accurate diagnosis and case selection for nonsurgical retreatment. What's clear from the prognosis literature is that correctable endodontic and restorative issues are readily and predictably treated via nonsurgical retreatment.[1,8] Generally, excellent candidates for nonsurgical retreatment are teeth with obvious but correctable causes for posttreatment disease, including teeth with sufficient remaining coronal tooth structure with leaking restorations or undertreated or untreated canal spaces (Fig 6-2). Patients presenting with root fractures, suspicion of extraradicular infections, or uncorrectable complications like instrument separation beyond the curvature of a canal space may not be good candidates for nonsurgical retreatment. Posttreatment disease resulting from causes that are not easily corrected may be more appropriately managed with other treatments, including surgical retreatment or extraction (Fig 6-3).

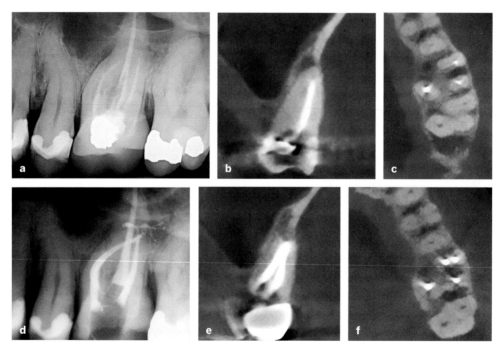

FIG 6-2 (a) Nonsurgical retreatment is an excellent treatment modality when untreated anatomy is noted as the etiology of recurrent or persistent apical periodontitis, like the untreated second mesio-buccal canal (ie, MB2) visible in the (b) coronal and (c) axial CBCT sections in this case. (d) Nonsurgical retreatment addressing this untreated anatomy resulted in complete healing of apical periodontitis, as seen at the 1-year follow-up with (e) coronal and (f) axial CBCT imaging.

Nonsurgical retreatment preferred	Nonsurgical retreatment contraindicated
• Untreated canal anatomy as likely etiology for pathology • Coronal leakage under existing restoration	• Adequate prior root canal fills • Large posts that are risky to remove • Obturation material that is extruded beyond the apex • Anatomy that cannot be accessed nonsurgically

FIG 6-3 Factors aiding in case selection for nonsurgical retreatment.

Coronal Disassembly

At its core, nonsurgical retreatment involves many of the same protocols as NSRCT. From anesthesia and dental dam isolation to canal location, obturation, and restorative care, the procedures by and large look very similar. That said, significant differences arise in the access phase, in the necessary removal of obturation material, and in considerations for intracanal medicaments. Access during nonsurgical retreatment is frequently referred to as coronal disassembly. Just as in NSRCT, access shapes are dictated by the shape of the tooth at the cementoenamel junction (CEJ) in order to facilitate canal location.[9] Rather than making access through pulp within a chamber, however, retreatment procedures involve making access through some form of restorative materials prior to reaching the canal spaces. In patients with leaking coronal restorations, the entirety of the restoration should be removed or the margins should be patched to facilitate the development of a leak-proof seal during treatment, with definitive restorative care to follow. If, however, retreatment is to be performed through a well-sealed crown, removal of the core material through an endodontic access is appropriate. Magnification with a surgical operating microscope is a crucial component of nonsurgical retreatment given the need for conservative removal of materials to preserve the remaining tooth structure. Once the restorative material is removed from the pulp chamber, the previously treated and untreated canal spaces can be located.

Post Removal

During the diagnosis and coronal disassembly process, posts may be found. In roots with well-sealed posts and the absence of apical pathology confirmed via CBCT imaging, the decision may be made to retain the existing post and perform selective retreatment on only the affected roots. When the coronal seal has been compromised or pathology is noted in the root containing the post, however, the post should be removed along with other obturation materials (Fig 6-4). Careful case selection should ensure that removal of the post does not compromise the tooth, and alternative treatments, including surgical retreatment or extraction, should be considered first (Fig 6-5).

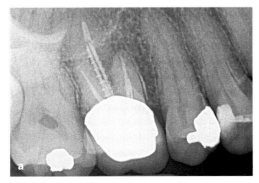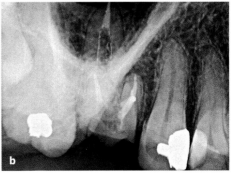

FIG 6-4 *(a and b)* Coronal disassembly refers to the removal of restorative material from the pulp chamber during nonsurgical retreatment. This may include the need for post removal along with complete removal of the coronal restorative materials, as in this maxillary right first molar where significant leakage was noted beneath the existing crown and resulted in the need for removal of the crown and the post to complete nonsurgical retreatment.

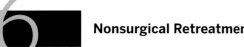

Is leakage noted under the core material surrounding the post?

Is apical pathology noted on the root with the post?

Is removal required to access a neighboring canal?

Does removal of the post present an undue risk of fracture or perforation?

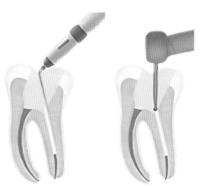

FIG 6-5 Treatment planning considerations for post removal.

FIG 6-6 Fiber post removal techniques.

Fiber posts can be removed with ultrasonic drills and standardized tips or with high-speed handpieces and surgical-length burs.[10] The challenge lies in discerning the post from the surrounding root structure, and a surgical operating microscope is necessary for this reason. Furthermore, ultrasonic instruments will often turn the fiber post black, making visibility a challenge. Frequent irrigation will enhance visibility and ensure that the ultrasonic instrument does not overheat the root or surrounding periodontal ligament (PDL) and bone (Fig 6-6).

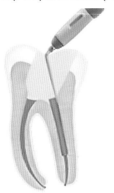

FIG 6-7 Metal posts are most readily removed with the use of ultrasonic drills.

Removal of metal posts can often be accomplished with similar techniques. Many metal posts can be removed readily with the vibration of an ultrasonic drill with standardized tips,[11] first targeting the cement surrounding the post and then the post itself (Fig 6-7). Specialized post removal ultrasonic tips are available, but many clinicians find that other tips in their armamentarium work just as well for this purpose. Longer and wider posts are usually more challenging to remove, as are parallel, cemented posts. Shorter, thinner, and threaded posts are often easily removed. Care must be taken to avoid thermal injury when post removal requires the use of ultrasonic energy instruments for long durations.[12,13] In some cases, posts are so tightly fitted into the canal space that the selective removal of root structure, referred to as *troughing*, must be performed with ultrasonic instruments.[11] The loss of radicular dentin by troughing may weaken the root and predispose it to fracture, so care must be taken to remove only the minimum amount of tooth structure.[12,13]

Obturation Material Removal

When pathology is noted in roots containing obturation material, the material needs to be removed. The removal of prior obturation materials must precede cleaning and reshaping. The ease of removal depends on the composition of the material that was used, including the sealer.[14,15] Removal can be accomplished by chemical and/or mechanical means and must be tailored to the type of obturation material within the canal system. This section reviews the methods and material considerations for obturation material removal.

Chemical removal of obturation materials

Solvents can be useful to soften existing obturation materials. Chloroform is generally considered the most effective solvent to soften gutta-percha–based filling materials.[16] Chloroform additionally possesses antibacterial properties,[17] enhancing its utility in nonsurgical retreatment (Fig 6-8). Care must be exercised with chloroform because it can also destroy other materials, including dental dam, and is harmful if in contact with soft tissues.[18] Certain paste-type obturation materials (often used outside of the United States) may require the use of alternative solvents, such as isopropyl alcohol or orange solvent.

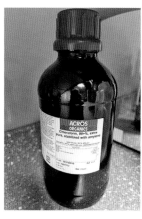

FIG 6-8 Chloroform is the most useful solvent for removing gutta-percha during endodontic retreatment but must be used judiciously because it will dissolve dental dam.

Mechanical removal of obturation materials

Both hand and rotary files used during cleaning and shaping of the root canal system can be employed in the removal of obturation materials.[19] Hedstrom files are useful for grabbing onto pieces of gutta-percha within a canal space, and a drop of chloroform solvent can give the Hedstrom file a purchase to grab pieces for removal. Gates Glidden drills may be used to remove gutta-percha in the coronal portions of wide and straight canals. Rotary instruments designed specifically for retreatment are also available from some manufacturers (Fig 6-9). Care must be taken to avoid creating canal wall defects or transporting canals, particularly with the use of the more aggressive retreatment-specific rotary instruments.[20] These instruments have an end-cutting design that can create pathways outside the canal space, leading to ledging, transportation, and even perforation. Beyond these traditional intracanal instruments, the heated downpacking implements of warm vertical obturation techniques can be used to soften and remove large pieces of gutta-percha.

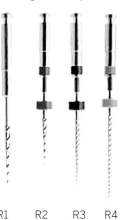

FIG 6-9 Traditional hand and rotary instruments, as well as retreatment-specific rotary instruments, can be used for the mechanical removal of obturation materials. (Shown here: EdgeFile XR Series, EdgeEndo.) R1   R2   R3   R4

Material considerations

Gutta-percha

Gutta-percha can be removed readily with a combination of solvents and rotary instruments.[19] Both traditional hand and rotary instruments, as well as retreatment-specific files, may be used. Clinicians often find that the coronal portion of gutta-percha can be removed easily with obturation heating implements, Gates Glidden drills, or larger rotary files, including retreatment files. Once the coronal gutta-percha is removed and a well exists within the canal space, a few drops of chloroform solvent[16–18,21] can be added into the coronal canal space to further facilitate removal, which can be completed with hand or rotary instruments.

Once the bulk of gutta-percha is removed, patency checks should be performed with no. 08 or no. 10 K files to an estimated length that is confirmed with an electronic apex locator (EAL). Even once patency is obtained, care should be taken to remove all gutta-percha remnants, both to ensure complete cleaning of the canal space and to eliminate the possibility of apical extrusion of debris. Chloroform combined with non-retreatment finishing files or Hedstrom hand files is useful for removing gutta-percha–based debris.

Carrier-based materials

There are additional removal considerations for carrier-based obturation materials. Though gutta-percha surrounding a metal or plastic carrier can be removed using the techniques already discussed, the carrier itself, whether plastic or metal, is impervious to solvent dissolution or direct instrumentation.[22] Carriers are often bound in the apical portions of the root and will sometimes separate upon manipulation. When retreating a tooth with carrier-based filling materials, clinicians should remove surrounding gutta-percha in a way that minimally disrupts the carrier to reduce the chance of its fracture or breakage. This generally involves adding a few drops of chloroform solvent and using narrow rotary instruments or hand files to create pathways for the introduction of additional solvent along opposing sides of the carrier.[23] Whenever rotary instruments are used, instrument separation is a risk, and gentle motions must be used with frequent visualization of the instrument to catch early signs of instrument fatigue.[24]

Once the surrounding gutta-percha is removed and the carrier is loosened, a few strategies exist for carrier removal. Loosened metal carriers may be removed with the use of an ultrasonic drill with a narrow tip (eg, Endo 3 or Endo 4 ProUltra Ultrasonic Tip, Dentsply Sirona). Loosened plastic carriers can sometimes be maneuvered out simply with the point of a DG16 double-ended explorer wedged into an accessible area of the carrier. If a carrier remains bound apically, narrow rotary devices can be used in a pecking motion at varying purchase points on opposing sides; however, this risks instrument separation alongside metal carriers. In some cases, plastic carriers will wrap around the rotary instrument for removal. In other cases, small Hedstrom hand files (ie, no. 10, 15, or 20) can be placed into similar paths alongside the carrier and then twisted around each other with the carrier inside to be removed all together, which is referred to as the braiding technique (Fig 6-10). Especially when

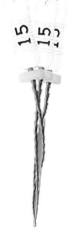

FIG 6-10 Braided Hedstrom files can be used to facilitate removal of plastic carriers.

using rotary instruments, care must be taken to remove the entire carrier without forcing any pieces into the extraradicular spaces, which would necessitate surgical access for removal.

Pastes

Paste-type fillings without a solid core include Sargenti-type materials, red pastes of eastern European and Asian origin, and white pastes from other parts of the world. Their radiographic appearance is typically lightly radiopaque in the pulp chambers and coronal one-third of roots, with apical spaces appearing unfilled (Fig 6-11). Paste composition varies significantly. When pastes are suspected, patients should be informed of the unknown nature of the material and that exploratory treatment is required for a better assessment.[25] Often, these materials are soft and cleaned easily with irrigation solutions, hand instruments, and rotary files, similar to initial NSRCT. Rarely, particularly in materials originating from eastern Europe, a hard cement may be encountered that is not responsive to solvents.[26] These materials require the use of ultrasonics and files under magnification for removal,[25,27] with extreme care taken to remove only filling materials and to preserve remaining tooth structure.

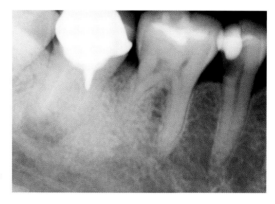

FIG 6-11 Paste-type filling materials have a typical radiographic appearance: lightly radiopaque in the pulp chambers and coronal one-third of roots, with apical spaces appearing unfilled. Their composition varies, and care must be taken during their removal.

Silver points

Silver point obturation materials are no longer used because they fall below the standard of care,[28] but clinicians may encounter silver points due to their historic usage. In the absence of pathology, prophylactic revision is not indicated, but recurrent or persistent infection may necessitate silver point removal[28] (Fig 6-12). As obturation materials, silver points suffer from high rates of failure and are challenging to remove. They are subject to corrosion in the presence of tissue fluids, and the toxic oxidative byproducts that are produced can allow leakage to occur within the canal space and directly degrade the silver points themselves.[29] This degradation can weaken the silver points so that they fracture when removal is attempted. In the best-case scenario, silver points may be loose within the canal, extending untrimmed into the chamber so that they can be removed with cotton pliers or Stieglitz-type forceps. In other cases, solvents and hand files may be required to first remove the sealer and gutta-percha surrounding the silver point, exposing a coronal portion that can be grabbed with cotton pliers, narrow Stieglitz forceps, or a modified Masserann technique in which a tube is inserted around the exposed coronal portion of the point (Fig 6-13).[30] Finally, silver points may be wedged within canals, requiring gentle vibration with a narrow, flame-tipped ultrasonic drill (eg, Endo 8 ProUltra Ultrasonic Tip) circumferentially to loosen the point until it comes out.[30] In these latter cases, if the silver point fractures and an apical segment cannot be bypassed or removed, apical microsurgery may be necessary.

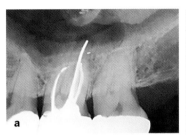 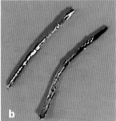 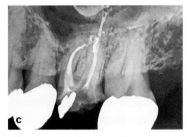

FIG 6-12 Special care is required when removing silver point obturation materials because they are often found to be corroded in the canal spaces *(a)* and have a high risk of fracture *(b)*. That said, successful retreatment *(c)* is often possible.

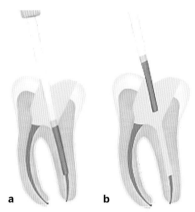

FIG 6-13 *(a and b)* The modified Masserann technique involves the insertion of a tube around the coronal portion of a post, silver point, or carrier in order to remove the entire apparatus.

Correcting Prior Treatment

One of the more frustrating aspects of nonsurgical retreatment is the correction of mishaps that may have occurred during the initial nonsurgical therapy. These mishaps may include ledge formation, instrument separation, and perforation, among others. All patients undergoing nonsurgical retreatment should be advised of the potential discovery of complications, as well as treatment strategies for these issues and the potential need for apical microsurgery if uncorrectable mishaps are discovered. A complete discussion of complications and their treatment strategies can be found in chapter 10.

Single- versus Multiple-Visit Therapy

The conversation surrounding one- or two-visit treatment in nonsurgical retreatment is grounded in an understanding of the microbiology of recurrent and persistent infection. Generally, these infections are associated with mature microbial communities that are colonized differently than primary endodontic infections.[31,32] They warrant aggressive antimicrobial treatment[3,33] and may resultantly require the use of intracanal medications. Consequently, nonsurgical retreatments are often performed as two-visit therapy, with the use of intracanal interappointment calcium hydroxide as previously described for NSRCT. That said, there is limited data to prove that interappointment medication serves to reduce the intracanal microbial load,[34–37] and prognosis data does not favor one methodology over another in terms of long-term success.[38] There is evidence, however, that for patients with persistent symptoms or drainage following calcium hydroxide interappointment medication, re-medication with antibiotic pastes may prove effective, as they often demonstrate superior antimicrobial efficacy over calcium hydroxide.[39]

References

1. de Chevigny, Dao TT, Basrani BR, et al. Treatment outcome in endodontics: The Torotono study—Phases 3 and 4: Orthograde retreatment. J Endod 2008;34:131–137.
2. Salehrabi R, Rotstein I. Endodontic treatment outcomes in a large patient population in the USA: An epidemiological study. J Endod 2004;30:846–850.
3. Sundqvist G, Figdor D, Persson S, Sjögren U. Microbiologic analysis of teeth with failed endodontic treatment and the outcome of conservative retreatment. Oral Surg Oral Med Oral Pathol Oral Radiol Endod 1998;85:86–93.
4. Lin LM, Skribner JE, Gaengler P. Factors associated with endodontic treatment failures. J Endod 1992;18:625–627.
5. Ricucci D, Siqueira JF Jr. Apical actinomycosis as a continuum of intraradicular and extraradicular infection: Case report and critical review on its involvement with treatment failure. J Endod 2008;34:1124–1129.
6. Saunders WP, Saunders EM. Prevalence of periradicular periodontitis associated with crowned teeth in an adult Scottish subpopulation. Br Dent J 1998;185:137–140.
7. Nudera WJ. Selective root retreatment: A novel approach. J Endod 2015;41:1382–1388.
8. Gorni FG, Gagliani MM. The outcome of endodontic retreatment: A 2-yr follow-up. J Endod 2004;30:1–4.
9. Krasner P, Rankow HJ. Anatomy of the pulp-chamber floor. J Endod 2004;30:5–16.
10. Lindemann M, Yaman P, Dennison JB, Herrero AA. Comparison of the efficiency and effectiveness of various techniques for removal of fiber posts. J Endod 2005;31:520–522.
11. Johnson WT, Leary JM, Boyer DB. Effect of ultrasonic vibration on post removal in extracted human premolar teeth. J Endod 1996;22:487–488.
12. Dominici JT, Clark S, Scheetz J, Eleazer PD. Analysis of heat generation using ultrasonic vibration for post removal. J Endod 2005;31:301–303.
13. Huttula AS, Tordik PA, Imamura G, Eichmiller FC, McClanahan SB. The effect of ultrasonic post instrumentation on root surface temperature. J Endod 2006;32:1085–1087.
14. Neelakantan P, Grotra D, Sharma S. Retreatability of 2 mineral trioxide aggregate-based root canal sealers: A cone-beam computed tomography analysis. J Endod 2013;39:893–896.
15. Hess D, Solomon E, Spears R, He J. Retreatability of a bioceramic root canal sealing material. J Endod 2011;37:1547–1549.
16. Kaplowitz GJ. Evaluation of gutta-percha solvents. J Endod 1990;16:539–540.
17. Edgar SW, Marshall JG, Baumgartner JC. The antimicrobial effect of chloroform on Enterococcus faecalis after gutta-percha removal. J Endod 2006;32:1185–1187.
18. Chutich MJ, Kaminski EJ, Miller DA, Lautenschlager EP. Risk assessment of the toxicity of solvents of gutta-percha used in endodontic retreatment. J Endod 1998;24:213–216.
19. Ferreira JJ, Rhodes JS, Ford TR. The efficacy of gutta-percha removal using ProFiles. Int Endod J 2001;34:267–274.
20. Shemesh H, Roeleveld AC, Wesselink PR, Wu MK. Damage to root dentin during retreatment procedures. J Endod 2011;37:63–66.
21. McDonald MN, Vire DE. Chloroform in the endodontic operatory. J Endod 1992;18:301–303.
22. Wilcox LR. Thermafil retreatment with and without chloroform solvent. J Endod 1993;19:563–566.
23. Bertrand MF, Pellegrino JC, Rocca JP, Klinghofer A, Bolla M. Removal of Thermafil root canal filling material. J Endod 1997;23:54–57.
24. Royzenblat A, Goodell GG. Comparison of removal times of Thermafil plastic obturators using ProFile rotary instruments at different rotational speeds in moderately curved canals. J Endod 2007;33:256–258.

25. Schwandt NW, Gound TG. Resorcinol-formaldehyde resin "Russian Red" endodontic therapy. J Endod 2003;29:435–437.
26. Vranas RN, Hartwell GR, Moon PC. The effect of endodontic solutions on resorcinol-formalin paste. J Endod 2003;29:69–72.
27. Krell KV, Neo J. The use of ultrasonic endodontic instrumentation in the re-treatment of a paste-filled endodontic tooth. Oral Surg Oral Med Oral Pathol 1985;60:100–102.
28. American Association of Endodontists. Use of Silver Points. AAE Position Statement. 2017. https://www.aae.org/specialty/wp-content/uploads/sites/2/2017/06/silverpointsstatement.pdf. Accessed 29 March 2023.
29. Seltzer S, Green DB, Weiner N, DeRenzis F. A scanning electron microscope examination of silver cones removed from endodontically treated teeth. Oral Surg Oral Med Oral Pathol 1972;33:589–605.
30. Krell KV, Fuller MW, Scott GL. The conservative retrieval of silver cones in difficult cases. J Endod 1984;10:269–273.
31. Love RM. Enterococcus faecalis—A mechanism for its role in endodontic failure. Int Endod J 2001;34:399–405.
32. Ricucci D, Candeiro GTM, Bugea C, Siqueira JF Jr. Complex apical intraradicular infection and extraradicular mineralized biofilms as the cause of wet canals and treatment failure: Report of 2 cases. J Endod 2016;42:509–515.
33. Molander A, Reit C, Dahlén G, Kvist T. Microbiological status of root-filled teeth with apical periodontitis. Int Endod J 1998;31:1–7.
34. Law A, Messer H. An evidence-based analysis of the antibacterial effectiveness of intracanal medicaments. J Endod 2004;30:689–694.
35. Xavier ACC, Martinho FC, Chung A, et al. One-visit versus two-visit root canal treatment: Effectiveness in the removal of endotoxins and cultivable bacteria. J Endod 2013;39:959–964.
36. Peters LB, Wesselink PR. Periapical healing of endodontically treated teeth in one and two visits obturated in the presence or absence of detectable microorganisms. Int Endod J 2002;35:660–667.
37. Vera J, Siqueira JF Jr, Ricucci D, et al. One- versus two-visit endodontic treatment of teeth with apical periodontitis: A histobacteriologic study. J Endod 2012;38:1040–1052.
38. Toia CC, Khoury RD, Corazza BJM, Orozco EIF, Valera MC. Effectiveness of 1-visit and 2-visit endodontic retreatment of teeth with persistent/secondary endodontic infection: A randomized clinical trial with 18 months of follow-up. J Endod 2022;48:4–14.
39. Vatankhah M, Khosravi K, Zargar N, Shirvani A, Nekoofar MH, Dianat O. Antibacterial efficacy of antibiotic pastes versus calcium hydroxide intracanal dressing: A systematic review and meta-analysis of ex vivo studies. J Conserv Dent 2022;5:463–480.

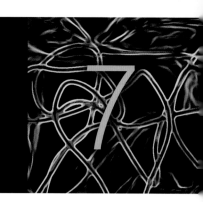

Apical Microsurgery

Apical microsurgery refers to the treatment of recurrent or persistent endodontic pathology, otherwise known as posttreatment pathology, via an apical approach. In general, this approach requires the exposure and removal of a soft tissue lesion, resection of the apex, retropreparation into the canal anatomy with ultrasonics, and placement of a biocompatible filling within the root apex. This differs significantly from historic surgical approaches that involved the use of bur retropreparations and amalgam or intermediate restorative (IRM) retrofillings (Fig 7-1). Though these historic techniques were markedly unpredictable, modern techniques and technology mean that the prognosis for surgical endodontics is now quite predictable, with reported success rates between 79% and 95%.[1,2]

FIG 7-1 (a) Historic apical microsurgery approaches involved bur retropreparations and amalgam or IRM retrofillings. (b) Modern apical microsurgery employs ultrasonic retropreparations and bioceramic retrofillings for a more exact result and improved predictability.

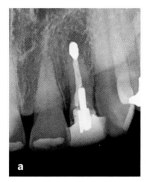
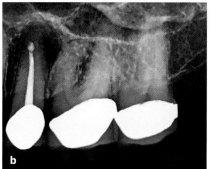

Apical microsurgery should be considered in lieu of nonsurgical retreatment if (1) prior nonsurgical root canal therapy (NSRCT) or nonsurgical retreatment appears adequate upon clinical and radiographic evaluation, (2) the removal of restorative materials, such as posts present in the canal spaces, would represent a significant risk of perforation or fracture, (3) prior treatment complications would render nonsurgical approaches unreliable or impossible, (4) obturation material is extruded beyond the apex and cannot be retrieved, or (5) the anatomy is not accessible without surgery[3] (Fig 7-2). In the case of unfilled canal anatomy or coronal leakage, however, nonsurgical care should be considered first (Fig 7-3).

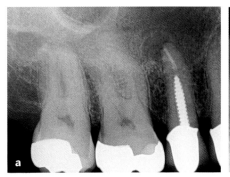 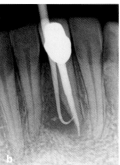

FIG 7-2 Recurrent or persistent pathology in teeth with large posts (a) or overextended obturation material (b) may be better addressed by apical microsurgery as opposed to nonsurgical retreatment.

Apical microsurgery preferred	Apical microsurgery contraindicated
• Adequate prior root canal fills • Large posts that would be risky to remove • Obturation material extruded beyond the apex • Anatomy cannot be accessed nonsurgically	• Untreated canal anatomy as likely etiology for pathology • Coronal leakage under existing restoration • Medical contraindications

FIG 7-3 Factors aiding in case selection for apical microsurgery.

Preoperative Evaluation

A thorough preoperative evaluation is essential for all patients, and it is of particular importance for surgical patients. When reviewing a patient's medical history, clinicians must be attentive to medications that may present bleeding risks, including anticoagulants like aspirin, warfarin, and newer medications like apixaban (Eliquis, Bristol-Myers Squibb).[4–6] Clinicians must also be aware of patients' use of nonprescription substances and medications that may increase bleeding risk, including garlic, ginseng, and ginger, among others. While the use of these medications does not represent a surgical contraindication, it may necessitate additional hemostatic measures during surgery.[6] Clinicians should also consider how medical conditions and medications might impact a patient's immune function. Conditions like diabetes mellitus, a history of smoking, and chemotherapy or immunosuppressant medications reduce immune function, which may increase the likelihood of postoperative infection or compromise the patient's ability to heal.[7] Consequently, these patients should undergo careful postoperative monitoring.

Also of concern in the surgical patient is the use of medications that impact bone metabolism, including both oral and intravenous bisphosphonates and other antiresorptive medications. These, among other medications, may increase the risk of jaw osteonecrosis.[8,9] Lastly, a history of radiation exposure to the head and neck for the treatment of oral cancers introduces the risk of osteoradionecrosis after dental surgery.[7] Consequently, intravenous bisphosphonates and a history of radiation are both contraindications to apical microsurgery in most outpatient settings (Fig 7-4).

The preoperative evaluation of surgical patients should also include CBCT imaging. Not only does this imaging modality inform the treating clinician about the dental anatomy that will be treated but, more importantly, it shows the maxillofacial anatomy as it relates to the surgical site, namely, the maxillary sinus, incisive canal, inferior alveolar nerve canal, and the mental foramen, among other structures[10] (Fig 7-5). When assessing surgical patients, it is important to note that sinus exposures during apical microsurgery largely do not impact the prognosis of the case.[11] That said, paresthesia caused by neural trauma may be permanent. Consequently, the preoperative CBCT evaluation is essential for obtaining true informed consent.

An oral rinse with chlorhexidine gluconate is generally advisable immediately prior to surgical endodontic treatment,[12,13] though controversy exists as to whether it is helpful to begin the course a few days prior to oral surgical procedures.[14]

Diabetes mellitus

History of smoking

Chemotherapeutics or immunosuppressants

Anticoagulant therapy

Medications that impact bone metabolism (eg, bisphosphonates) or other immune modulators

Radiation to the head and neck

FIG 7-4 Medical history considerations for apical microsurgery patients. Diabetes, a history of smoking, and chemotherapeutics can impact healing but do not represent contraindications to surgery. Similarly, anticoagulants can create challenges with hemostasis but do not represent an absolute contraindication to apical microsurgery. Patients with a history of intravenous bisphosphonate use or radiation to the head and neck are poor surgical candidates.

FIG 7-5 Preoperative CBCT assessment is essential for apical microsurgery, particularly because it accurately demonstrates the location of pathology relative to vital structures like the maxillary sinus (a) and incisive canal (b), among others.

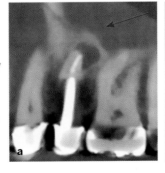
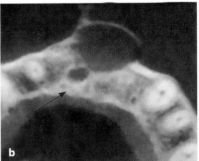

Surgical Anesthesia and Pain Control

On the day of surgery, adequate local anesthesia (described in chapter 4) is essential for a comfortable patient experience. Local anesthetics may also serve as hemostatic agents and adjuncts to postoperative pain control. In patients without medical contraindications, anesthetics containing a higher concentration of epinephrine (1:50,000) may be used to aid in hemostasis. Long-acting local anesthetics (namely, bupivacaine) should

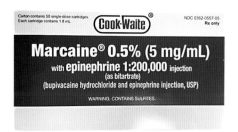

FIG 7-6 Long-acting local anesthetics like bupivacaine (Marcaine, Pfizer) should be used during apical microsurgery. These medications not only provide local anesthesia during the procedure but significantly improve pain control postoperatively.

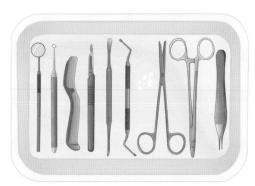

FIG 7-7 Surgical armamentarium includes a mouth mirror, micromirrors, retractors, scalpel, elevators, spoon excavators and scalers, scissors, needle holders, and cotton pliers or forceps.

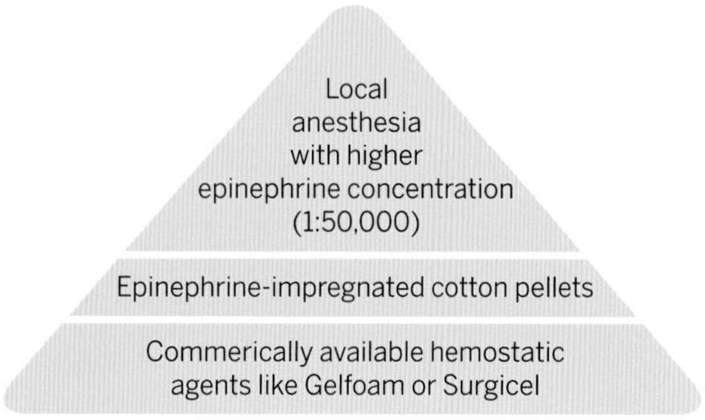

Local anesthesia with higher epinephrine concentration (1:50,000)

Epinephrine-impregnated cotton pellets

Commerically available hemostatic agents like Gelfoam or Surgicel

FIG 7-8 Adjunctive hemostatic measures in apical microsurgery.

also be considered to aid in postoperative pain control (Fig 7-6).[15] These medications provide local anesthesia of extended duration to allow patients to consume oral pain medications and have also been shown to significantly decrease postoperative pain for several days following the procedure, even after anesthesia wears off.[16,17]

Surgical Visibility: Magnification and Hemostasis

Excellent visualization of the surgical field is necessary for successful outcomes, and both magnification and hemostasis are essential components of visualization, in addition to the rest of the tools in the surgical armamentarium (Fig 7-7).[18,19] Minimally, loupes are necessary to provide magnification during surgery. That said, evidence in the literature suggests that apical microsurgery performed with microscopes for magnification as opposed to loupes is associated with greater predictability.[18]

Hemostasis is the other arm of visualization. Good hemostatic control in the surgical site both permits clinicians to see the structures in question and aids in material manipulation. Having a well-positioned, knowledgeable surgical assistant to provide directed suction is the best means of hemostatic control during surgery. As previously mentioned, local anesthetics with higher epinephrine concentrations can also be used to enhance hemostasis in the operative field.[20] Epinephrine-impregnated cotton pellets (Racellet Pellets, Pascal International) can also be used to aid hemostasis, as can other commercially available hemostatic agents, like Gelfoam (Pfizer) or Surgicel (Ethicon)[6,19,21] (Fig 7-8). None of these materials affect postsurgical healing, and postoperative hemostasis can be achieved by careful reapproximation of the flap and appropriately applied pressure to the surgical site.

Surgical Flap Design

Flap design should allow for complete visualization of the relevant anatomy and will often include both horizontal and vertical incisions. A single vertical incision produces a triangular flap, and two vertical incisions will produce a rectangular flap (Fig 7-9). In either case, a full-thickness flap should be reflected to fully expose the underlying bone.

FIG 7-9 *(a)* Triangular flaps are produced with a horizontal incision and a single vertical incision. *(b)* Rectangular flaps are produced with a horizontal incision and two vertical incisions.

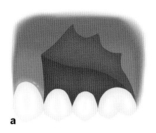
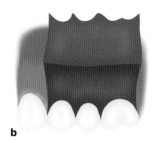

a   b

Clinicians must ensure that incisions are not made over the existing pathology or anticipated osteotomy site to avoid the development of significant soft tissue defects postoperatively. The most common horizontal incisions used for apical microsurgery include intrasulcular incisions, papilla-preserving incisions, and submarginal incisions (Fig 7-10). Intrasulcular incisions allow for the greatest degree of root visibility and should be considered if an apicomarginal bony defect is suspected based on clinical or radiographic findings and especially when clinicians suspect root fracture.[22] That said, intrasulcular incisions are associated with the greatest risk of gingival recession post-operatively.[23] Papilla-preserving incisions should be considered in cases where visibility of the entire root surface from the alveolar crest to the apex is needed but the clinician wishes to lessen the risk of recession.[24,25] Submarginal incisions can be considered when sufficient attached tissue is present with minimal risk of recession.[22] Vertical incisions should be oriented vertically as opposed to diagonally to keep them parallel to the blood vessels within the soft tissue.[22] These incisions should not be placed over bony or root prominences because scarring or tearing is more likely in these areas.

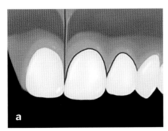
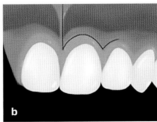
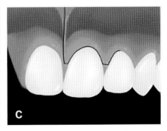

a   b   c

FIG 7-10 Common horizontal incisions for apical microsurgery include the intrasulcular incision *(a)*, the submarginal incision *(b)*, and the papilla-preserving incision *(c)*.

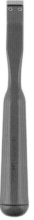

FIG 7-11 Retractors are used to keep the soft tissue flap out of the bony surgical site to aid visibility. Retractors should be placed on bone to avoid crushing soft tissues. (Shown here: Leetrac Retractor, courtesy of B&L Biotech.)

Excellent soft tissue management also involves maintaining flap hydration during the surgical procedure to avoid excessive swelling and challenges with reapproximation when the procedure is finished. This can be accomplished with sterile gauze moistened with sterile saline. Furthermore, flaps should be kept away from the surgical site with appropriate retraction. The retractor should be placed on bone as opposed to soft tissue to avoid crushing the flap (Fig 7-11).

The Surgical Osteotomy

In cases where apical pathology has perforated the cortex or when the relevant anatomy is readily visible, a direct osteotomy can be performing with a carbide bur under sterile saline irrigation to expose the entire diameter of the lesion[26] (Fig 7-12). Clinicians should be aware of the location of the root apices and pathology prior to surgery, particularly when CBCT imaging is used during presurgical planning. If CBCT imaging is not available, an intraoperative radiograph can be used to confirm accuracy prior to performing the osteotomy. Using anatomical landmarks and preoperative radiographs to estimate the cortical plate proximal to the root apex and lesion, the carbide bur under sterile saline irrigation can be used to make a small concavity. A 1-mm-diameter piece of radiopaque foil, most conveniently obtained from traditional radiographic films, should be pushed into the cortical plate concavity, and an intraoperative periapical image should then be taken (Fig 7-13). Adjustments can then be made prior to drilling to reach the targeted location for surgical access.

If surgery is to be performed in the posterior maxilla, patients should be advised of the potential for sinus communication following osteotomy and/or lesion excision. In the event of a sinus exposure, clinicians should attempt to keep the sinus membrane intact and be exceptionally careful not to dislodge surgical materials into the sinus. Membrane placement can be considered, though it is not necessary in many cases. Patients should be advised that most cases of sinus exposure heal well with proper postoperative care.

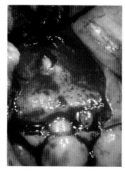
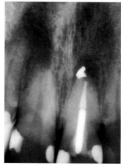

FIG 7-12 An osteotomy through the alveolar bone to the root apex should be performed with carbide or diamond burs under sterile saline irrigation.

FIG 7-13 When CBCT imaging is not available, 2D films with radiographic foil can be used to determine the accuracy of osteotomy placement prior to drilling.

Lesion Excision and Biopsy

Removal of the lesion will permit visualization of the entirety of the root apex. The lesion should be removed whole if possible and placed into a formalin solution for histopathologic evaluation (Fig 7-14). These formalin containers should be available from oral pathology services. Pathologic evaluation should be considered the standard of care. The pathology report may indicate atypical findings that would necessitate further treatment or referral. The most common pathologic findings include odontogenic cysts and granulomas, and uncommon findings include actinomycosis, nonodontogenic cysts, and benign or malignant odontogenic or nonodontogenic tumors.

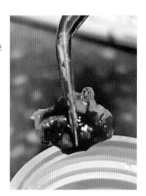

FIG 7-14 During endodontic microsurgery, lesions should be removed and submitted for pathologic evaluation. Formalin specimen containers can be obtained from oral pathology services.

Apical Management: Resection, Retropreparation, and Retrofilling

The apex should be evaluated for fractures or other anomalies. Micromirrors can be used for enhanced visualization during this process (Fig 7-15), and hemostatic agents can be useful to mitigate bleeding that may mask findings. The use of dyes, including methylene blue or vegetable-based dye (eg, To Dye For, Roydent), can facilitate fracture detection.[27] After careful inspection, the apex should be resected with a carbide or diamond bur under sterile saline irrigation.[28] The resection should run parallel to the occlusal plane of the tooth rather than at an angle to avoid excess exposure of dentinal tubules.[29] A minimum of 3 mm of resection should be completed to facilitate removal of the majority of the lateral canal anatomy (Fig 7-16).[30]

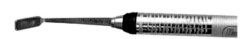

FIG 7-15 The use of micromirrors can enhance visualization and assessment during apical microsurgery.

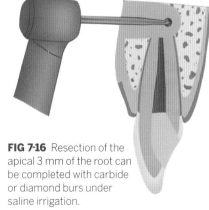

FIG 7-16 Resection of the apical 3 mm of the root can be completed with carbide or diamond burs under saline irrigation.

Retropreparation of the canal anatomy within the resected apex, including isthmuses between canals on molar or premolar teeth, should be performed with an appropriate ultrasonic tip, like Jetips (B&L Biotech), under sterile saline irrigation (Fig 7-17).[25,31] Dyes can also be used at this stage to enhance detection of both untreated canals and isthmus anatomy and to detect apical fractures. Micromirrors remain useful to enhance visualization of the preparation. The preparation depth should reach 3 mm,[32] and surgical ultrasonic tips are often fabricated to facilitate these preparation depths (Fig 7-18). Radiographs may be considered to confirm preparation depth and adequacy. Retrofillings should be placed in the retropreparation after sterile paper points are used to dry the space. Bioceramic materials (eg, mineral trioxide aggregate [MTA] and EndoSequence BC Root Repair Material Fast Set Putty [Brasseler USA]) should be used for retrofillings as these are associated with the most favorable healing responses following endodontic microsurgery.[33–36] Placement of the retrofilling should be confirmed with a radiograph (Fig 7-19).

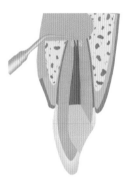 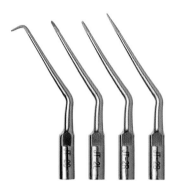 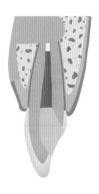

FIG 7-17 Retropreparation involves the removal of gutta-percha from the apical 3 mm of the canal space following resection.

FIG 7-18 Ultrasonic tips designed for apical microsurgery develop preparations with parallel walls at a depth of 3 mm into the canal and isthmus spaces. (Shown here: Jetips, courtesy of B&L Biotech.)

FIG 7-19 Retrofilling involves the placement of a bioceramic restoration material into the prepared apical canal space.

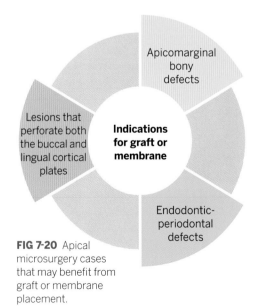

FIG 7-20 Apical microsurgery cases that may benefit from graft or membrane placement.

Grafting

Many apical microsurgery cases do not require the routine placement of membranes or grafts prior to flap replacement,[37] though their use may be beneficial in several clinical situations. These include cases where apicomarginal bony defects are present, cases with lesions that perforate both the buccal and lingual or palatal cortex, and endodontic-periodontal defects (Fig 7-20).[38–40] In these cases, resorbable membranes are appropriate, as are allograft- or xenograft-type bony materials.[40]

Flap Replacement and Suturing

The flap should be repositioned passively in its original orientation prior to suturing. This can be achieved by applying gentle pressure to the flap with a saline-soaked gauze sponge. Tension-free closure is essential for ensuring primary healing of the surgical incision. Sutures should be placed along the incision. Simple interrupted sutures are advisable over continuous sutures to avoid flap reopening in the event of suture tearing (Fig 7-21). Sling sutures can also be considered with intrasulcular incisions. In areas where muscular tension is of concern, vertical or horizontal mattress sutures can be used in conjunction with simple interrupted sutures. Monofilament synthetic sutures should be used due to their biocompatibility and healing profiles. These are preferable over silk sutures, which are associated with bacterial wicking.[22] Size 5-0 and 6-0 sutures are associated with excellent durability and have minimal impact on soft tissue esthetics.

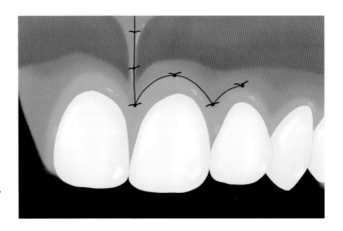

FIG 7-21 Simple interrupted sutures are appropriate for many apical microsurgery cases. Ideally, small-diameter monofilament sutures should be used.

Postoperative Care

Postoperative care instructions should advise patients on what to expect after surgery and how to properly care for themselves. Patients must be advised not to disturb the surgical site, which could result in suture or flap tearing. Similarly, patients should be advised to avoid crunchy foods and drinking through a straw because both activities could lead to similar tears. Patients should be encouraged to keep the surgical area clean by rinsing with warm salt water but to avoid tooth brushing and flossing near the surgical site. Patients should also be advised that minimal bleeding is likely during the first 24 hours postoperatively and that they should contact their clinician if excessive bleeding occurs that is uncontrollable with pressure or tea bag application. Additional instructions should focus on pain control, namely the scheduled use of a combination of ibuprofen and acetaminophen during the first 48 hours postoperatively. Without evidence of disseminated infection, postoperative antibiotics are not often recommended following apical microsurgery.[11,41,42] Patients should be advised that ice should be used during the first 24 hours postoperatively both for pain control and to minimize swelling (Fig 7-22).

Surgical Aftercare Instructions

<u>Discomfort</u>: Some mild to moderate discomfort is not uncommon. For this reason, you have been given instructions for over-the-counter pain medication. **Please take the first dose before your anesthesia wears off.** Take only as instructed. Do not mix Tylenol (acetaminophen) with alcohol.

<u>Swelling</u>: Most discomfort after a surgical procedure is due to swelling of the affected tissues. Application of ice can minimize swelling and discomfort. **Place the ice pack on the area for 20 minutes, then remove it for 10 minutes.** Repeat this cycle during waking hours for the first 24 hours post surgery.

<u>Bleeding</u>: Slight bleeding or oozing is normal for the first 24 hours. If bleeding persists or is excessive, please call the office.

<u>Bruising</u>: Bruising may develop and persist for several days following your procedure. Application of ice can lessen the severity of bruising. As above, ice should be used vigilantly for the first few hours, at 20 minutes on/10 minutes off intervals.

<u>Food</u>: For your comfort, try to eat on the side opposite the surgery. Eat a soft diet (jello, ice cream, pudding, yogurt, or whatever feels comfortable) and drink **plenty** of fluids. Avoid foods that can particulate into sharp pieces, such as potato chips or hard, crusty breads. If eating is difficult, a diet supplement (such as Ensure or Nutrament) is recommended. Do not drink through a straw.

<u>Oral Hygiene</u>: Use a soft toothbrush in all areas **except** directly around the surgical site until after the sutures are removed. You may rinse your mouth with warm salt water to help keep your mouth clean. After 48 hours, you may use Peridex mouth rinse, if prescribed by the doctor, to keep your mouth clean.

<u>Activity</u>: Avoid strenuous activity for 24–48 hours. This includes running, aerobics, weightlifting, etc.

<u>Don'ts</u>: **Do not** disturb the area. Do not lift up your lip to get a better look. **Do not** spit, smoke, or drink through a straw. **Do not** use any commercial mouth rinses, peroxide, or any "Waterpik" type devices.

<u>Do</u>: Call us with any concerns. Please report any unusual symptoms such as excessive bleeding, swelling, or elevated temperature immediately.

<u>Problems</u>: If you have any problems or questions, call the office as soon as possible.

Please call your provider immediately with any concerns.

FIG 7-22 Postoperative instructions.

In the event of sinus exposures during surgery or other sinus-related concerns, patients should be advised to follow specific precautions. These include avoiding behaviors that could lead to abrupt pressure changes within the sinus. Patients should be advised to sneeze with their mouths open and to use decongestants. Antibiotics may be considered for these patients, though research does not demonstrate a clear and definitive benefit.[28] Patients should be advised that sinus communications usually heal well, often without grafting or membrane placement; however, monitoring is advised. If sinus symptoms develop, referral to an otolaryngologist or oral and maxillofacial surgeon should be considered.

Sutures should be removed after 48 to 96 hours.[22] In the vast majority of cases, infiltration anesthesia is not necessary for patient comfort. Topical anesthetics, either 20% benzocaine or 5% lidocaine, are preferred and should be applied directly to the incision prior to suture removal. The biopsy report obtained from the pathologist's evaluation of the apical tissues can be reviewed with the patient at the suture removal appointment or later over the phone.

Follow-up

Follow-up is essential after all endodontic treatments, including apical microsurgery. Both clinical and radiographic follow-ups are indicated at a minimum of 1 year postoperatively, though some clinicians may choose to recall their patients earlier. Long-term follow-up may be indicated to evaluate for late failure or slow healing. Clinical follow-up should assess for signs and symptoms of recurrent pathology. Although traditional 2D radiographs are appropriate in most cases, clinicians can also use CBCT imaging to confirm the approximation of alveolar bone to the cut surface of the root (Fig 7-23), which is considered the benchmark of successful endodontic microsurgery in newer publications.

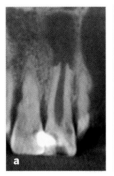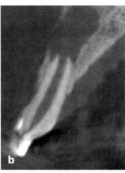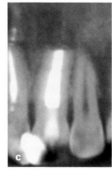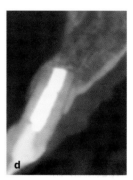

FIG 7-23 Follow-up is essential after apical microsurgery, and CBCT imaging can be considered for this purpose, especially because it demonstrates bone growth across the cut root surface. *(a and b)* Preoperative CBCT images. *(c and d)* CBCT images from the 1-year follow-up.

References

1. Rubinstein RA, Kim S. Long-term follow-up of cases considered healed one year after apical microsurgery. J Endod 2002;28:378–383.
2. Huang S, Chen NN, Yu VSH, Lim HA, Liu JN. Long-term success and survival of endodontic microsurgery. J Endod 2020;46:149–157.e4.
3. Iqbal MK, Kratchman SI, Guess GM, Karabucak B, Kim S. Microscopic periradicular surgery: Perioperative predictors for postoperative clinical outcomes and quality of life assessment. J Endod 2007;33:239–244.
4. Kaplovitch E, Dounaevskaia V. Treatment in the dental practice of the patient receiving anticoagulation therapy. J Am Dent Assoc 2019;150:602–608.
5. Lin S, Hoffman R, Nabriski O, Moreinos D, Dummer PMH. Management of patients receiving novel antithrombotic treatment in endodontic practice: Review and clinical recommendations. Int Endod J 2021;54:1754–1768.
6. Witherspoon DE, Gutmann JL. Haemostasis in periradicular surgery. Int Endod J 1996;29:135–149.
7. Little JW, Miller D, Rhodus NL, Falace D (eds). Little and Falace's Dental Management of the Medically Compromised Patient, ed 9. St Louis: Mosby, 2016.
8. Ruggiero SL, Dodson TB, Assael LA, et al. American Association of Oral and Maxillofacial Surgeons position paper on bisphosphonate-related osteonecrosis of the jaws—2009 update. J Oral Maxillofac Surg 2009;67:2–12.
9. McLeod NM, Brennan PA, Ruggiero SL. Bisphosphonate osteonecrosis of the jaw: A historical and contemporary review. Surgeon 2012;10:36–42.
10. Kovisto T, Ahmad M, Bowles WR. Proximity of the mandibular canal to the tooth apex. J Endod 2011;37:311–315.
11. Rud J, Rud V. Surgical endodontics of upper molars: Relation to the maxillary sinus and operation in acute state of infection. J Endod 1998;24:260–261.
12. Martin MV, Nind D. Use of chlorhexidine gluconate for pre-operative disinfection of apicectomy sites. Br Dent J 1987;162:459–461.
13. Kim S, Pecora G, Rubinstein RA. Color Atlas of Microsurgery in Endodontics. Philadelphia: Saunders, 2001.

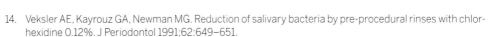

14. Veksler AE, Kayrouz GA, Newman MG. Reduction of salivary bacteria by pre-procedural rinses with chlorhexidine 0.12%. J Periodontol 1991;62:649–651.

15. Keiser K, Hargreaves KM. Building effective strategies for the management of endodontic pain. Endod Topics 2002;3:93–105.

16. Gordon SM, Dionne RA, Brahim J, Jabir F, Dubner R. Blockade of peripheral neuronal barrage reduces postoperative pain. Pain 1997;70:209–215.

17. Jebeles JA, Reilly JS, Gutierrez JF, Bradley EL Jr, Kissin I. Tonsillectomy and adenoidectomy pain reduction by local bupivacaine infiltration in children. Int J Pediatr Otorhinolaryngol 1993;25:149–154.

18. von Arx T, Peñarrocha M, Jensen S. Prognostic factors in apical surgery with root-end filling: A meta-analysis. J Endod 2010;36:957–973.

19. Gutmann JL. Parameters of achieving quality anesthesia and hemostasis in surgical endodontics. Anesth Pain Control Dent 1993;2:223–226.

20. Buckley JA, Ciancio SG, McMullen JA. Efficacy of epinephrine concentration in local anesthesia during periodontal surgery. J Periodontol 1984;55:653–657.

21. Vickers FJ, Baumgartner JC, Marshall G. Hemostatic efficacy and cardiovascular effects of agents used during endodontic surgery. J Endod 2002;28:322–323.

22. Velvart P, Peters CI. Soft tissue management in endodontic surgery. J Endod 2005;31:4–16.

23. Kramper BJ, Kaminski EJ, Osetek EM, Heuer MA. A comparative study of the wound healing of three types of flap design used in periapical surgery. J Endod 1984;10:17–25.

24. Velvart P, Ebner-Zimmermann U, Ebner JP. Comparison of long-term papilla healing following sulcular full thickness flap and papilla base flap in endodontic surgery. Int Endod J 2004;37:687–693.

25. Del Fabbro M, Corbella S, Sequeira-Byron P, et al. Endodontic procedures for retreatment of periapical lesions. Cochrane Database Syst Rev 2016;10:CD005511.

26. Nicoll BK, Peters RJ. Heat generation during ultrasonic instrumentation of dentin as affected by different irrigation methods. J Periodontol 1998;69:884–888.

27. Cambruzzi JV, Marshall FJ, Pappin JB. Methylene blue dye: An aid to endodontic surgery. J Endod 1985;11:311–314.

28. Kim S, Kratchman S. Microsurgery in Endodontics. Hoboken, NJ: Wiley-Blackwell, 2017.

29. Gilheany PA, Figdor D, Tyas MJ. Apical dentin permeability and microleakage associated with root end resection and retrograde filling. J Endod 1994;20:22–26.

30. Block RM, Bushell A, Rodrigues H, Langeland K. A histopathologic, histobacteriologic, and radiographic study of periapical endodontic surgical specimens. Oral Surg Oral Med Oral Pathol 1976;42:656–678.

31. de Lange J, Putters T, Baas E, van Ingen JM. Ultrasonic root-end preparation in apical surgery: A prospective randomized study. Oral Surg Oral Med Oral Pathol Oral Radiol Endod 2007;104:841–845.

32. Mattison GD, von Fraunhofer JA, Delivanis PD, Anderson AN. Microleakage of retrograde amalgams. J Endod 1985;11:340–345.

33. Song M, Kim E. A prospective randomized controlled study of mineral trioxide aggregate and super ethoxy–benzoic acid as root-end filling materials in endodontic microsurgery. J Endod 2012;38:875–879.

34. Torabinejad M, Higa RK, McKendry DJ, Pitt Ford TR. Dye leakage of four root end filling materials: Effects of blood contamination. J Endod 1994;20:159–163.

35. Baek SH, Plenk H Jr, Kim S. Periapical tissue responses and cementum regeneration with amalgam, SuperEBA, and MTA as root-end filling materials. J Endod 2005;31:444–449.

36. Damas BA, Wheater MA, Bringas JS, Hoen MM. Cytotoxicity comparison of mineral trioxide aggregates and EndoSequence bioceramic root repair materials. J Endod 2011;37:372–375.

37. Garrett K, Kerr M, Hartwell G, O'Sullivan S, Mayer P. The effect of a bioresorbable matrix barrier in endodontic surgery on the rate of periapical healing: An in vivo study. J Endod 2002;28:503–506.

38. Douthitt JC, Gutmann JL, Witherspoon DE. Histologic assessment of healing after the use of a bioresorbable membrane in the management of buccal bone loss concomitant with periradicular surgery. J Endod 2001;27:404–410.

39. Lin L, Chen MYH, Ricucci D, Rosenberg PA. Guided tissue regeneration in periapical surgery. J Endod 2010;36:618–625.

40. Tsesis I, Rosen E, Tamse A, Taschieri S, Del Fabbro M. Effect of guided tissue regeneration on the outcome of surgical endodontic treatment: A systematic review and meta-analysis. J Endod 2011;37:1039–1045.

41. Lin L, Chance K, Shovlin F, Skribner J, Langeland K. Oroantral communication in periapical surgery of maxillary posterior teeth. J Endod 1985;11:40–44.

42. Walton RE. Iatrogenic maxillary sinus exposure during maxillary posterior root-end surgery. Oral Surg Oral Med Oral Pathol Oral Radiol Endod 2004;97:3.

Vital Pulp Therapy

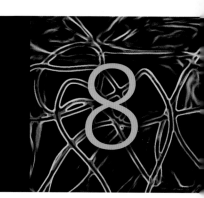

Historically, a diagnosis of asymptomatic irreversible pulpitis, defined by a carious pulp exposure without symptoms, was associated with a blanket recommendation for nonsurgical root canal therapy (NSRCT). Given the widespread availability of pulp-biocompatible dental materials, however, this recommendation has changed. Previously routine for immature permanent teeth, vital pulp therapy is now recommended even for mature permanent teeth with asymptomatic carious exposures.[1-3] As the name implies, vital pulp therapy aims to leave the apical portion of the pulp tissue intact. In immature permanent teeth, vital pulp therapy is also referred to as *apexogenesis* because it promotes continued apical development. Vital pulp therapy is the treatment of choice for both immature permanent teeth with vital pulp tissue and for many instances of carious or traumatic exposures in mature permanent teeth[1,3] (Figs 8-1 and 8-2).

New data on the success of vital pulp therapy procedures suggest that it may represent definitive care in the absence of apical pathology, especially when bioceramic materials are used and treatment is performed according to updated protocols.[1] The broadening of applications for vital pulp therapy in mature permanent teeth stems from a body of literature referencing particular protocols and materials associated with predictable success in teeth at all stages of development. This literature highlights the necessity of strict infection control protocols, including the use of dental dam isolation, and the use of bioceramic family calcium silicate cements as restorative materials placed adjacent to the pulp.[1] Alternative materials, including calcium hydroxide, glass-ionomer cements, and resins,

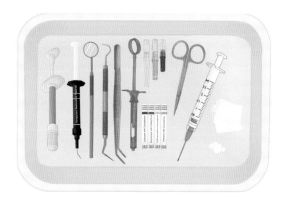

FIG 8-1 Armamentarium for vital pulp therapy should include local anesthetic armamentarium (syringes, needles, drugs), a mouth mirror, cotton pliers, explorer, periodontal probe, pluggers and plastic instruments, scissors, irrigation needles and solution, bioceramic materials, and either temporary or definitive restorative materials.

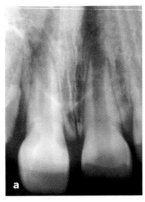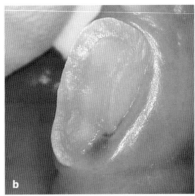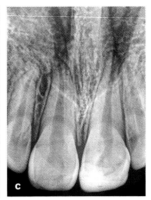

FIG 8-2 Vital pulp therapy is the treatment of choice for vital immature permanent teeth and is referred to as *apexogenesis*. *(a and b)* This patient experienced a complicated crown fracture on the maxillary left central incisor, which was treated with a calcium hydroxide pulp capping agent. *(c)* At the 3-year follow-up, the pulp remained vital and complete apical closure was noted.

are associated with less predictable outcomes, and thus their use is no longer routinely advised.[1] Treatment modalities that fall under vital pulp therapy include indirect pulp caps, direct pulp caps, and pulpotomies.

Indirect Pulp Capping

The indirect pulp cap is a technique wherein a thin layer of carious dentin is left behind during the course of caries removal in order to prevent pulp exposure.[2] Indirect pulp caps are only indicated in asymptomatic teeth without evidence of pulpitis or periapical disease.[2] That said, complete caries removal is essential to eliminate infected tissues and visualize pulp tissue conditions under magnification when pulpal exposures occur.[1] Given the widespread availability of bioceramic materials and their predictability when used as direct pulp capping agents, clinicians may consider other approaches to treating deep caries.

Historic approaches to indirect pulp capping followed a two-step protocol involving the placement of a medicated restorative material, such as calcium hydroxide, with appropriate temporary restorative materials at the first visit and a second visit for complete caries removal once pulpal bridging occurred, with the bridge protecting the pulp from carious exposure. The current consensus is that this staged approach does not offer improved outcomes[4] over selective caries removal in a single step,[5] and it risks failure if patients are lost to follow-up.

As a result, modern indirect pulp capping entails a single visit for caries removal, leaving a thin layer of carious dentin behind.[6] Pulp capping materials, including hard-setting calcium hydroxide preparations like Dycal (Dentsply Sirona), bioceramics, and resin-modified glass-ionomer cements, are then placed directly over the remaining caries, with appropriate coronal restoration to immediately follow (Fig 8-3). Of note, carious tooth structure from the periphery of the lesion should be removed to ensure a complete coronal seal overlying the preparation. Rubber dam isolation is imperative for these procedures to ensure proper and thorough disinfection. Follow-up includes close monitoring for signs or symptoms of pulpal involvement or radiographic pathology and for maintenance of pulp sensitivity responses. If there is evidence of pulpal inflammation or degeneration, NSRCT is indicated.

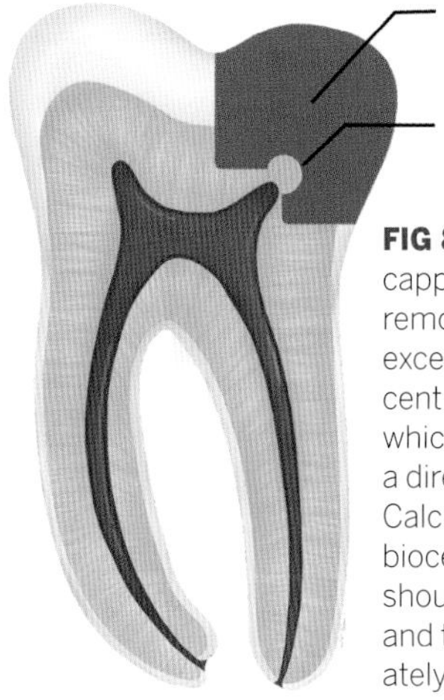

Though the indirect pulp cap is theoretically a less invasive procedure than direct pulp capping or pulpot-

Restorative material

Bioceramic material or calcium hydroxide

FIG 8-3 Indirect pulp capping involves the removal of all caries except a thin layer adjacent to the pulp tissue, which is meant to prevent a direct pulp exposure. Calcium hydroxide or bioceramic materials should then be placed and the tooth appropriately restored.

omy treatment, leaving infected dentin behind is not without risks, including the chance for recurrent caries and the development of endodontic pathology. Direct visualization of pulp tissues during complete caries excavation also allows for the most accurate assessment of pulp viability because vital tissue can be directly distinguished from necrotic tissues.[1] Furthermore, bonding may be unfavorable when caries remain, leading to coronal leakage.[7,8] Given the high reliability of direct pulp capping procedures with bioceramics, complete caries removal, even when it leads to a pulp exposure, is advisable.[1]

Direct Pulp Capping

The direct pulp cap aims to cover a mechanical, carious, or traumatic vital pulp exposure without pulp extirpation. It is a well-accepted method for repairing traumatic or mechanical pulp exposures, especially when the exposures are repaired within the 48-hour window before progressive inflammation normally occurs.[9] Though the technique has been used for many years in primary and immature permanent teeth with good success, the introduction of bioceramic materials and their associated improved outcomes has more recently allowed the procedure to be considered even for mature permanent teeth with asymptomatic or symptomatic carious pulp exposures.[1,2]

Ultimately, direct pulp caps may be considered for teeth with vital pulp tissue as confirmed by reliable pulp sensitivity tests or direct visualization. Patients should be informed that the succsss rate of these procedures is comparable to that of NSRCT when proper protocols are followed.[10–13] That said, patients must also be counseled on the need for careful follow-up after these procedures and the potential need for additional endodontic (and restorative) care if pulpal inflammation progresses.[1]

Direct pulp capping procedures should be performed under dental dam isolation.[1,2] Following complete caries removal using a water-cooled high-speed drill, the preparation should be rinsed with sodium hypochlorite.[1] This may be done with gentle syringe irrigation or with a cotton pellet soaked in the solution. Recommended protocols advise an irrigation routine with 5 to 10 minutes of tissue contact for hemostasis and disinfection.[1]

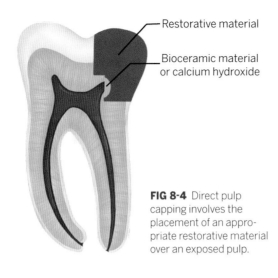

FIG 8-4 Direct pulp capping involves the placement of an appropriate restorative material over an exposed pulp.

Labels: Restorative material; Bioceramic material or calcium hydroxide

Hemostasis must be achieved prior to the application of restorative material. If hemostasis cannot be achieved, pulp tissue removal by pulpotomy or pulpectomy is necessary. A bioceramic material should be placed in direct contact with the pulp according to the manufacturer's directions (Fig 8-4), and a definitive restoration should be placed. When using bioceramic materials, clinicians should alert patients that coronal staining is possible.[14]

Given the greatly improved success rates with bioceramic materials, calcium hydroxide pulp caps are used less frequently.[1,15] However, they represent a reasonable alternative to delaying care because immediate placement of a pulp cap is the best predictor of success.[16] Additionally, because calcium hydroxide poses little risk of the coronal staining that can occur with the use of bioceramics, it may be the material of choice where esthetics are a high priority.[14] Placement of calcium hydroxide pulp caps follows a similar protocol to that of using bioceramics. A calcium hydroxide preparation, such as Dycal, should be placed directly over the exposed pulp following disinfection and topped with a resin-based seal to mitigate washout. Following this, appropriate coronal restorative care should be completed (Fig 8-5).

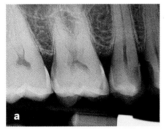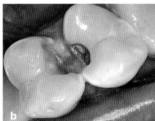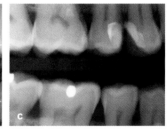

FIG 8-5 *(a and b)* A carious exposure was noted on the maxillary right second premolar. Vital pulp therapy was performed, wherein a bioceramic direct pulp cap was placed on the affected tooth, along with caries management on the distal aspect of the maxillary right first premolar. *(c)* Indirect ceramic onlays were placed to definitively restore the teeth.

Pulpotomy

A pulpotomy involves removal of the coronal portion of the vital pulp in an effort to preserve the vitality of the radicular pulp. The pulpotomy procedure was historically reserved for primary or immature permanent teeth. However, the use of bioceramic materials has improved its predictability in mature permanent teeth as well.[1,11,17–20] Of note, formocresol should never be used for pulpotomy procedures due to the carcinogenic properties of its formaldehyde component.[1,21]

Pulpotomy treatment is performed in cases of larger carious or traumatic exposures when pulpal bleeding cannot be easily controlled from the site of exposure. A *complete pulpotomy* refers to removal of the entirety of the coronal portion of the pulp to the level of the canal orifice. A *partial pulpotomy* removes only a small portion of the coronal pulp to preserve whatever healthy tissue remains within the pulp chamber[22,23] (Fig 8-6). The decision to perform a full or partial pulpotomy is made intraoperatively based on the clinician's ability to achieve hemostasis of the remaining tissue.

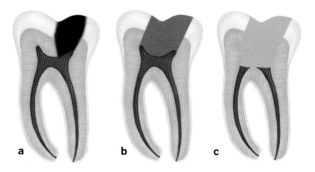

FIG 8-6 Pulpotomy treatment is appropriate for teeth with large carious exposures (*a*) or more extensive pulpal inflammation. In this technique, the entire pulp chamber roof is removed under dental dam isolation (*b*), and the coronal pulp tissue is removed to the level of the canal orifices in cases of full pulpotomy (*c*) or only partially in cases of partial pulpotomy treatment.

A pulpotomy should always be completed under dental dam isolation. The tooth should be accessed according to the protocols used during NSRCT and the pulp chamber unroofed. Tissue should be removed gently with either a round bur in a slow-speed handpiece or a sharp spoon excavator. Once healthy tissue is visualized, pulp extirpation can stop. The exposed pulp should be gently disinfected with a sodium hypochlorite rinse, dried with a sterile cotton pellet, and covered with a bioceramic material. The coronal restoration should follow best restorative practices (Fig 8-7). Because this procedure is often performed in children, a full-coverage restoration may take the form of a stainless steel crown or another interim restoration. In adults warranting full-coverage restorative care, extended provisionalization allows for early assessment of pulpal recovery so that NSRCT can be completed without undue consequences in case of early failures. Careful follow-up for signs and symptoms of apical pathology is crucial because progressive disease warrants immediate intervention.

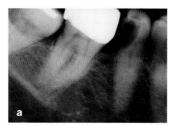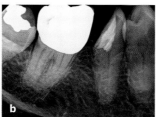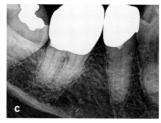

FIG 8-7 (*a*) The mandibular right second premolar with a preoperative diagnosis of asymptomatic irreversible pulpitis had a carious exposure that required a pulpotomy to obtain hemostasis. (*b*) A bioceramic material (EndoSequence BC Root Repair Material Fast Set Putty, Brasseler USA) was used to fill the pulp chamber, and (*c*) the tooth was definitively restored with a crown.

References

1. American Association of Endodontists, Vital Pulp Therapy. AAE Position Statement. 2021. https://www. aae.org/wp-content/uploads/2021/05/VitalPulpTherapyPositionStatement_v2.pdf. Accessed 30 March 2023.
2. Duncan HF, Galler KM, Tomson PL, et al. European Society of Endodontology position statement: Management of deep caries and the exposed pulp. Int Endod J 2019;52:923–934.
3. Wolters WJ, Duncan HF, Tomson PL, et al. Minimally invasive endodontics: A new diagnostic system for assessing pulpitis and subsequent treatment needs. Int Endod J 2017;50:825–829.
4. Maltz M, Koppe B, Jardim JJ, et al. Partial caries removal in deep caries lesions: A 5-year multicenter randomized controlled trial. Clin Oral Investig 2018;22:1337–1343.
5. Asgary S, Hassanizadeh R, Torabzadeh H, Eghbal MJ. Treatment outcomes of 4 vital pulp therapies in mature molars. J Endod 2018;44:529–535.
6. Dhar V, Pilcher L, Fontana M, et al. Evidence-based clinical practice guideline on restorative treatments for caries lesions: A report from the American Dental Association. J Am Dent Assoc 2023;154:551-566.e51.
7. Nakajima M, Sano H, Burrow MF, et al. Tensile bond strength and SEM evaluation of caries-affected dentin using dentin adhesives. J Dent Res 1995;74:1679–1688.
8. Yoshiyama M, Tay FR, Torii Y, et al. Resin adhesion to carious dentin. Am J Dent 2003;16:47–52.
9. American Association of Endodontists. Recommended Guidelines of the American Association of Endodontists for the Treatment of Traumatic Dental Injuries. 2013. https://www.aae.org/specialty/clinical-resources/treatment-planning/traumatic-dental-injuries/.
10. Asgary S, Eghbal MJ. Treatment outcomes of pulpotomy in permanent molars with irreversible pulpitis using biomaterials: A multi-center randomized controlled trial. Acta Odontol Scand 2013;71:130–136.
11. Asgary S, Eghbal MJ, Bagheban AA. Long-term outcomes of pulpotomy in permanent teeth with irreversible pulpitis: A multi-center randomized controlled trial. Am J Dent 2017;30:151–155.
12. Awawdeh L, Al-Qudah A, Hamouri H, Chakra RJ. Outcomes of vital pulp therapy using mineral trioxide aggregate or biodentine: A prospective randomized clinical trial. J Endod 2018;44:1603–1609.
13. Kundzina R, Stangvaltaite L, Eriksen HM, Kerosuo E. Capping carious exposures in adults: A randomized controlled trial investigating mineral trioxide aggregate versus calcium hydroxide. Int Endod J 2017;50:924–932.
14. Beatty H, Svec T. Quantifying coronal tooth discoloration caused by Biodentine and Endosequence root repair material. J Endod 2015;41:2036–2039.
15. Li Z, Cao L, Fan M, Xu Q. Direct pulp capping with calcium hydroxide or mineral trioxide aggregate: A meta-analysis. J Endod 2015;41:1412–1417.
16. Bergenholtz G. Advances since the paper by Zander and Glass (1949) on the pursuit of healing methods for pulpal exposures: Historical perspectives. Oral Surg Oral Med Oral Pathol Oral Radiol Endod 2005;100:S102–S108.
17. Tan SY, Yu VSH, Lim KH, et al. Long-term pulpal and restorative outcomes of pulpotomy in mature permanent teeth. J Endod 2020;46;383–390.
18. Linsuwanont P, Wimonsutthikul K, Pothimoke U, Santiwong B. Treatment outcomes of mineral trioxide aggregate pulpotomy in vital permanent teeth with carious pulp exposure: The retrospective study. J Endod 2017;43:225–230.
19. Taha NA, Khazali MA. Partial pulpotomy in mature permanent teeth with clinical signs indicative of irreversible pulpitis: A randomized clinical trial. J Endod 2017;43:1417–1421.
20. Uesrichai N, Nirunsittirat A, Chuveera P, Srisuwan T, Sastraruji T, Chompu-Inwai P. Partial pulpotomy with two bioactive cements in permanent teeth of 6- to 18-year-old patients with signs and symptoms indicative of irreversible pulpitis: A noninferiority randomized controlled trial. Int Endod J 2019;52:749–759.
21. American Association of Endodontists. Concerning Paraformaldehyde-Containing Endodontic Filling Materials and Sealers. AAE Position Statement. 2017. https://www.aae.org/specialty/wp-content/uploads/sites/2/2017/06/paraformaldehydefillingmaterials.pdf. Accessed 30 March 2023.
22. Cvek M. A clinical report on partial pulpotomy and capping with calcium hydroxide in permanent incisors with complicated crown fracture. J Endod 1978;4:232–237.
23. American Association of Endodontists. Glossary of Endodontic Terms, ed 10. 2020. https://www.aae.org/specialty/clinical-resources/glossary-endodontic-terms/. Accessed 30 March 2023.

Treatment of Immature Necrotic Teeth

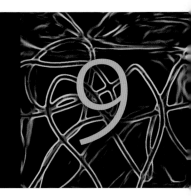

While vital pulp therapy is the treatment of choice for vital immature permanent teeth, necrotic immature teeth require a different approach. Immature teeth are generally defined as those with apical diameters greater than 1 mm.[1] Immature teeth cannot undergo routine endodontic procedures for several reasons. The lack of an apical stop in these teeth renders normal gutta-percha and sealer obturation difficult, if not impossible, and their thin radicular walls result in a poor long-term prognosis due to risks of root fracture. Treatment modalities for managing immature necrotic teeth include calcium hydroxide apexification, bioceramic apexification, and regenerative endodontic therapy. Each of these modalities is associated with predictable success, and treatment selection should reflect a comprehensive understanding of the individual patient and tooth at the time of diagnosis.[2] Even in cases where treatment may be considered less predictable or when restorative factors are less than ideal, clinicians may consider providing apexification treatment to maintain a compromised tooth in a young patient to facilitate growth and development of the alveolus (Fig 9-1). Follow-up is especially crucial in these cases to monitor for signs of recurrent or persistent infection that could necessitate immediate extraction.

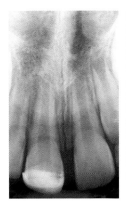

FIG 9-1 In cases where treatment may be considered less predictable or restorative factors less than ideal, clinicians may consider providing apexification treatment to maintain a compromised tooth and facilitate growth and development of the alveolus, like in this patient with a crown-root fracture that extended to the crestal bone on the palatal surface of the tooth.

Apexification

The purpose of apexification treatment is to develop a barrier at the apex of an immature necrotic tooth to facilitate obturation of the canal space. In general, the technique involves a pulpectomy followed by barrier development either immediately with bioceramic materials or with long-term calcium hydroxide.[2,3] While this is certainly a predictable treatment modality in the short term, there is a long-term higher risk of cervical fracture due to the thinness of the remaining dentinal walls[4,5] (Fig 9-2).

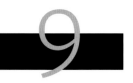

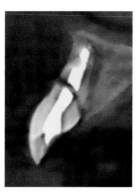

FIG 9-2 The long-term risk of apexification is fracture of the thin dentinal walls. This patient presented with a horizontal root fracture through an apexified central incisor due to secondary trauma.

Bioceramic apexification

Also called the *artificial barrier technique* of apexification, the bioceramic apexification procedure involves the use of bioceramic material to create a barrier at the apical terminus. Under many circumstances, this can be completed in a single visit, which is advantageous when compliance is of concern.[6,7] That said, both single- and multivisit bioceramic apexification are associated with predictable success.[6,7]

Apexification procedures begin with a pulpectomy completed according to protocols similar to those used during nonsurgical root canal therapy (NSRCT), including local anesthesia, dental dam isolation, and access opening (Fig 9-3). Because the canal space or spaces should be readily accessible in these immature teeth, canal scouting is straightforward. Working lengths should be estimated with preoperative images, and electronic apex locators are often accurate. If readings are inconsistent, as in the case of very wide, open apices, working length radiographs should be taken until confident working length measurements are attained. Conservative instrumentation should be performed, focused on the removal of necrotic pulp debris and minimizing forces on or removal of radicular dentin to conserve what remains. Irrigation should be performed with 1.5% sodium hypochlorite and ethylenediaminetetraacetic acid (EDTA), as with NSRCT, though extreme care should be taken to never extrude sodium hypochlorite into the apical spaces.

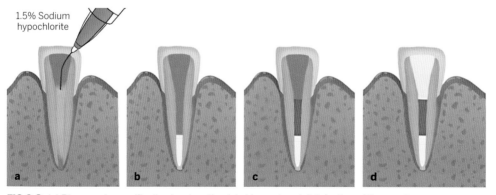

1.5% Sodium hypochlorite

FIG 9-3 *(a)* Bioceramic apexification involves the debridement and disinfection of the canal space with instruments and 1.5% sodium hypochlorite. *(b)* Following this, a 3- to 5-mm-thick layer of bioceramic material is compacted to the apex with or without a resorbable collagen plug placed at the periapex. *(c)* The coronal canal space is then filled with gutta-percha, and *(d)* the coronal access is definitively restored.

The apical barrier can then be placed at the terminus of the cleaned canal space. Clinicians can consider placement of a resorbable collagen plug at the apex to facilitate compaction of the bioceramic material into the apical tooth structure. This is particularly useful in teeth with very wide apices. The collagen can be placed into the apex with premeasured pluggers. Whether or not collagen is used, the bioceramic material should be placed in increments of 2 mm with the use of premeasured obturation pluggers or with a cut gutta-percha cone used as a compaction device (Fig 9-4). A radiograph should be used to confirm appropriate placement

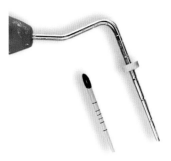

FIG 9-4 Bioceramic barriers can be apically compacted with premeasured pluggers or with cut gutta-percha cones.

of this apical barrier prior to filling the remaining canal with either bioceramic cement or gutta-percha and sealer placed with a backfill device (Fig 9-5). In esthetic zones, gutta-percha is preferred over bioceramics, which may cause staining. Clinical and radiographic follow-up appointments are recommended at 6-month intervals for at least 1 year following treatment.

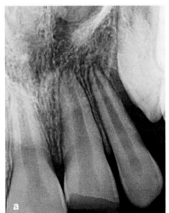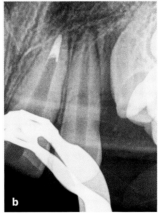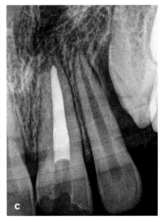

FIG 9-5 (a) Dental trauma led to pulp necrosis in the maxillary right central incisor, managed with bioceramic apexification. (b) A bioceramic barrier was compacted to the apex, and (c) the remaining canal space was filled with gutta-percha and sealer, followed by temporization.

Though the bioceramic apexification procedure is classically performed in a single visit, a modified version wherein intracanal calcium hydroxide is placed as an interappointment medicament may be performed in certain clinical situations. For example, if preoperative swelling, a sinus tract, or significant drainage is noted, or if a patient is scheduled for emergency treatment and there is not enough time to properly develop the apical barrier, two-stage therapy with intracanal medication may be beneficial.

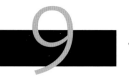

Calcium hydroxide apexification

Unlike bioceramic apexification, where apical barriers are created with artificial materials, calcium hydroxide apexification involves the use of the medicament to stimulate apical stem cells to develop a barrier substantial enough to withstand gutta-percha compaction for an apical seal.[8] Calcium hydroxide–based procedures are time-consuming and require patient (and parent) compliance over multiple visits spanning several months to over 1 year.[9,10] Prior research suggested that long-term calcium hydroxide might predispose roots to fracture. However, newer evidence suggests that this is not necessarily true.[4,5] Rather, the calcium hydroxide–based procedures most likely result in less root thickening than the alternatives, which itself increases the risk of root fracture.[4] Though bioceramic apexification procedures are preferred, calcium hydroxide–based procedures may still be considered for certain patients.

Ultimately, these procedures follow the same protocols as bioceramic apexification procedures until immediately following the completion of the pulpectomy. Following this, calcium hydroxide is introduced to the working length. Paste-type calcium hydroxide products alone can be associated with washout, so preparation of a hard pack should be considered. This can be made by mixing powdered calcium hydroxide with commercially available paste calcium hydroxide formulations that contain radiopacifiers (eg, UltraCal, Ultradent). The hardpack can be transferred into the canal space with a Lentulo spiral or plugger and condensed into the canal space with a plugger equipped with a stopper to the working length, similar to the technique used to place the bioceramic apical barrier (Fig 9-6). A radiograph should be taken to confirm appropriate placement of the calcium hydroxide to the apical tissues.

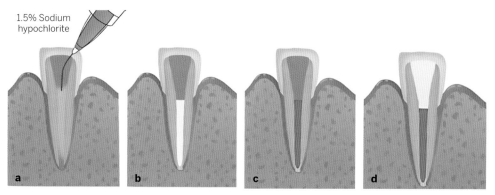

1.5% Sodium hypochlorite

a   b   c   d

FIG 9-6 *(a)* Calcium hydroxide apexification involves the debridement and disinfection of the canal space with instruments and 1.5% sodium hypochlorite. *(b)* Calcium hydroxide is then introduced into the canal space and left until a radiographic barrier becomes apparent at the apex. *(c)* Once the barrier forms, gutta-percha is compacted into the canal space, and *(d)* the coronal access is definitively restored.

Patients should be recalled at 3-month intervals, or sooner if symptoms develop.[11] Clinical signs and symptoms should be absent, and radiographs should be used to monitor for intact calcium hydroxide and continued apical closure. The tooth should be re-accessed for replacement of calcium hydroxide according to the same protocol if signs of calcium hydroxide breakdown are evident. Once there is evidence of apical closure wherein the apical diameter is less than 1 mm across, the calcium hydroxide can be removed, and the tooth can be obturated with gutta-percha according to NSRCT protocols (Fig 9-7).

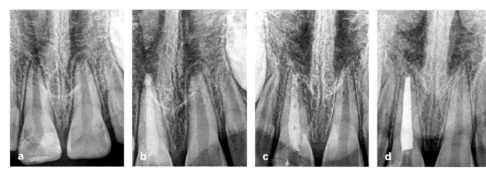

FIG 9-7 *(a)* This patient with an immature, necrotic maxillary right central incisor was treated with calcium hydroxide apexification. *(b)* A pulpectomy was completed, and a hard pack of calcium hydroxide was placed and confirmed radiographically. *(c)* The patient was recalled at 3-month intervals, and an apical barrier was radiographically detected 9 months after treatment was initiated. *(d)* The calcium hydroxide was removed, and the canal space was obturated with gutta-percha and sealer.

Regenerative Endodontics

Regeneration of the dental pulp has long been sought after as the ideal means to manage teeth with endodontic pathology. Research on immature necrotic teeth has proven that at least in this cohort of patients, regeneration of tissue permitting continued dental development is possible. Regenerative endodontic procedures originate from the idea that immature teeth have the ability to recover from injury based on their robust apical blood supply and bank of stem cells within the apical papilla.[1] These stem cells, along with growth factors and scaffolds produced by blood clots, are the requisites for tissue engineering[11–15] (Fig 9-8). Treatment protocols aim to maximize the survival and utility of all of the above. Currently, successful adaptation of these procedures is limited to cases of pulpal necrosis in immature teeth,[16] but broader use is an active area of research.[17–19]

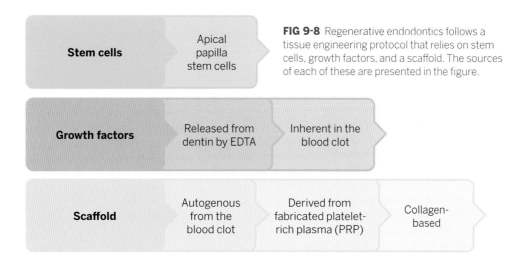

FIG 9-8 Regenerative endodontics follows a tissue engineering protocol that relies on stem cells, growth factors, and a scaffold. The sources of each of these are presented in the figure.

Stem cells	Apical papilla stem cells		
Growth factors	Released from dentin by EDTA	Inherent in the blood clot	
Scaffold	Autogenous from the blood clot	Derived from fabricated platelet-rich plasma (PRP)	Collagen-based

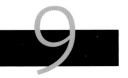

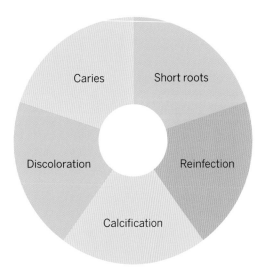

FIG 9-9 Risks associated with regenerative endodontics.

Regenerative endodontic procedures are indicated for patients with immature necrotic teeth when patient and parent compliance permit the procedure to be performed as prescribed. The necessity of two-visit care may make single-visit bioceramic apexification a better alternative in cases where returning for a second visit may be problematic. The procedure is contraindicated in cases where post placement will be needed within the canal space or if allergies or medical contraindications exist to any component of the procedure.[20,21] Patients and parents must be informed of the risks of the procedure, including the risk of coronal staining related to bioceramic material[20,21]; however, this staining may be responsive to internal bleaching procedures if it occurs[22] (see chapter 10). Furthermore, patients and parents should be advised of the risk of treatment failure (Fig 9-9) and that apexification represents an alternative treatment should failure of the regenerative procedure occur.

In general, regenerative endodontic therapy requires two visits, including a modified intratreatment cleaning protocol followed by placement of an intracanal, interappointment medicament for further disinfection following the first visit. The second visit entails stimulation of apical bleeding, bringing the stem cell and growth factor–rich blood clot scaffold into the radicular structure.[13,21] The second visit is completed with placement of a bioceramic material directly over the blood clot to complete the scaffold, followed by definitive restorative care[23,24] (Fig 9-10). The bioceramic material is a crucial component of regenerative endodontic procedures due to its biocompatibility and ability to seal, even in the presence of moisture.[25–27]

More specifically, the first visit of the regenerative endodontic procedure begins with anesthesia, dental dam isolation, and access into the pulp space.[20] Once the necrotic pulp stump is visualized within the pulp chamber, the protocol diverges greatly from other orthograde endodontic procedures because mechanical cleaning in these teeth is contraindicated in order to minimize disruption of the radicular walls, which serve as a future scaffold.[24] Working length should be estimated radiographically to ensure that irrigants are not introduced past the apex (Fig 9-11). Chemical cleaning should be performed with dilute 1.5% sodium hypochlorite followed by 17% EDTA as a gentle stream over the pulp stump under constant surgical suction, each dosed at 20 mL/canal over the course of 5 minutes.[20,21,28–31] Notably, much research has investigated the specifics of these irrigation protocols, including both their efficacy and potential cytotoxicity to apical stem cells. Alterations to the protocol adversely affect both; therefore, the use of alternative irrigation solutions such as chlorhexidine[28] or higher concentrations of sodium hypochlorite are contraindicated.[32]

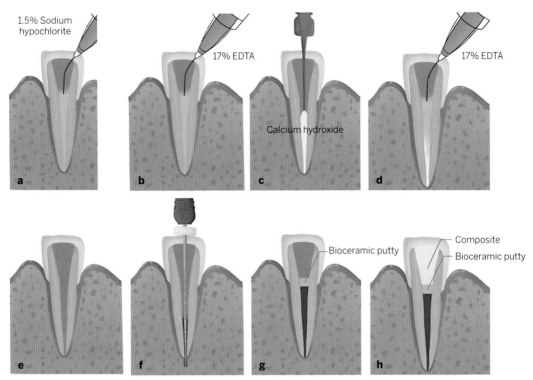

FIG 9-10 *(a)* Regenerative endodontic procedures involve the disinfection of the canal space and pulp stump with sodium hypochlorite but not instrumentation. *(b)* Irrigation with 17% EDTA follows to release growth factors from dentin. *(c)* Calcium hydroxide is used as an intracanal medicament placed over the remaining disinfected pulp stump. *(d)* At the second visit, 17% EDTA is used to irrigate the calcium hydroxide. *(e)* The canal space is then dried. *(f)* A sterile file is then introduced into the periapex to stimulate bleeding. *(g)* A bioceramic material is placed over the blood clot, and *(h)* the coronal access is definitively restored.

Following initial disinfection, the canal space is dried to the level of the remaining necrotic tissue, and an intracanal medicament is placed directly over the pulp stump.[20] While historically, antibiotic pastes were used, calcium hydroxide is now considered the medicament of choice for regenerative endodontics. Calcium hydroxide balances minimal toxicity with widespread availability and does not pose the risk of staining that is associated with antibiotic pastes containing tetracycline family drugs.[33–35] After application of the calcium hydroxide medicament, the access should be sealed with a resin-modified glass-ionomer–based temporary restorative material.

After 1 to 4 weeks, the patient should return for the second treatment visit, at which time resolution of clinical signs and symptoms can be assessed.[20] At this visit, epinephrine-free local anesthesia should be used to

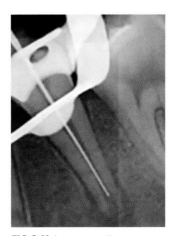

FIG 9-11 In regenerative endodontic procedures, the working length should be estimated radiographically to ensure that irrigants are not extruded past the apex.

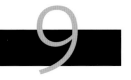

avoid vasoconstriction that could affect the apical blood supply.[20,21] Dental dam isolation and re-access should be followed by a rinse of 5 mL of 17% EDTA in order to remove the intracanal calcium hydroxide.[20] Sodium hypochlorite rinses should be avoided at this second visit due to potential cytotoxic effects. Once the calcium hydroxide is fully removed, clinicians should induce bleeding into the canal space. This can be accomplished with the introduction of a no. 10 K file into the periapical tissues.[20] Bleeding should fill the intraradicular canal space to a level below the cementoenamel junction (CEJ), creating a stable blood clot within a few minutes. A 2-mm bioceramic plug should be placed over the blood clot and the placement confirmed radiographically.[20,36] The tooth may be temporized as before, or an immediate definitive restoration can be placed.

Follow-up at 6 months, 12 months, and 24 months is advised with clinical and radiographic assessments of healing[20] (Fig 9-12). Success is defined by both the resolution of apical pathology and increases in the length and width of the roots.[37] Some authors also suggest that retesting for return of pulp sensitivity responses might indicate the reformation of organized pulp tissue; however, this return to sensitivity is rare and does not appear to have an effect on outcomes, so negative responses should not be deemed failures.[20,38] Any evidence of failure, including lack of continued root development, failed healing, or new apical pathology or root resorption, should prompt immediate intervention, likely in the form of apexification.[20]

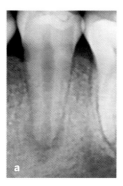 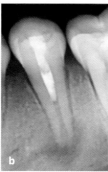 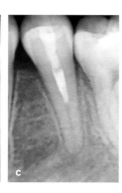

FIG 9-12 *(a)* This necrotic and immature mandibular left second premolar underwent regenerative endodontic therapy, including *(b)* placement of a bioceramic plug over the blood clot and definitive restoration. *(c)* An 8-month follow-up revealed signs of apical closure and the resolution of apical periodontitis.

References

1. Kling M, Cvek M, Mejare I. Rate and predictability of pulp revascularization in therapeutically reimplanted permanent incisors. Endod Dent Traumatol 1986;2:83–89.
2. Jeeruphan T, Jantarat J, Yanpiset K, Suwannapan L, Khewsawai P, Hargreaves KM. Mahidol study 1: Comparison of radiographic and survival outcomes of immature teeth treated with either regenerative endodontic or apexification methods: A retrospective study. J Endod 2012;38:1330–1336.
3. Pace R, Giuliani V, Nieri M, Di Nasso L, Pagavino G. Mineral trioxide aggregate as apical plug in teeth with necrotic pulp and immature apices: A 10-year case series. J Endod 2014;40:1250–1254.
4. Kahler SL, Shetty S, Andreasen FM, Kahler B. The effect of long-term dressing with calcium hydroxide on the fracture susceptibility of teeth. J Endod 2018;44:464–469.
5. Cvek M. Prognosis of luxated non-vital maxillary incisors treated with calcium hydroxide and filled with gutta-percha. Endod Dent Traumatol 1992;8:45–55.
6. Simon S, Rilliard F, Berdal A, Machtou P. The use of mineral trioxide aggregate in one-visit apexification treatment: A prospective study. Int Endod J 2007;40:186–197.
7. Witherspoon DE, Ham K. One-visit apexification: Technique for inducing root-end barrier formation in apical closures. Pract Proced Aesthet Dent 2001;13:455–460.

8. Frank AL. Therapy for the divergent pulpless tooth by continued apical formation. J Am Dent Assoc 1966;72:87–93.

9. Kleier DJ, Barr ES. A study of endodontically apexified teeth. Endod Dent Traumatol 1991;7:112–117.

10. Shabahang S. Treatment options: Apexogenesis and apexification. J Endod 2013;39:S26–S29.

11. Finucane D, Kinirons MJ. Non-vital immature permanent incisors: Factors that may influence treatment outcome. Endod Dent Traumatol 1999;15:273–277.

12. Nygaard-Ostby B, Hjortdal O. Tissue formation in the root canal following pulp removal. Scand J Dent Res 1971;79:333–349.

13. Banchs F, Trope M. Revascularization of immature permanent teeth with apical periodontitis: New treatment protocol? J Endod 2004;30:196–200.

14. Langer R, Vacanti JP. Tissue engineering. Science 1993;260:920–926.

15. Lovelace TW, Henry MA, Hargreaves KM, Diogenes A. Evaluation of the delivery of mesenchymal stem cells into the root canal space of necrotic immature teeth after clinical regenerative endodontic procedure. J Endod 2011;37:133–138.

16. Diogenes A, Ruparel NB, Shiloah Y, Hargreaves KM. Regenerative endodontics: A way forward. J Am Dent Assoc 2016;147:372–380.

17. He L, Kim SG, Gong Q, et al. Regenerative endodontics for adult patients. J Endod 2017;43:S57–S64.

18. Saoud TMA, Mistry S, Kahler B, Sigurdsson A, Lin LM. Regenerative endodontic procedures for traumatized teeth after horizontal root fracture, avulsion, and perforating root resorption. J Endod 2016;42:1476–1482.

19. Santiago CN, Pinto SS, Sassone LM, Hirata R Jr, Fidel SR. Revascularization technique for the treatment of external inflammatory root resorption: A report of 3 cases. J Endod 2015;41:1560–1564.

20. AAE Clinical Considerations for a Regenerative Procedure Revised 5/18/2021. https://www.aae.org/specialty/wp-content/uploads/sites/2/2021/08/ClinicalConsiderationsApprovedByREC062921.pdf. Accessed 31 March 2023.

21. Law AS. Considerations for regeneration procedures. J Endod 2013;39:S44–S56.

22. Kirchhoff AL, Raldi DP, Salles AC, Cunha RS, Mello I. Tooth discolouration and internal bleaching after the use of triple antibiotic paste. Int Endod J 2015;48:1181–1187.

23. Mente J, Leo M, Panagidis D, et al. Treatment outcome of mineral trioxide aggregate in open apex teeth. J Endod 2013;39:20–26.

24. Hargreaves KM, Giesler T, Henry M, Wang Y. Regeneration potential of the young permanent tooth: What does the future hold? J Endod 2008;34(7 Suppl):S51–S56.

25. Parirokh M, Torabinejad M. Mineral trioxide aggregate: A comprehensive literature review—Part I: Chemical, physical, and antibacterial properties. J Endod 2010;36:16–27.

26. Torabinejad M, Parirokh M. Mineral trioxide aggregate: A comprehensive literature review—Part II: Leakage and biocompatibility investigations. J Endod 2010;36:190–202.

27. Parirokh M, Torabinejad M. Mineral trioxide aggregate: A comprehensive literature review—Part III: Clinical applications, drawbacks, and mechanism of action. J Endod 2010;36:400–413.

28. Trevino EG, Patwardhan AN, Henry MA, et al. Effect of irrigants on the survival of human stem cells of the apical papilla in a platelet-rich plasma scaffold in human root tips. J Endod 2011;37:1109–1115.

29. Pang NS, Lee SJ, Kim E, et al. Effect of EDTA on attachment and differentiation of dental pulp stem cells. J Endod 2014;40:811–817.

30. Zeng Q, Nguyen S, Zhang H, et al. Release of growth factors into root canal by irrigations in regenerative endodontics. J Endod 2016;42:1760–1766.

31. Smith AJ, Duncan HF, Diogenes A, Simon S, Cooper PR. Exploiting the bioactive properties of the dentin-pulp complex in regenerative endodontics. J Endod 2016;42:47–56.

32. Martin DE, De Almeida JFA, Henry MA, et al. Concentration-dependent effect of sodium hypochlorite on stem cells of apical papilla survival and differentiation. J Endod 2014;40:51–55.

33. Ruparel NB, Teixeira FB, Ferraz CCR, Diogenes A. Direct effect of intracanal medicaments on survival of stem cells of the apical papilla. J Endod 2012;38:1372–1375.

34. Nagata JY, Soares AJ, Souza-Filho FJ, et al. Microbial evaluation of traumatized teeth treated with triple antibiotic paste or calcium hydroxide with 2% chlorhexidine gel in pulp revascularization. J Endod 2014;40:778–783.

35. Althumairy RI, Teixeira FB, Diogenes A. Effect of dentin conditioning with intracanal medicaments on survival of stem cells of apical papilla. J Endod 2014;40:521–525.

36. Petrino JA, Boda KK, Shambarger S, Bowles WR, McClanahan SB. Challenges in regenerative endodontics: A case series. J Endod 2010;36:536–541.

37. Lenzi R, Trope M. Revitalization procedures in two traumatized incisors with different biological outcomes. J Endod 2012;38:411–414.

38. Saoud TM, Martin G, Chen YHM, et al. Treatment of mature permanent teeth with necrotic pulps and apical periodontitis using regenerative endodontic procedures: A case series. J Endod 2016;42:57–65.

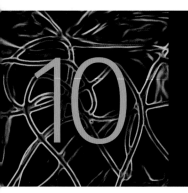

Emergency Treatment and Complication Management

Endodontics is a specialty that often involves managing patients experiencing pain and infection. As a result, clinicians must be at the ready to provide emergency care with the same care and concern as in nonemergency situations. This chapter discusses both emergency treatment and the intraoperative and postoperative complications unique to endodontics, including their diagnosis and management.

Emergency Treatment

Endodontic emergencies are defined by severe pain, swelling, and trauma. This chapter focuses on emergencies associated with pain and swelling. Chapter 14 discusses trauma management. While the diagnosis and treatment of endodontic emergencies doesn't necessarily differ from nonemergency cases, the urgency can result in added stress for provider and patient, making these cases unduly challenging. Staff members should be trained to triage emergencies appropriately and schedule patients based on perceived severity. Patients reporting facial swelling, for example, should be seen immediately for assessment and management given the risk of dangerous infections, including cellulitis and infections adjacent to the airway or ocular structures. Patients reporting unstimulated pain, loss of sleep, or a lack of response to medications should also be seen immediately. Discomfort that is controllable with medication may be considered less urgent (Fig 10-1).

More urgent	Less urgent
• Facial swelling • Systemic symptoms of infection (fever, malaise, lymphadenopathy) • Pain that is unresponsive to medication • Sleeplessness due to dental pain	• Pain that is controllable with medication • Pain that does not interfere with the patient's ability to function

FIG 10-1 Triage of endodontic emergencies.

Neither the unscheduled nature of these issues nor the potentially limited time providers may have in their schedule to appropriately diagnose and treat these patients should interfere with the objective to alleviate symptoms. The expedient provision of an accurate pulpal and periapical diagnosis is necessary to determine the most appropriate treatment, and care for emergency patients should include both the provision of treatment as well as adjunctive medical management. Treatment can include incision and drainage, pulpotomy, or pulpectomy (Fig 10-2). Adjunctive medical care can include oral analgesics, antibiotics, or appropriate medical referral.

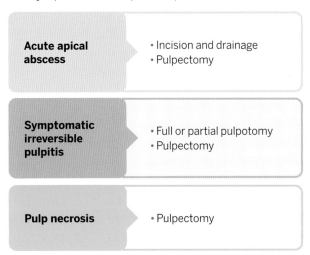

Acute apical abscess
• Incision and drainage
• Pulpectomy

Symptomatic irreversible pulpitis
• Full or partial pulpotomy
• Pulpectomy

Pulp necrosis
• Pulpectomy

FIG 10-2 Emergency treatment modalities by diagnosis.

Incision and drainage

The periapical diagnosis of an acute apical abscess is defined by swelling. Intraoral incision and drainage is appropriate in cases of fluctuant swelling, both to relieve the painful pressure in the swelling and to increase blood flow to the area. Incision and drainage may also be considered in areas of indurated swelling to shift an anaerobic environment to an aerobic one (Fig 10-3). Profound anesthesia should be attained prior to the incision and drainage. Larger areas of cellulitis or facial swellings may require more extensive surgical debridement necessitating referral to an oral and maxillofacial surgery specialist for management.

A sharp scalpel blade is used to incise into the vertex of the swelling down to the periosteum (Fig 10-4). Drainage of purulence and/or blood should initially be managed with surgical suction. As drainage slows, the area can be packed with guaze until hemostasis is achieved or drainage slows significantly. Placement of physical drains is contraindicated because the wound will remain open until drainage ceases, and consequently, the insertion of a foreign body is an unnecessary

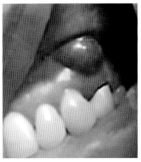

FIG 10-3 Incision and drainage should be performed in areas of fluctuant swelling, as well as for more indurated swellings.

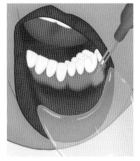

FIG 10-4 To perform an incision and drainage procedure, a sharp scalpel blade should be inserted into the vertex of the swelling down to the periosteum.

step. Postoperative rinsing with warm salt water is indicated as a nonirritating means of cleansing the wound. It is disputed whether incision and drainage of swelling aids healing when performed concomitantly with pulpectomy procedures.[1]

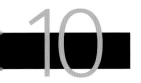

Pulpotomy

Patients with a pulpal diagnosis of symptomatic irreversible pulpitis present with heightened and lingering responses to pulp sensitivity tests and may report spontaneous, unremitting discomfort. For these patients, removal of inflamed pulp tissue will provide significant relief. When time or clinician experience limits a provider's ability to complete nonsurgical root canal therapy (NSRCT), pulpotomy procedures can provide as much relief as full pulpectomy procedures.[2]

Completion of an emergency pulpotomy begins with profound local anesthesia. Dental dam isolation should be used when drilling to access the canal space. Caries and restorative materials should be removed with a water-cooled, high-speed handpiece and the pulp chamber fully unroofed. The pulpotomy may involve debridement of the full chamber or take the form of a partial pulpotomy, in which only the visibly hyperemic tissue is removed[3] (Fig 10-5). Removal of pulp tissue can be completed with a round bur or sharp spoon excavator with sodium hypochlorite irrigation. Pulp tissue must be removed to a level where hemostasis can be achieved. Hemostasis may be aided by applying pressure in the chamber with a sterile cotton pellet soaked in sodium hypochlorite or sterile saline. If hemostasis cannot be achieved in 10 minutes with pressure application, additional pulp tissue should be removed.

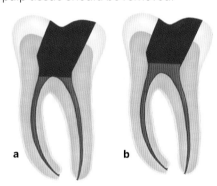

FIG 10-5 Full or partial pulpotomy treatment can be considered in patients presenting with a diagnosis of symptomatic irreversible pulpitis. *(a)* Full pulpotomy treatment involves the removal of the entirety of the pulp tissue within the pulp chamber to the level of the chamber floor. *(b)* Partial pulpotomy treatment entails removal of a portion of the coronal pulp tissue to a level where hemostasis can be achieved.

When performing a pulpotomy for emergency purposes, calcium hydroxide or eugenol dressings can be used over the remaining pulp tissues. Materials including formaldehyde in their makeup, such as formocresol, are well-known to be carcinogens and should never be used for pulpotomy procedures.[4,5] If commercially available preparations (eg, UltraCal, Ultradent) are available, they may be directly dispensed. Otherwise, powdered calcium hydroxide and water may be mixed to a paste consistency and directly applied. The tooth may be temporized with cotton and an appropriate temporary seal until definitive care is delivered. Occlusal reduction may be considered both for patient comfort and to avoid interferences that might contribute to occlusal trauma or fracture while treatment is in progress.[6]

Pulpectomy

Pulpectomy is defined as the complete removal of the pulp tissue. Pulpectomy treatment is indicated for patients with a pulpal diagnosis of symptomatic irreversible pulpitis where hemostasis of the pulp tissue within the chamber or root canal spaces cannot be achieved and for patients with a pulpal diagnosis of necrosis or a periapical diagnosis of acute apical abscess. Pulpectomy procedures should follow the same protocols as two-visit NSRCT (see chapter 5).

Adjunctive medical management

Endodontic emergencies are defined by pain and/or infection, and adjunctive medical management may be required to treat both concerns. Pain management can take the form of local anesthetics or oral medications. Long-acting anesthetics, namely bupivacaine, provide an excellent means of both supplemental intraoperative anesthesia and postoperative analgesia in cases of painful pulpitis or acute apical abscess. Oral medications should include nonsteroidal anti-inflammatory drugs (NSAIDs) and acetaminophen, as outlined in chapter 4. Opioid medications are rarely indicated, despite their widespread provision by emergency room physicians for dental emergencies.[7]

The use of antibiotics as adjunctive medical management should follow the American Association of Endodontists (AAE) prescribing guidelines.[8] Antibiotics are only indicated for acute apical abscesses when there are signs of systemic spread, the patient is immunocompromised, or definitive treatment by pulpectomy and/or incision and drainage cannot be initiated immediately. Appropriate prescription includes prescribing the correct drug with adequate dosing at appropriate intervals to ensure therapeutic levels for the drug to achieve efficient and optimal efficacy (Fig 10-6).

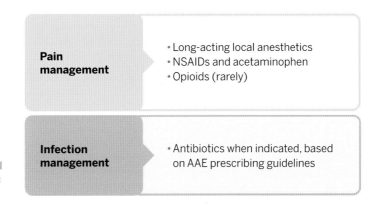

Pain management
- Long-acting local anesthetics
- NSAIDs and acetaminophen
- Opioids (rarely)

Infection management
- Antibiotics when indicated, based on AAE prescribing guidelines

FIG 10-6 Adjunctive medical management for endodontic emergency care.

Complication Management

Despite every effort to avoid their occurrence, complications can and will occur during the provision of endodontic care. Preventing complications should be at the forefront of every clinican's mind before and during endodontic treatment. Using a tool like the AAE Case Difficulty Assessment Form[9] to ensure that clinician skill level is matched to the individual tooth and patient can significantly diminish the likelihood of complications. Maintaining one's armamentarium and skillset can do the same.

The possibility of complications should be discussed during the informed consent process. Patients must be made aware of the potential for intra- and postoperative complications, as well as their potential impact on the short- and long-term prognoses of endodontic treatment. Moreover, if complications do occur during treatment, patients must be made

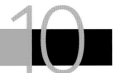

aware of their occurrence, as well as any needed follow-up. Ultimately, well-managed complications do not necessarily result in failure of the endodontic treatment.

Ledging

Ledges are created when inaccurate length control results in internal surface irregularities (steps) that can prevent the passage of instruments to the working length within an otherwise patent canal space[10] (Fig 10-7). Their complexity is often increased by debris packed within the canal space. Ledges may be caused by an under-extended access; when noncurved stainless steel files are used and instruments are forced into the canal space; by erroneous working length determination; and by insufficient irrigation, among other things.[10] Ledges are of clinical significance because they prevent instrumentation to the working length, impeding cleaning and shaping of the canal system and ultimately resulting in recurrent or persistent endodontic infections. Attempts to correct ledges can result in perforations, transportation, and instrument separation.[10] Therefore, clinicians must attempt to prevent ledge development. Use of the electronic apex locator (EAL) with every instrument introduced into the canal space, recapitulation and EAL confirmation between rotary instruments, and copious irrigation are key for prevention.

Ledges are diagnosed when a hard stop is felt within the root canal space that is not explained by instrument separation or other causes. Furthermore, EALs will no longer read within the canal space.[10] Ledges are corrected by bypassing them with small-diameter hand files (eg, no. 06 or no. 08) with sharp apical curvatures (Fig 10-8). These instruments should be wound past the ledge and then used carefully. Instrument size should be incrementally increased to a minimum of a no. 15 hand file before rotary instruments are introduced into the canal[10] (Fig 10-9).

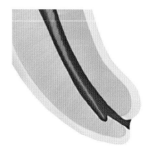

FIG 10-7 Ledges are created when inaccurate length control results in internal surface irregularities within an otherwise patent canal space.

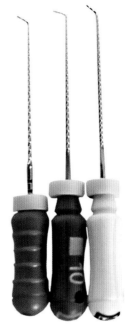

FIG 10-8 Correction of ledges is completed by bypassing them with small-diameter hand files with sharp apical curvatures, which are incrementally increased in size.

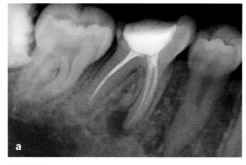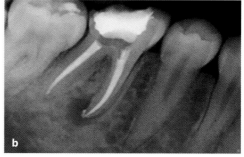

FIG 10-9 Ledges, including ledges in previously treated cases like this mandibular right first molar (a), can be readily corrected in many instances (b).

Transportation

Transportation occurs when instrumentation is performed asymmetrically on one side of the canal, changing its pathway and shape. These instrumentation errors typically arise in the apical half of the canal space. Extensive transportation may result in ledge formation or perforation. Transportation often develops secondary to the improper use or overuse of large, noncurved hand instruments. Modern rotary instruments with shape memory may reduce the tendency toward transportation and strip perforations (Fig 10-10).

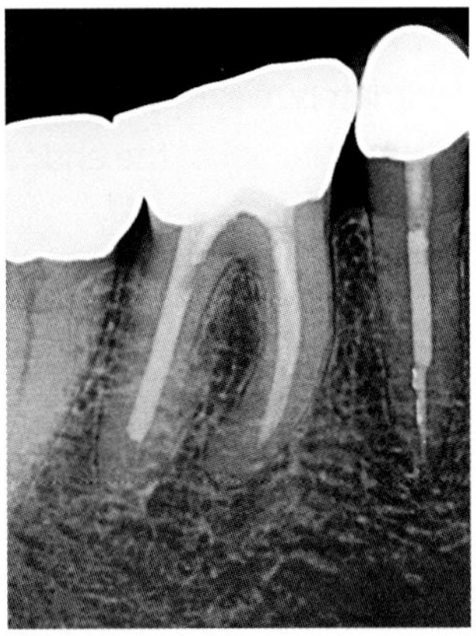

Preventing transportation is essential because once it develops, it cannot be corrected. Asymmetric removal of intracanal dentin can increase the risk of root fractures, and strip perforations can lead to infections and associated bone loss, both of which can result in tooth loss. Areas of significant transportation may benefit from restoration with a bioceramic material, similar to the treatment of other iatrogenic root perforations.[11,12]

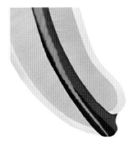

FIG 10-10 Transportation of the mesial canals of the mandibular left first molar is apparent. The obturation material is out of line with the root curvature. This instrumentation error will result in difficult recapturing of the true canal anatomy if nonsurgical retreatment becomes necessary. Separated instrument fragments are also visible in the second premolar. (Photo courtesy of Dr David Baker.)

Apical zipping

Apical zipping occurs when a file extends through the apical foramen and transports its outer wall, resulting in an oval or elliptical shape at the foramen (Fig 10-11). Zipping is of clinical significance due to its impact on obturation. The aberrant apical shape limits tugback with round gutta-percha cones. Furthermore, significant enlargement of the canal space may limit the ability of the provider to safely obturate with gutta-percha and sealer and may necessitate the creation of a bioceramic apical barrier using techniques similar to apexification strategies. Zipping may be prevented by careful adherence to defined working lengths with frequent reconfirmation using an EAL to ensure that files aren't being passed through the apical foramen. Though patency checks are appropriate, they should only be done with files smaller than a no. 10 and with care to avoid active cutting of the extraforaminal space.[13]

FIG 10-11 Apical zipping occurs when a file extends through the apical foramen and transports its outer wall, resulting in an oval- or elliptical-shaped apical foramen.

Instrument separation

Instrument separation refers to the fracture of a portion of an endodontic instrument in the canal space. Any instrument can separate, including hand and rotary files, burs, and ultrasonic tips. Nickel-titanium (NiTi) rotary instruments have a greater risk of instrument separation than hand instruments, which is related to their reduced resistance to cyclic

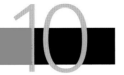
fatigue,[14] manifested as flexural failure at the point of greatest canal curvature. Prior to instrument fracture, files may be seen unwinding or distorting (Fig 10-12). Visualization of each rotary instrument under a surgical operating microscope allows for detection of signs of instrument fatigue and imminent instrument separation. Separation is of clinical significance because it may prevent adequate cleaning and shaping of the canal space, resulting in recurrent or persistent endodontic pathology. Furthermore, attempts at retrieving separated instruments may lead to root perforations or weaken canal structures, resulting in an increased risk of root fracture.

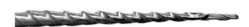

FIG 10-12 Prior to instrument fracture, files may be seen unwinding or distorting. Files must always be monitored for the development of this unwinding.

A diagnosis of instrument separation may be suspected when a click is heard during rotary instrumentation, when a hard stop is felt on recapitulation, and of course, when a shorter file is seen. For this reason, rotary instruments should be measured with a ruler both before and after entry into the canal. Separation may also be diagnosed radiographically by visualizing the separated instrument fragment within the canal space. This fact alone makes radiographic imaging of all teeth with previously initiated endodontic therapy essential during the diagnostic work-up.

When an instrument does separate, removal efforts must balance maintenance of the canal anatomy and minimal removal of radicular structure. Magnification, particularly with a surgical operating microscope, is a crucial component in any attempt at instrument removal.[15] Ultrasonic instruments with narrow tips may be used to vibrate instrument fragments loose or to trough around them to create a platform for removal[16,17] (Fig 10-13). If the area of instrument separation is accessible, several systems are available that use a Masserann technique to lock on to the exposed tip of a separated instrument, including syringe tips bonded with cement and commercially available loop instruments (Fig 10-14).

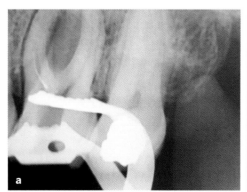
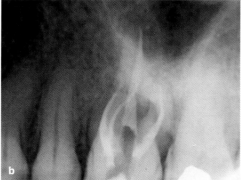

FIG 10-13 *(a)* Ultrasonic instruments with narrow tips may be used to vibrate instruments loose or trough around them to create a platform for their removal. *(b)* This allows for complete cleaning and disinfection of the canal space.

FIG 10-14 Commercially available kits, including ultrasonic tips and loop devices like the Terauchi File Retrieval Kit (PlanBdental) can be used to retrieve separated instrument fragments.

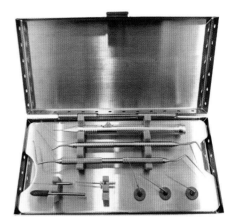

In certain cases, the instrument may not be removed but rather bypassed to allow for cleaning of more apical spaces (Fig 10-15). Surgical access may be necessary when blockages cannot be bypassed. Ultimately, the better the quality of the root fill despite instrument separation and the less damage that occurs in attempts at fragment removal, the better the expected prognosis is for a tooth.[18–20] Managing this complication often requires creativity and care, as well as the understanding that careful monitoring is crucial in cases where the instrument cannot be removed.

FIG 10-15 In cases where separated instrument fragments cannot be retrieved (a), the instrument should be bypassed to permit additional cleaning and disinfection of the canal space and then incorporated into the root canal obturation material (b).

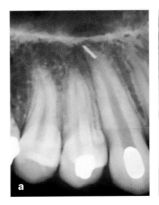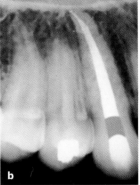

Instrument separation is often preventable. The reuse of endodontic files is not advised for reasons of infection control,[21] and even new instruments should be inspected prior to their introduction into the canal space to alert the clinician to areas of stress or unwinding so that the instrument can be replaced. Used clinical instruments should be monitored for signs of unwinding. Minimal force should be used with hand instruments, and rotary instruments should only be introduced into a canal space with an established glide path and while using gentle motion and the appropriate torque and speed settings per the manufacturer.

Perforations

Perforation refers to the development of a communication between the pulp space and the external tooth surface.[22] Perforations can be iatrogenic or pathologic in nature.

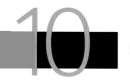

Iatrogenic perforations are caused by errors during access and instrumentation, whereas pathologic perforations present at the time of diagnosis and occur secondary to caries or resorptive pathology. Aberrant endodontic access can lead to both lateral perforations through coronal tooth structure or furcal perforations (Fig 10-16). Poor instrumentation techniques can lead to both apical and strip perforations (Fig 10-17).

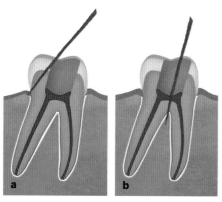

FIG 10-16 *(a and b)* Perforations can include those that occur laterally through the coronal tooth structure and those that occur through the furcation during access

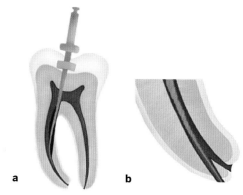

FIG 10-17 Strip *(a)* and apical *(b)* perforations often develop due to improper or aggressive instrumentation techniques.

Perforations are of concern because they facilitate the spread of microbial contaminants and foreign bodies into the periodontal ligament (PDL) space, which can activate inflammatory pathways and result in bone loss similar to apical periodontitis.[23] Smaller perforations and those located entirely within bone are associated with a better prognosis.[23,24] Once pocketing or periodontal defects are noted adjacent to a perforation, outcomes are poor.[12,24] The prognosis of perforations also relates to the rapidity with which they are diagnosed and treated. If a perforation is noted, immediate repair with a bioceramic material offers the best chance for a successful outcome.[11,12,24–26] Any delays or microbial contamination of the perforation will adversely affect the prognosis[23,27] (Fig 10-18).

Better prognosis
- Smaller perforations
- Perforations located entirely within alveolar bone
- Immediate diagnosis and repair

Poorer prognosis
- Larger perforations
- Perforations associated with periodontal pockets
- Delayed diagnosis and repair

FIG 10-18 Several factors can impact the prognosis of perforations and their repair.

Perforations can be diagnosed visually, with instruments, and radiographically. Unexpected bleeding often is the first indication of a possible perforation. For example, unexpected bleeding during access of a tooth diagnosed with pulp necrosis warrants a pause in treatment so the clinician can confirm that the space accessed is indeed the pulp chamber or canal rather than a perforation. Teeth with pulpitis will often exhibit significant bleeding upon initial access, which can be difficult to differentiate from bleeding secondary to a furcal perforation.[23] Because sodium hypochlorite should never contact periradicular

tissues, including those exposed by a root perforation, if one is at all suspected, saline or distilled water should be used as the irrigation solution. In addition to bleeding, perforations themselves may be visible, particularly with the aid of a surgical operating microscope (Fig 10-19). Endodontic instruments can also be used to diagnose perforations. EALs can detect contact of a file with the PDL space. When perforations are present, the EALs will immediately read past the apex when the file contacts the defect. Essentially, an extraradicular reading will occur as soon as the file is introduced into the perforation.[23]

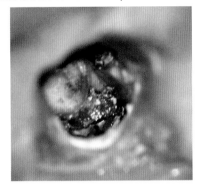

FIG 10-19 Perforations like this one in a maxillary premolar can be diagnosed visually, particularly with surgical operating microscopes. (Photo courtesy of Dr Stephanie Jue.)

Both 2D and 3D radiography can be used to diagnose perforations (Fig 10-20). To differentiate a canal space from a furcal perforation, a small file may be introduced and a periapical radiograph exposed for direct visualization. Previously treated or initiated teeth should be assessed preoperatively for the presence of perforations, which are often visible on bitewing or periapical radiographs, or with CBCT imaging. Prior iatrogenic perforations may present with bone loss adjacent to the perforation site and can easily be recognized with CBCT imaging.[28] These perforations have a poor prognosis for repair and represent a contraindication to nonsurgical retreatment.

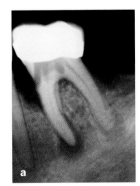
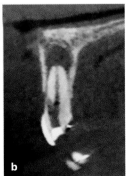

FIG 10-20 (a and b) Both 2D radiographs, like periapicals and bitewings, and 3D CBCT imaging can be used in perforation diagnosis.

Upon recognition, most perforations should be treated nonsurgically, though surgical intervention may be indicated under certain circumstances. If bone loss develops following nonsurgical repair of iatrogenic perforations or if significant material extrusion develops during nonsurgical repair, surgical repair is possible when performed according to the general principles of apical and periodontal surgery. Surgical procedures must be considered on a case-by-case basis and take into account surgical accessibility, the need for grafting material or membranes, and the overall expected prognosis of treatment.

Treatment also differs based on the location of the perforation. Supracrestal perforations should be sealed immediately given the risks of sodium hypochlorite leakage into the gingival space during treatment. Saliva leakage or bleeding within these perforations can pose difficulties in drying that can be overcome with surgical suction or the careful application of cotton pellets. For supracrestal perforations that are also supragingival, direct or indirect restorations are appropriate. For subgingival supracrestal perforations, the placement of resin-modified glass-ionomer repairs is advised according to the manufacturer's recommendations due to the risk of bioceramic washout in these areas.[29] Any signs of leakage during further treatment warrants immediate replacement. Large supracrestal perforations can pose restorative difficulties in the long term and may require additional procedures, such as crown-lengthening surgery, for effective management and restoration.

Perforations within the crestal bone are managed with bioceramic materials. Repairs should be completed under dental dam isolation, ideally prior to the continuation of nonsurgical endodontic procedures that require the use of sodium hypochlorite irrigation.

Subcrestal perforations should be gently rinsed with saline or sterile water and dried with a cotton pellet. The bioceramic material should be placed according to manufacturer instructions in direct contact with the periodontal ligament, with care taken to ensure that the entire area is sealed.[11,12,24–26] Because bioceramic materials are subject to washout, if any further instrumentation or irrigation is required during the same visit, a resin-modified glass-ionomer cement or resin seal can be placed on top of the bioceramic perforation repair[23,27] (Fig 10-21).

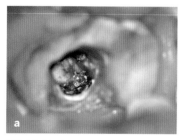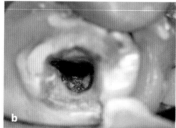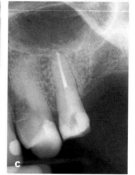

FIG 10-21 *(a to c)* Perforations should be sealed immediately with bioceramic materials. This perforation was sealed immediately with a bioceramic material and liner. (Case courtesy of Dr Stephanie Jue.)

Perforations within the canal space, including strip perforations that develop secondary to overinstrumentation of root curvatures, are challenging to manage because of likely contamination of the perforation from within the canal space, expected difficulties in effectively cleaning the root canal space without the use of sodium hypochlorite, and challenges in placing bioceramic materials within the canal space. That said, these perforations must be treated similarly to subcrestal perforations, including with the placement of a bioceramic filling material.

Prevention of perforations requires careful access and instrumentation techniques. Assessment of case difficulty is crucial when choosing whether to treat a tooth or refer out for specialized care. The use of magnification (especially a surgical operating microscope) and ultrasonic drills can minimize the risk of perforations, and intimate knowledge of tooth and root anatomy both in general and specific to the tooth in question is crucial prior to the initiation of endodontic access. Constant attention must be paid to anatomical landmarks and color changes in tooth structure as one approaches and moves away from calcified chamber anatomy. Radiographs should be used to confirm access angulation. Should a perforation develop, early recognition and management is key.

Sodium hypochlorite accident

Sodium hypochlorite accidents result from the spread of irrigant into the periradicular tissues. This spread causes severe pain and sudden onset tissue necrosis.[30] It most frequently occurs due to the binding of irrigation syringes in the canal spaces or in the presence of open apices or perforations. Sodium hypochlorite accidents are characterized by immediate, severe pain despite adequate anesthesia, profuse intracanal bleeding, swelling, and edema of the affected tissues.[31] Swelling can spread rapidly depending on the amount of sodium hypochlorite extruded and the local anatomy.[32] Sodium hypochlorite accidents are of clinical relevance because tissue necrosis may lead to nerve injury, and prolonged anesthesia and paresthesia may be late sequelae (Fig 10-22).[32] Furthermore, in the immediate aftermath of a sodium hypochlorite accident, swelling in areas adjacent to the airway can lead to its compromise. In these instances, care must be taken to monitor a patient's vital signs and to activate emergency medical services as needed.[32]

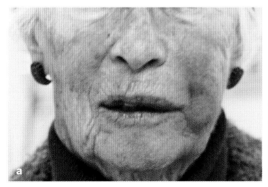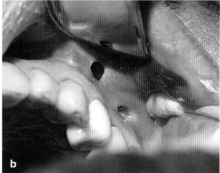

FIG 10-22 Rapid recognition and treatment of sodium hypochlorite accidents is essential to prevent long-term dysfunction. (a) This patient experienced an unrecognized hypochlorite accident and sought care several days later. By that time, swelling, numbness, and paralysis of the left facial musculature was present. (b) Severe infection along with tissue damage led to the opening of her alveolar mucosa in two places.

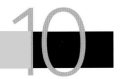

Immediate recognition of a sodium hypochlorite accident is critical. Emergency treatment should focus on controlling pain and diluting the sodium hypochlorite remaining in the affected area. The canal should be immediately irrigated with saline and local anesthetics, and additional local anesthetic can be injected. The area should be monitored to assess for compromise of vital structures. Pain control during the initial time frame should include oral analgesics and cold compresses.[32] After 24 hours, patients may switch to warm compresses to promote circulation. The use of steroids, though often suggested, is controversial and should be considered on a case-by-case basis depending on the extent of swelling and inflammation.[31] Daily monitoring of symptoms is recommended because late sequelae include infection and paresthesia.[31,32] Antibiotics are only indicated if signs and symptoms of infection arise, though they may be prescribed prophylactically in high-risk patients following consultation with their managing physician (Fig 10-23). Symptoms usually resolve within 1 month following a sodium hypochlorite accident.[33]

Immediate treatment	Follow-up care
• Irrigate tooth with saline or local anesthetic • Add additional local anesthetic in the surrounding soft tissues • Assess for compromise of vital structures and patient decompensation	• Cold packs to reduce swelling, followed by heat to promote circulation • Pain medication and potentially steroids • Antibiotics as needed • Daily follow-up

FIG 10-23 Proper care for a sodium hypochlorite accident.

Sodium hypochlorite accidents can be prevented by the use of side-vented needles (Fig 10-24), gentle irrigation pressure, and the cautious use of sodium hypochlorite near open apices or perforations. Generally, completion of the root canal therapy procedure that incited the sodium hypochlorite accident is possible; however, use of an alternative irrigation solution such as saline or chlorhexidine is advised due to remaining risk factors for a repeat sodium hypochlorite accident and the risks to already damaged tissues suffering further injury.

Material extrusion beyond the apex

Extrusion of intracanal medicaments and obturation materials can occur in any patent canal and becomes more likely in procedures performed without appropriate length control.[34] Most modern endodontic

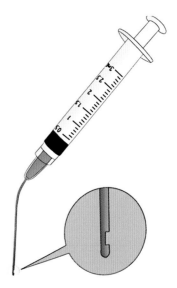

FIG 10-24 Side-vented needles should be used for endodontic irrigation to minimize the likelihood of sodium hypochlorite accidents.

materials will not cause long-lasting sequelae if extruded beyond the apex unless they contact at-risk anatomical structures, including the maxillary sinus, mental foramen, or inferior alveolar nerve canal.[34,35] Extrusion of materials into these vital structures cause serious consequences, including infection and paresthesia, and should be duly avoided.[34,36] Calcium hydroxide used as an intracanal medicament can cause localized tissue necrosis regardless of location, so care and attention to length control is imperative during its placement.[35]

Minimal extrusion of materials, including sealer puffs, has not been associated with negative sequelae (Fig 10-25). However, controversy exists as to whether or not material extrusion poses a risk of foreign body reactions.[37–40] Endodontic sealers of the lowest toxicity possible should be used in all circumstances, especially when proximal to susceptible spaces. For example, because eugenol-based endodontic sealers are known to both support certain fungal infections in the maxillary sinus[41] and contribute to nerve

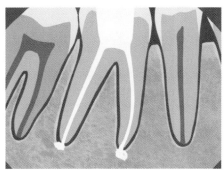

FIG 10-25 Minimal extrusion of materials and sealer puffs is not associated with negative sequelae.

toxicity when in contact with the inferior alveolar and mental nerves,[42] they should be avoided in the posterior maxilla and the posterior mandible.[43,44]

Treatment of significant extrusion is outside the scope of endodontic care and often requires referral to appropriate medical and oral surgical specialists. If materials are extruded into the inferior alveolar nerve canal, immediate referral for microsurgical removal is indicated.[34,45,46] Repairs performed within 24 to 48 hours have markedly improved success rates in the resolution of sensory neuropathies, whereas delays beyond this time frame result in poorer outcomes. Referral to otolaryngology specialists is advised if materials are extruded into the maxillary sinus.

Prevention of material extrusion is paramount. Early recognition and management of root perforations and careful working length control, especially in the case of open apices, are crucial to avoid these incidents.[34] Intracanal medicaments such as calcium hydroxide should be placed carefully within the confines of root canal anatomy and without any forceful injection into a canal space. This is of particular importance when using injectable medications where plastic or metal dispensing tips may be inadvertently bound in the root, forcing materials beyond the apices.[34] Care must be taken to place these medications without binding of the dispensing tip or with the use of a premeasured Lentulo spiral as an effective means to ensure introduction of the medication to the appropriate working length.

Thermal injury

Thermal injury to the periodontium is possible from procedures that generate heat within the canal that can be transferred to the root surface. This is true particularly with the use of ultrasonic instruments, high-speed handpieces, and heated devices for obturation.[47]

Using ultrasonics without coolant within the root for more than 20 seconds can dangerously raise root surface temperature.[48] Controlled heat sources used for obturation, such as the System B Heat Source (Kerr Dental) used below 250°F,[49] are considerably safer than noncontrolled heat sources and instruments heated by flame.[50]

Excessive heat from these sources can cause localized soft tissue necrosis and bone necrosis, along with significant discomfort and secondary infection. Necrosis can occur immediately during the procedure, or it may become visible in the several days postoperatively (Fig 10-26). If thermal injuries occur, management is case dependent and may involve consultation with outside specialists like oral surgeons or periodontists. Short-term management is palliative with analgesics and, potentially, antibiotics to prevent infection. Soft tissue necrosis and even bone necrosis may recover with palliative treatment to avoid infection, though certain injuries may require surgical debridement and result in permanent structural damage, including tooth loss (Fig 10-27).

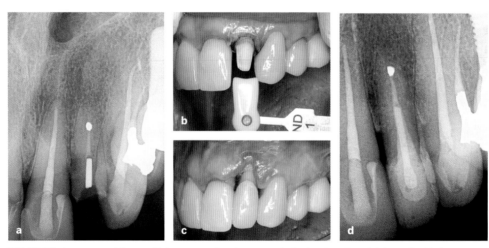

FIG 10-26 A presumed thermal injury secondary to removal of a fractured post *(a)* resulted in immediate irritation of the surrounding gingiva *(b)* that progressed to necrosis of the associated bone and sloughing of the overlying tissues 2 weeks later *(c and d)*.

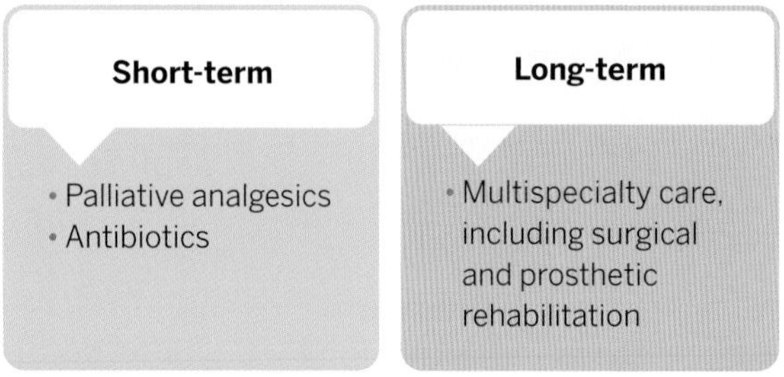

Short-term
- Palliative analgesics
- Antibiotics

Long-term
- Multispecialty care, including surgical and prosthetic rehabilitation

FIG 10-27 Management of thermal injuries.

The risk of thermal injuries increases with increased temperatures and the duration of application. As with all intraoperative complications, prevention of thermal injuries is key. Prevention strategies for thermal injuries secondary to nonsurgical endodontics include the use of cooling irrigants with ultrasonic and high-speed drills, taking breaks when using instruments like ultrasonics for long periods of time, and avoiding high or uncontrolled heat sources in obturation units.[49] Irrigation is also able to minimize uncontrolled heat from high-speed drills for osteotomy and root preparation during apical microsurgery[51] and from perforating drills used for intraosseous anesthesia.[52]

Flare-up

Flare-ups do not refer to normal postoperative pain. Rather, these involve an acute exacerbation of periradicular pathology. Flare-ups are thought to occur secondary to chemical, mechanical, and microbial insults generated during the endodontic procedure.[53] Flare-ups classically develop later than typical postoperative pain, often approximately 48 hours after treatment. They are characterized by worsening pain and possibly swelling, usually prompting a phone call or unscheduled visit to the clinician.[54] Flare-ups have a relatively low incidence, occurring in about 8% of cases after nonsurgical endodontics.[53] They most frequently occur in patients with high levels of preoperative pain and analgesic use.[55,56] Suggested associations with preoperative apical periodontitis or single versus multiple visits have not been definitively determined.[55,57–59] Flare-ups cannot be prevented with preemptive antibiotic use.[60,61]

All patients should be instructed about the possible occurrence of a flare-up during the informed consent process and in the postoperative instructions, with special emphasis for patients presenting with greater preoperative symptoms or analgesic use. Patients should be counseled that flare-ups are a rare postoperative complication and are not the result of poor care, and that their occurrence should have no undue effects on the completion of treatment or its prognosis.[60,62,63] Preemptive discussions about the possibility of a postoperative flare-up during consent and postoperative conversations and the provision of emergency contacts to the patient in case a flare-up occurs are part and parcel to their management.

When they develop, flare-ups require palliative management, typically with analgesics; operative care to reopen the tooth for recleaning and medication; or incision and drainage if swelling is present. Systemic antibiotics are only indicated if swelling develops or spreads rapidly, is accompanied by systemic signs of infection, or presents in an immunocompromised individual.[64] Combination therapy analgesia with ibuprofen and acetaminophen up to the maximum recommended daily dosages is advised until flare-up symptoms pass.[65–67] Patients should be monitored via phone or in-person examination as appropriate until symptoms subside to ensure that needed interventions occur in case of progressive infections[68] (Fig 10-28).

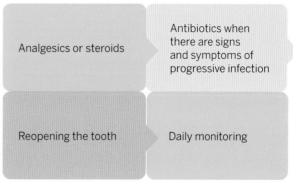

FIG 10-28 Treatment strategies for flare-ups.

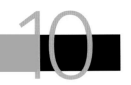

Paresthesia

Paresthesia refers to altered sensation, namely "pins and needles," pricking, or tingling, in the distribution of an injured nerve. Paresthesia in endodontics is most often associated with local anesthetic use, overextension of instruments and materials into the periapical tissues in close proximity to neural structures, and surgical intervention. Though a low risk of paresthesia exists with the administration of local anesthetics, provision of endodontic care does not pose any unique risks compared to anesthetics administered for other dental procedures. Generally, paresthesia is noted more commonly with the use of higher concentration anesthetic solutions, particularly 4% prilocaine and articaine administered via inferior alveolar nerve block.[69–71] The 4% solutions are presumed to exhibit a higher rate of neurotoxicity compared to lower concentration solutions, and their use is therefore not advised for block anesthesia. Even avoiding the use of high concentration solutions, postoperative paresthesia is possible whenever block anesthesia is delivered.[72] Some clinicians advise the use of oral corticosteroids to reduce inflammation that might contribute to paresthesia. However, limited evidence exists to support this practice over that of careful monitoring.

Paresthesia is also associated with the overextension of obturation materials, medicaments, and irrigants into the periapical tissues leading to nerve damage.[73,74] When obturation materials or medicaments are extruded into the inferior alveolar nerve canal or in close proximity to the mental foramen, patients should be immediately referred for oral surgical consultation because there is some evidence that rapid removal of the materials and decompression leads to better long-term outcomes[75] (Fig 10-29). Finally, paresthesia may be associated with surgical intervention. Transient paresthesia may occur following apical microsurgery given the potential for severance of superficial neural structures within the flap. If major nerve bundles are not damaged, the spontaneous recovery of nerve sensibility can be expected within weeks or months.[76] Less than 1% of affected patients will experience permanent sensory deficits.[77] If there is any suspicion of damage to any major nerve bundles, immediate referral to a specialist capable of microsurgical nerve repair is indicated. Otherwise, close clinical follow-up with mapping of sensory deficits can be performed to monitor recovery.[76]

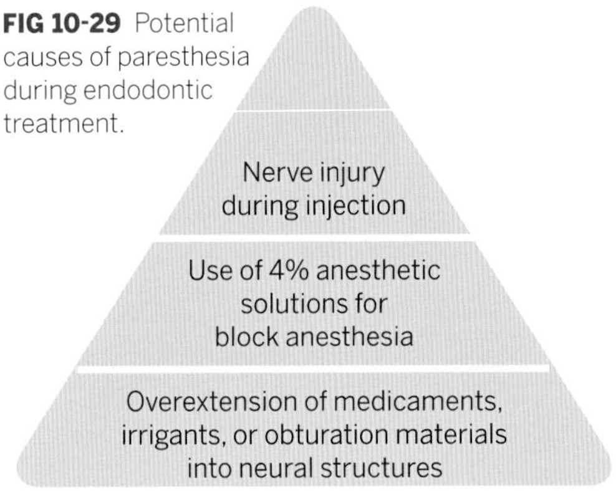

FIG 10-29 Potential causes of paresthesia during endodontic treatment.

Nerve injury during injection

Use of 4% anesthetic solutions for block anesthesia

Overextension of medicaments, irrigants, or obturation materials into neural structures

Persistent pain

Postoperative discomfort is normal in endodontics and lasts an average of 2 days following treatment. Pain that persists beyond 7 days following endodontic therapy is atypical.[78] That said, pain that persists more than 6 months postoperatively occurs in about 5% of patients and is referred to as persistent pain.[79] Certain factors are associated with an increased risk for persistent pain, including female sex, comorbid chronic pain disorders, and the presence of preoperative pain, particularly preoperative mechanical allodynia (ie, percussion tenderness).[80]

Patients experiencing persistent pain should be carefully examined to determine the cause of symptoms. First and foremost, complications secondary to the endodontic treatment should be ruled out. In some cases, persistent pain is representative of a preoperative misdiagnosis or secondary diagnosis, including incomplete endodontic treatment. In others, the persistent pain is truly idiopathic.[81,82] Clinicians must be willing to question their own initial diagnostics and treatment just as they would other clinicians'. Careful diagnostics following the same principles and practice as recommended preoperatively should be followed to ensure that symptoms are indeed secondary to the tooth in question rather than the result of referred pain. Therefore, neighboring teeth in the affected quadrant and opposing arch should be examined. Occlusal trauma should be ruled out and necessary adjustments made. CBCT imaging can rule out obvious causes of endodontic failure, including untreated anatomy, enlarging periapical pathology, and evidence of root fracture.

If no other etiologies, sources of infection, or comorbid diagnoses can be determined, pain is presumed idiopathic until something else presents.[82] The term *idiopathic pericementitis* may be used to describe the persistent inflammation that occurs following complete endodontic therapy in the absence of other causes. Essentially, the PDL is presumed to be inflamed because of the inciting endodontic pathology, the trauma of endodontic therapy, or some combination of both. In many cases, this inflammation is self-limiting and will resolve on its own. In others, the tooth may remain symptomatic in perpetuity. Oral corticosteroid medications, including methylprednisolone dose packs or dexamethasone, are often suggested for their anti-inflammatory action, but in practice, the relief they provide is inconsistent (Fig 10-30).

Patients suffering from persistent pain sometimes find solace in the work-up to rule out obvious sources of pathology with known interventions, and they are often understanding of a tooth that feels "different" than neighboring teeth. These patients should be monitored in case further symptoms or pathology lead to a more definitive diagnosis that warrants intervention. Other patients may have severe enough symptoms that they instead elect to have a persistently symptomatic tooth extracted.

Any suspicion of alternative odontogenic or nonodontogenic sources of pain should be thoroughly investigated. Ruling out neuropathic pain is imperative to ensure that patients do not needlessly suffer. Special attention to rule out persistent dentoalveolar pain disorder will ensure that patients will

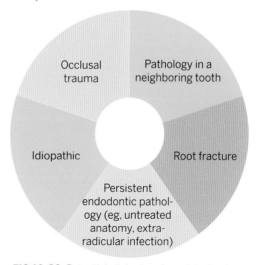

FIG 10-30 Potential etiologies of persistent pain following endodontic treatment.

not have persistent pain even following an extraction.[83] Regardless of the patient's ultimate decision, all choices must involve a confident diagnosis.

Discoloration treated with internal bleaching

Internal bleaching involves the use of chemical oxidizing agents within the coronal portion of an endodontically treated tooth to remove staining caused by internal discoloration of the dentin.[84] Case selection and counseling is especially important when considering internal bleaching. All patients should be counseled about the need for full-coverage restorative care if bleaching is unsuccessful. Organic staining caused by necrotic pulp tissue, infectious debris, and incomplete tissue removal are generally more susceptible to bleaching than inorganic stains caused by metal-containing restorative materials.[85,86] Intrinsic staining, such as that attributed to the childhood use of tetracycline family drugs, may also be less treatable than staining from topical agents, such as with triple antibiotic pastes[87] or mineral trioxide aggregate filling materials[88] (Fig 10-31).

Most susceptible	Moderately susceptible	Least susceptible
• Organic staining caused by blood byproducts, necrotic tissue debris, or bacteria	• Stains caused by the application of antibiotic pastes • Stains caused by bioceramic materials	• Stains caused by metal restorative materials • Intrinsic staining due to the use of antibiotics during childhood

FIG 10-31 Causes of stains that are more and less susceptible to internal bleaching.

The safe and recommended protocol for internal bleaching is called *walking bleach*.[89] Preoperative photos, ideally taken in natural light, should be available for ready comparison of treatment progress (Fig 10-32). Though anesthesia is not usually necessary for internal bleaching, dental dam placement is required, and the rest of the required armamentarium for internal bleaching is shown in Fig 10-33. Access should expose the full extent of the pulp chamber, and all restorative materials in contact with the dentinal walls should be removed. Any remaining tissue fragments within pulp horns should also be removed, along with overextensions of gutta-percha within the exposed portion of the crown, so that the bleaching agent can reach all extensions and fins of the pulp chamber. Gutta-percha should be removed to a level below the cementoenamel junction (CEJ), and placement of a resin-modified glass-ionomer base is advisable over the gutta-percha to the height of the CEJ to minimize the long-term risk of cervical resorption, though certainly this risk has decreased with newer bleaching protocols.[89]

FIG 10-32 Before *(a and b)* and after *(c and d)* photographs are helpful to monitor progress during internal bleaching treatment.

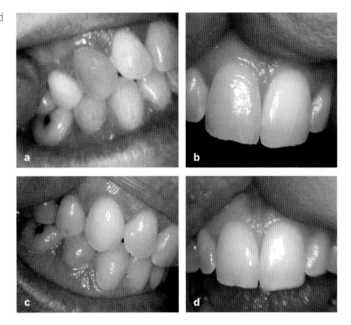

FIG 10-33 Armamentarium for internal bleaching should include a mouth mirror, explorer, periodontal probe, cotton pliers, spoon excavator, amalgam carrier, plastic instrument, Schilder pluggers or similar gutta-percha pluggers, irrigation needles and saline or sterile water, sodium perborate, paper points, and temporary restorative materials.

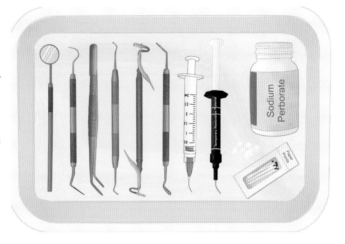

The bleaching agent is then introduced into the pulp chamber. Commercially available internal bleaching agents can be used, but sodium perborate is considered both safe and effective (Fig 10-34). Though improved bleaching can be attained with thermocatalytic bleaching techniques that combine heat and oxidizing agents or stronger agents such as Superoxol, these agents are known to cause external cervical resorption.[90–92] Thus, escalating bleaching efforts with these agents is ill-advised. The sodium perborate should be mixed with a small amount of saline or sterile water and placed into the pulp chamber with an amalgam carrier or spoon excavator. Excess moisture should be dried with an absorbent paper point, and 2 to 3 mm of temporary restorative material should be used to seal the access.

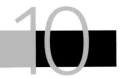

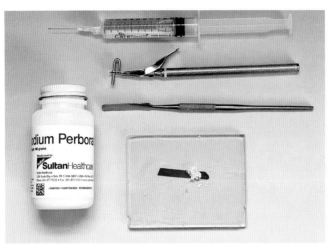

FIG 10-34 A combination of sodium perborate and saline is a safe and effective means for the provision of internal bleaching. The mixture can easily be applied to a tooth using an amalgam carrier or spoon excavator.

After 7 to 10 days, the patient should return for clinical assessment. Follow-up photography in similar lighting conditions can be used to evaluate color change. Patients should be involved in the decision to stop or continue bleaching, with the aid of a mirror during discussions. If clinician and patient are satisfied with the esthetic result, the tooth should be isolated with a dental dam, re-accessed, and the chamber rinsed clean of the bleaching agent with sterile water or saline. The chamber should be dried, and a temporary or immediate definitive restoration can be placed. If continued bleaching is desired, the sodium perborate protocol should be repeated following rinsing of the expired material. The bleaching process can be repeated several times, though diminishing returns are expected. Patients should be informed that regression of bleaching is possible, warranting consideration of future rebleaching. Of course, when satisfactory results are not achievable following safe protocols for internal bleaching, full-coverage ceramic restorations remain the best alternative.

References

1. Beus H, Fowler S, Drum M, et al. What is the outcome of an incision and drainage procedure in endodontic patients? A prospective, randomized, single-blind study. J Endod 2018;44:193–201.
2. Asgary S, Eghbal MJ. The effect of pulpotomy using a calcium-enriched mixture cement versus one-visit root canal therapy on postoperative pain relief in irreversible pulpitis: A randomized clinical trial. Odontology 2010;98:126–133.
3. Elmsmari F, Ruiz XF, Miró Q, Feijoo-Pato N, Durán-Sindreau F, Olivieri JG. Outcome of partial pulpotomy in vicariously exposed posterior permanent teeth: A systematic review and meta-analysis. J Endod 2019; 45:1296.e3–1306.e3.
4. Pashley EL, Myers DR, Pashley DH, Whitford GM. Systemic distribution of 14C-formaldehyde from formocresol-treated pulpotomy sites. J Dent Res 1980;59:602–608.
5. Concerning paraformaldehyde-containing endodontic filling materials and sealers. AAE Position Statement. American Association of Endodontists, 2017. https://www.aae.org/specialty/wp-content/uploads/sites/2/2017/06/paraformaldehydefillingmaterials.pdf. Accessed 31 March 2023.
6. Rosenberg PA, Babick PJ, Schertzer L, Leung A. The effect of occlusal reduction on pain after endodontic instrumentation. J Endod 1998;24:492–496.
7. Roberts RM, Bohm MK, Bartoces MG, Fleming-Dutra KE, Hicks LA. Chalmers NI. Antibiotic and opioid prescribing for dental-related conditions in emergency departments. J Am Dent Assoc 2020;151:174.e1–181.e1.

8. Johnson M. Antibiotics and the treatment of dental infections. Endodontics: Colleagues for Excellence. American Association of Endodontists, Fall 2019.

9. Case Assessment Tools. American Association of Endodontists, 2022. https://www.aae.org/specialty/clinical-resources/treatment-planning/case-assessment-tools/. Accessed 31 March 2023.

10. Jafarzadeh H, Abbott PV. Ledge formation: Review of a great challenge in endodontics. J Endod 2007;33:1155–1162.

11. Mente J, Leo M, Panagidis D, Saure D, Pfefferle T. Treatment outcome of mineral trioxide aggregate: Repair of root perforations—Long-term results. J Endod 2014;40:790–796.

12. Siew K, Lee AHC, Cheung GSP. Treatment outcome of repaired root perforation: A systematic review and meta-analysis. J Endod 2015;41:1795–1804.

13. Goldberg F, Massone EJ. Patency file and apical transportation: An in vitro study. J Endod 2002;28:510–511.

14. Iqbal MK, Kohli MR, Kim JS. A retrospective clinical study of incidence of root canal instrument separation in an endodontics graduate program: A PennEndo database study. J Endod 2006;32:1048–1052.

15. Suter B, Lussi A, Sequeira P. Probability of removing fractured instruments from root canals. Int Endod J 2005;38:112–123.

16. Madarati AA, Hunter MJ, Dummer PMH. Management of intracanal separated instruments. J Endod 2013;39:569–581.

17. Ward JR, Parashos P, Messer HH. Evaluation of an ultrasonic technique to remove fractured rotary nickel-titanium endodontic instruments from root canals: An experimental study. J Endod 2003;29:756–763.

18. Fu M, Zhang Z, Hou B. Removal of broken files from root canals by using ultrasonic techniques combined with dental microscope: A retrospective analysis of treatment outcome. J Endod 2011;37:619–622.

19. Crump MC, Natkin E. Relationship of broken root canal instruments to endodontic case prognosis: A clinical investigation. J Am Dent Assoc 1970;80:1341–1347.

20. Spili P, Parashos P, Messer HH. The impact of instrument fracture on outcome of endodontic treatment. J Endod 2005;31:845–850.

21. Smith A, Dickson M, Aitken J, Bagg J. Contaminated dental instruments. J Hosp Infect 2002;51:233–235.

22. Glossary of Endodontic Terms, ed 10. American Association of Endodontists, 2020. https://www.aae.org/specialty/clinical-resources/glossary-endodontic-terms/. Accessed 31 March 2023.

23. Fuss Z, Trope M. Root perforations: Classification and treatment choices based on prognostic factors. Endod Dent Traumatol 1996;12:255–264.

24. Gorni FG, Ionescu AC, Ambrogi F, Brambilla E, Gagliani MM. Prognostic factors and primary healing on root perforation repaired with MTA: A 14-year longitudinal study. J Endod 2022;48:1092–1099.

25. Pitt Ford TR, Torabinejad M, McKendry DJ, Hong CU, Kariyawasam SP. Use of mineral trioxide aggregate for repair of furcal perforations. Oral Surg Oral Med Oral Pathol Oral Radiol Endod 1995;79:756–763.

26. Lee SJ, Monsef M, Torabinejad M. Sealing ability of a mineral trioxide aggregate for repair of lateral root perforations. J Endod 1993;19:541–544.

27. Seltzer S, Sinai I, August D. Periodontal effects of root perforations before and during endodontic procedures. J Dent Res 1970;49:332–339.

28. Shemesh H, Cristescu RC, Wesselink PR, Wu MK. The use of cone-beam computed tomography and digital periapical radiographs to diagnose root perforations. J Endod 2011;37:513–516.

29. Dragoo MR. Resin-ionomer and hybrid-ionomer cements: Part II, human clinical and histologic wound healing responses in specific periodontal lesions. Int J Periodontics Restorative Dent 1997;17:75–87.

30. Sabala CL, Powell SE. Sodium hypochlorite injection into periapical tissues. J Endod 1989;15:490–492.

31. Guivarc'h M, Ordioni U, Ahmed HMA, Cohen S, Catherine JH, Bukiet F. Sodium hypochlorite accident: A systematic review. J Endod 2017;43:16–24.

32. Hülsmann M, Hahn W. Complications during root canal irrigation—Literature review and case reports. Int Endod J 2000;33:186–193.

33. Kleier DJ, Averbach RE, Mehdipour O. The sodium hypochlorite accident: Experience of diplomates of the American Board of Endodontics. J Endod 2008;34:1346–1350.

34. Berman LH, Gluskin AH. Endodontics and neurovascular injury. Endodontics: Colleagues for Excellence. American Association of Endodontists, Fall 2021.

35. De Moor RJG, De Witte AMJC. Periapical lesions accidentally filled with calcium hydroxide. Int Endod J 2002;35:946–958.

36. Rowe AH. Damage to the inferior dental nerve during or following endodontic treatment. Br Dent J 1983;155:306–307.

37. Schilder H. Filling root canals in three dimensions. Dent Clin North Am 1967:723–744.

38. Sjögren U, Ohlin A, Sundqvist G, Lerner UH. Gutta-percha-stimulated mouse macrophages release factors that activate the bone resorptive system of mouse calvarial bone. Eur J Oral Sci 1998;106:872–881.

39. Sjögren U, Sundqvist G, Nair PN. Tissue reaction to gutta-percha particles of various sizes when implanted subcutaneously in guinea pigs. Eur J Oral Sci 1995;103:313–321.

40. Seltzer S, Soltanoff W, Smith J. Biologic aspects of endodontics. V. Periapical tissue reactions to root canal instrumentation beyond the apex and root canal fillings short of and beyond the apex. Oral Surg Oral Med Oral Pathol 1973;36:725–737.
41. Giardino L, Pontieri F, Savoldi E, Tallarigo F. Aspergillus mycetoma of the maxillary sinus secondary to overfilling of a root canal. J Endod 2006;32:692–694.
42. Kozam G. The effect of eugenol on nerve transmission. Oral Surg Oral Med Oral Pathol 1977;44:799–805.
43. Kang SH, Kim BS, Kim Y. Proximity of posterior teeth to the maxillary sinus and buccal bone thickness: A biometric assessment using cone-beam computed tomography. J Endod 2015;41:1839–1846.
44. Pagin O, Centurion BS, Rubira-Bullen IRF, Alvares Capelozza AL. Maxillary sinus and posterior teeth: Accessing close relationship by cone-beam computed tomographic scanning in a Brazilian population. J Endod 2013;39:748–751.
45. Pogrel MA. Damage to the inferior alveolar nerve as the result of root canal therapy. J Am Dent Assoc 2007;138:65–69.
46. Rosen E, Goldberger T, Taschieri S, Del Fabbro M, Corbella S, Tsesis I. The prognosis of altered sensation after extrusion of root canal filling materials: A systematic review of the literature. J Endod 2016;42:873–879.
47. Eriksson AR, Albrektsson T. Temperature threshold levels for heat-induced bone tissue injury: A vital-microscopic study in the rabbit. J Prosthet Dent 1983;50:101–107.
48. Davis S, Gluskin AH, Livingood PM, Chambers DW. Analysis of temperature rise and the use of coolants in the dissipation of ultrasonic heat buildup during post removal. J Endod 2010;36:1892–1896.
49. Floren JW, Weller RN, Pashley DH, Kimbrough WF. Changes in root surface temperatures with in vitro use of the system B HeatSource. J Endod 1999;25:593–595.
50. Lee FS, Van Cura JE, BeGole E. A comparison of root surface temperatures using different obturation heat sources. J Endod 1998;24:617–620.
51. Nicoll BK, Peters RJ. Heat generation during ultrasonic instrumentation of dentin as affected by different irrigation methods. J Periodontol 1998;69:884–888.
52. Woodmansey KF, White RK, He J. Osteonecrosis related to intraosseous anesthesia: Report of a case. J Endod 2009;35:288–291.
53. Tsesis I, Faivishevsky V, Fuss Z, Zukerman O. Flare-ups after endodontic treatment: A meta-analysis of literature. J Endod 2008;34:1177–1181.
54. Walton RE. Interappointment flare-ups: Incidence, related factors, prevention, and management. Endod Topics 2002;3:67–76.
55. Torabinejad M, Kettering JD, McGraw JC, Cummings RR, Dwyer TG, Tobias TS. Factors associated with endodontic interappointment emergencies of teeth with necrotic pulps. J Endod 1988;14:261–266.
56. Walton R, Fouad A. Endodontic interappointment flare-ups: A prospective study of incidence and related factors. J Endod 1992;18:172–177.
57. Iqbal M, Kurtz E, Kohli M. Incidence and factors related to flare-ups in a graduate endodontic programme. Int Endod J 2009;42:99–104.
58. Trope M. Flare-up rate of single-visit endodontics. Int Endod J 1991;24:24–26.
59. Eleazer PD, Eleazer KR. Flare-up rate in pulpally necrotic molars in one-visit versus two-visit endodontic treatment. J Endod 1998;24:614–616.
60. Walton RE, Chiappinelli J. Prophylactic penicillin: Effect on posttreatment symptoms following root canal treatment of asymptomatic periapical pathosis. J Endod 1993;19:466–470
61. Pickenpaugh L, Reader A, Beck M, Meyers WJ, Peterson LJ. Effect of prophylactic amoxicillin on endodontic flare-up in asymptomatic, necrotic teeth. J Endod 2001;27:53–56.
62. Sjögren U, Hagglund B, Sundqvist G, Wing K. Factors affecting the long-term results of endodontic treatment. J Endod 1990;16:498–504.
63. Friedman S, Abitbol S, Lawrence HP. Treatment outcome in endodontics: The Toronto Study. Phase 1: Initial treatment. J Endod 2003;29:787–793.
64. Johnson M. Antibiotics and the treatment or dental infections. Endodontics: Colleagues for Excellence. American Association of Endodontists, Fall 2019.
65. Richards D. The Oxford Pain Group League table of analgesic efficacy. Evid Based Dent 2004;5:22–23.
66. Menhinick KA, Gutmann J, Regan JD, Taylor SE, Buschang PH. The efficacy of pain control following nonsurgical root canal treatment using ibuprofen or a combination of ibuprofen and acetaminophen in a randomized, double-blind, placebo-controlled study. Int Endod J 2004;37:531–541.
67. Derry CJ, Derry S, Moore RA. Single dose oral ibuprofen plus paracetamol (acetaminophen) for acute postoperative pain. Cochrane Database Syst Rev 2013;2013:CD010210.
68. Shemesh A, Yitzhak A, Ben Itzhak J, Azizi H, Solomonov M. Ludwig angina after first aid treatment: Possible etiologies and prevention—Case report. J Endod 2019;45:79–82.
69. Gaffen AS, Haas DA. Retrospective review of voluntary reports of nonsurgical paresthesia in dentistry. J Can Dent Assoc 2009;75:579.
70. Haas DA, Lennon D. A 21-year retrospective study of reports of paresthesia following local anesthetic administration. J Can Dent Assoc 1995;61:319–320, 323–326, 329–330.

71. Garisto GA, Gaffen AS, Lawrence HP, Tenenbaum HC, Haas DA. Occurrence of paresthesia after dental local anesthetic administration in the United States. J Am Dent Assoc 2010;141:836–844.
72. Pogrel MA, Thamby S. Permanent nerve involvement resulting from inferior alveolar nerve blocks. J Am Dent Assoc 2000;131:901–907.
73. Ahlgren FKEK, Johannessen AC, Hellem S. Displaced calcium hydroxide paste causing inferior alveolar nerve paraesthesia: Report of a case. Oral Surg Oral Med Oral Pathol Oral Radiol Endod 2003;96:734–737.
74. Matthews J, Merrill RL. Sodium hypochlorite-related injury with chronic pain sequelae. J Am Dent Assoc 2014;145:553–555.
75. Gluskin AH. Anatomy of an overfill: A reflection on the process. Endod Topics 2009;16:64–81.
76. Kim S, Pecora G. Color Atlas of Microsurgery in Endodontics. Philadelphia: Saunders, 2001.
77. Wesson CM, Gale TM. Molar apicectomy with amalgam root-end filling: Results of a prospective study in two district general hospitals. Br Dent J 2003;195:707–714.
78. Law AS, Nixdorf DR, Rabinowitz I, et al. Root canal therapy reduces multiple dimensions of pain: A national dental practice-based research network study. J Endod 2014;40:1738–1745.
79. Nixdorf DR, Moana-Filho EJ, Law AS, McGuire LA, Hodges JS, John MT. Frequency of persistent tooth pain after root canal therapy: A systematic review and meta-analysis. J Endod 2010;36:224–230.
80. Polycarpou N, Ng YL, Canavan D, Moles DR, Gulabivala K. Prevalence of persistent pain after endodontic treatment and factors affecting its occurrence in cases with complete radiographic healing. Int Endod J 2005;38:169–178.
81. Nixdorf DR, Moana-Filho EJ, Law AS, McGuire LA, Hodges JS, John MT. Frequency of nonodontogenic pain after endodontic therapy: A systematic review and meta-analysis. J Endod 2010;36:1494–1498.
82. Vena DA, Collie D, Wu H, et al. Prevalence of persistent pain 3 to 5 years post primary root canal therapy and its impact on oral health-related quality of life: PEARL Network findings. J Endod 2014;40:1917–1921.
83. Malacarne A, Spierings ELH, Lu C, Maloney GE. Persistent dentoalveolar pain disorder: A comprehensive review. J Endod 2018;44:206–211.
84. Spasser H. A simple bleaching technique using sodium perborate. NYS Dent J 1961;27:332–334.
85. Glockner K, Hulla H, Ebeleseder K, Städtler P. Five-year follow-up of internal bleaching. Braz Dent J 1999;10:105–110.
86. Walton RE, O'Dell NL, Lake FT, Shimp RG. Internal bleaching of tetracycline-stained teeth in dogs. J Endod 1983;9:416–420.
87. Kirchhoff AL, Raldi DP, Salles AC, Cunha RS, Mello I. Tooth discolouration and internal bleaching after the use of triple antibiotic paste. Int Endod J 2015;48:1181–1187.
88. Belobrov I, Parashos P. Treatment of tooth discoloration after the use of white mineral trioxide aggregate. J Endod 2011;37:1017–1020.
89. Friedman S. Internal bleaching: Long-term outcomes and complications. J Am Dent Assoc 1997;128(suppl):51S–55S.
90. Nutting EB, Poe GS. Chemical bleaching of discolored endodontically treated teeth. Dent Clin North Am 1967:655–662.
91. Madison S, Walton R. Cervical root resorption following bleaching of endodontically treated teeth. J Endod 1990;16:570–574.
92. Lou EK, Cathro P, Marino V, Damiani F, Heithersay GS. Evaluation of hydroxyl radical diffusion and acidified thiourea as a scavenger during intracoronal bleaching. J Endod 2016;42:1126–1130.

PART III

Adjunctive Endodontic Diagnoses and Treatments

The specialty of endodontics is grounded in the diagnosis and treatment of orofacial pain and infection. While the pulpal and periapical diagnoses discussed in part I and the treatment strategies discussed in part II address the most common presentations of endodontic pathology, adjunctive diagnoses are also frequently encountered in the field. This section discusses the most common adjunctive diagnoses and their treatments, including fractures, resorptive dental diseases, periodontal-endodontic infections, and dental trauma.

Fractures

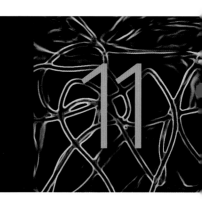

C racks and fractures are direct and indirect contributors to endodontic pathology.[1] They may lead to pulpal exposure or simply expose deeper recesses of the tooth to microbial irritants, causing associated inflammatory changes that can progress from pulpitis to necrosis.[2,3] Cracks are typically described as more shallow than fractures, but there is no consensus on the threshold dividing the two terms. The American Association of Endodontist's (AAE) Glossary of Endodontic Terms divides dental fractures into traumatic fractures that originate in the crown structure and root fractures that extend horizontally or vertically within the root structure.[4] Traumatic fractures include infractions, enamel fractures, enamel-dentin fractures, enamel-dentin-pulp fractures, and crown-root fractures. Despite using the term "traumatic" to describe them, these fractures do not always occur secondary to acute dental trauma but may result from more chronic occlusal forces. Compared to terminology defined in the AAE's trauma guidelines,[5,6] these fractures overlap in definition with *crown fractures* and *crown-root fractures*. Root fractures include horizontal root fractures and longitudinal fractures, including vertical root fractures and split roots (Fig 11-1). Unseparated fractures, wherein there is a fracture line but no loss of tooth structure, do not fit into this classification system well and will be discussed separately. The AAE glossary classification system differs from that of the AAE trauma guidelines.

Traumatic fractures	Root fractures

• Infractions
• Enamel fractures
• Enamel-dentin fractures
• Enamel-dentin-pulp fractures
• Crown-root fractures
	• Horizontal root fractures
	• Longitudinal root fractures
	  – Vertical root fractures
	  – Split roots

FIG 11-1 AAE Glossary of Endodontic Terms fracture classification.[4]

Consequently, the diagnosis and management of traumatic fractures is discussed in chapter 14.

In general, fractures are identified clinically. Certain diagnostic tools are more useful than others for the detection of fractures. Beyond direct visualization, the use of magnification, methylene blue or vegetable dyes, and transillumination may aid the clinician in directly observing fractures.[7,8] Photography can be useful for documentation, especially to establish a baseline for follow-up. Thermal and biting tests can be particularly useful to determine the potential pulpal effects of a suspected fracture. The periodontal examination, namely the measurement of periodontal probing depths, is an essential tool in determining root fracture involvement because attachment loss will follow the fracture line.

Typically, only large and separated fractures are visible with 2D radiographic examination. Unseparated fractures must sit within four degrees of the plane of the image to be seen with 2D imaging[9] (Fig 11-2). As a result, fractures can be detected more frequently with CBCT imaging. That said, resolution issues coupled with artifacts caused by radiopaque restorative materials, including posts and obturation material, may limit the utility of CBCT imaging in visualizing fracture lines.[10] CBCT imaging is often more useful to detect periradicular changes associated with fracture extension to the root structure. These findings include localized crestal bony defects, mid-root bone loss without adjacent coronal or apical bone loss, defects that are present on opposite walls of the tooth because of pathology developing on either end of a fracture line, and loss of the entire buccal plate or a space between the buccal or lingual plate and the root surface[11,12] (Fig 11-3).

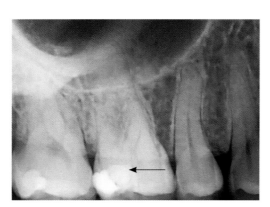

FIG 11-2 To be visualized with 2D imaging, the fracture line must sit within 4 degrees of the x-ray beam.

Localized crestal bony defects

Mid-root bone loss without adjacent coronal or apical bone loss

Defects that appear 180 degrees to one another

Loss of the entire buccal plate

Space between the buccal or lingual cortical plate and the root surface

FIG 11-3 CBCT findings associated with root fractures.

It is important to note that these fracture diagnoses must be added to the pulpal and periapical endodontic diagnoses. Teeth subject to fracture may develop pulpally mediated disease due to the fracture itself or another comorbid injury.

Traumatic Fractures

In the context of fracture diagnosis, traumatic fractures are breaks in the tooth structure that occur either due to acute dental trauma, discussed in chapter 14, or causes related to heavily restored teeth combined with acute or chronic damage from occlusion. The type of fracture resulting depends on the extent of the injury.

Infractions, also called *craze lines*, exist as cracks in the enamel without any loss of tooth structure. Enamel fractures also exist only in the enamel but involve additional structural loss. Both infractions and enamel fractures are generally asymptomatic. Enamel-dentin fractures involve loss of tooth structure extending into dentin and are referred to as *uncomplicated crown fractures* in the AAE trauma guidelines and other references.[5,6] Enamel-dentin-pulp fractures involve a loss of tooth structure that exposes the pulp and are also called *complicated crown fractures*. Based on the extent of damage, thermal sensitivity and other pulpal symptoms may result from any of these more extensive fractures. Crown-root fractures involve enamel, dentin, and cementum, with or without pulpal exposure. These fractures have a variable presentation but often result in greater pulpal and periapical symptomatology depending on their extension.

Management of each type of traumatic fracture depends on the extent of tooth structure loss. Restorative care is warranted to replace lost tooth structure for all fracture types except infractions. The need for endodontic management is variable and may involve vital pulp therapy or nonsurgical root canal therapy (NSRCT), particularly when posts are part of the restorative plan. Interdisciplinary treatment planning is often required due to the complexity of crown-root fractures. Unlike fractures resulting from traumatic dental injuries, follow-up needs for fractures of other causes are generally less involved. For more details on the diagnosis and treatment of coronal fractures occurring secondary to traumatic dental injuries, refer to chapter 14.

Root Fractures

The AAE Glossary of Endodontic Terms divides root fractures into horizontal root fractures and longitudinal root fractures.[4] Most horizontal root fractures are traumatic in origin and are therefore discussed in detail in chapter 14. That said, clinicians should be aware that horizontal root fractures may also develop secondary to occlusal trauma or parafunction.[13,14] These horizontal root fractures are more often found in older patients with comorbid periodontal disease (Fig 11-4).[13]

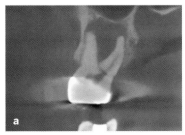 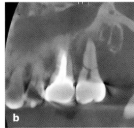 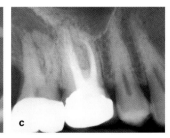

FIG 11-4 Horizontal root fractures in posterior teeth are frequently associated with bruxism and comorbid periodontal disease as opposed to acute dental trauma. These are often visible on coronal (*a*) and sagittal (*b*) sections of CBCT images as opposed to periapical (*c*) images, like with this fractured maxillary right second molar.

Fractures

Unlike horizontal root fractures, longitudinal fractures extend through the vertical plane of the tooth.[4] Fractures may be oriented buccolingually, mesiodistally, or obliquely and may originate either coronally or apically. Longitudinal root fractures most commonly occur in previously endodontically treated teeth[15] but may also occur in minimally restored or even unrestored teeth secondary to anatomical predispositions or parafunctional habits.[16] Longitudinal fractures in endodontically treated teeth are frequently, though not exclusively, associated with posts, particularly those that are large or long for the root into which they are fitted, resulting in excessive thinning of root dentin.[15,17] Longitudinal fractures in non-endodontically treated teeth invariably create a communication with pulpal tissues and frequently present with a pulpal diagnosis of necrosis[18] (Fig 11-5).

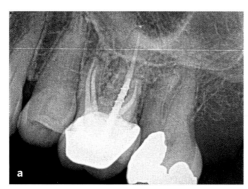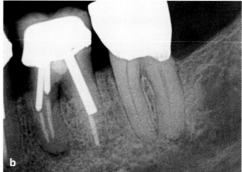

FIG 11-5 *(a and b)* Posts, particularly screw-type posts and wide posts that thin the root dentin, are associated with the development of longitudinal fractures.

The current terminology differentiates longitudinal root fractures into vertical root fractures and split roots, with the former describing incomplete longitudinal fractures that have not yet extended from crown to apex. Vertical root fractures are therefore narrower than split roots. Split roots are complete, longitudinally oriented fractures from crown to apex. Not infrequently, separation of fragments is radiographically visible and mobility is present between the halves of the split tooth (Fig 11-6).

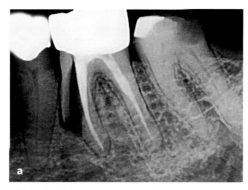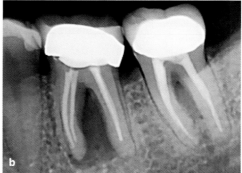

FIG 11-6 *(a)* Split roots involve the complete separation of fragments throughout the root. *(b)* Vertical root fracture involves incomplete separation.

Longitudinal fractures are problematic due to their invariable contamination with bacteria resulting in bone loss along the length of the fracture line.[19–21] This bone loss causes several typical findings, including the pathognomonic presentation of a narrow and isolated periodontal probing defect of greater than 5 mm depth adjacent to the fracture line.[15,19] Patients often present with multiple areas of drainage adjacent to the fracture line, manifesting as one or more sinus tracts. Sinus tracts associated with fracture are often more coronally positioned than the more apically positioned sinus tracts caused by apical periodontitis[15,19] (Fig 11-7). When this drainage is present, these fractures are often minimally or mildly symptomatic, with correspondingly minimal sensitivity to periapical tests expected. Pulp sensitivity tests will elicit responses consistent with the current pulp status.

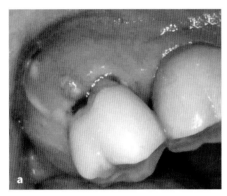 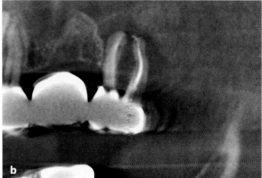

FIG 11-7 *(a)* Sinus tracts associated with teeth with vertical root fractures are often more coronally positioned, and multiple sinus tracts are often present. *(b)* This more coronal position reflects the drainage pathway via the apicomarginal bony defects noted on periapical radiographs or CBCT images.

The radiographic examination of teeth with longitudinal fractures does not often reveal fracture lines themselves. More often, fractures are suspected on radiograph based on the classical J-shaped or halo-like radiolucency seen in the adjacent periradicular bone.[12,20–22] CBCT imaging may be more useful in fracture detection, though posts and other radiodense root canal filling materials often found in teeth with longitudinal fractures can create beam-hardening artifacts that render these images nondiagnostic.[23,24] In the absence of artifacts, CBCT imaging is of particular utility in demonstrating the periradicular bony changes caused by fractures and can be helpful in determining fracture depth.[11,25] Radiographic halos in bone are often seen on opposing sides of a root, representative of inflammatory bone loss on opposing ends of the fracture, even if the fracture line itself is not visible. Periradicular bony defects often extend just to the terminal end of a post. Subcortical bone breakdown or a space between the root and the buccal or lingual cortical plate are also typical findings[11] (Fig 11-8).

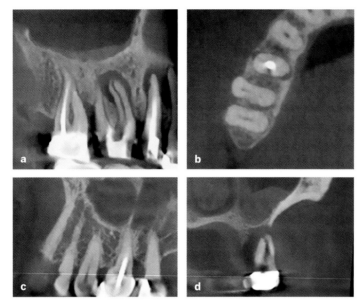

FIG 11-8 *(a)* CBCT images show fracture lines more frequently than periapical images. Even if visible fracture lines are absent, periradicular bony changes are commonly seen. These include *(b)* radiographic halos on opposing sides of a root, *(c)* bony defects extending to the apical end of a post, and *(d)* J-shaped lesions.

Whether incomplete, as vertical root fractures, or complete, as split roots, teeth with longitudinal root fractures require extraction. As of now, there is no material that can reinforce a fractured root without destruction of attachment tissues. Heroic procedures such as root amputations or hemisections leave behind weak structures that are subject to the same forces that resulted in the original fracture. Maintenance of these teeth leads not only to patient morbidity due to pain and infection but also to extensive bone loss that can negatively affect future replacement options.

Unseparated Fractures

Unseparated coronal fractures are common clinical findings. These may or may not be associated with symptoms. The diagnosis of unseparated fractures aims to understand the depth of these fracture lines as a crucial factor in both management and prognosis (Fig 11-9). Clinical examination of these teeth should include an exploration of the fracture for separation and a careful evaluation of the periodontal tissues, especially the probing depths surrounding the tooth.[20] 2D radiographs of these teeth will not often depict the fracture lines themselves or their concomitant bony changes. CBCT imaging more accurately depicts the periradicular changes that develop when fractures extend into root structure[11] (Fig 11-10).

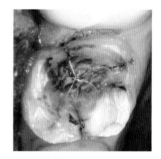

FIG 11-9 The diagnosis of teeth with unseparated fractures, like those depicted here, aims to account for both pulp status and fracture depth.

FIG 11-10 Unseparated fractures that extend into root structure will cause periradicular bony changes visible on CBCT imaging. *(a)* In sagittal sections, these changes amount to narrow angular bony defects. *(b)* In axial sections, semicircular interruptions in the periodontal ligament (PDL) space are visible.

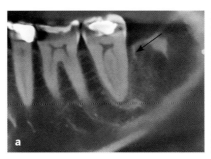
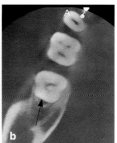

These clinical and radiographic findings aid clinicians' understanding of fracture depth, which directly impacts treatment planning. Fractures extending into root structure negatively impact the long-term prognosis of a tooth.[18,26,27] Additional factors associated with poor prognosis of fractured teeth include the presence of a periodontal probing measurement deeper than 6 mm adjacent to the fracture line,[28] a fracture involving the distal marginal ridge of a posterior tooth, a preoperative diagnosis of pulpal necrosis or an abnormal periapical diagnosis, and the presence of radiographically detectable marginal bone loss adjacent to the clinical fracture line[29] (Fig 11-11).

Periodontal probing depth > 6 mm

Pulpal necrosis

Fractures involving the distal marginal ridge

Radiographically visible marginal bone loss

FIG 11-11 Factors associated with poor prognosis for teeth with unseparated fractures.

Clinicians should develop their treatment recommendations for these teeth based on the pulpal and periapical diagnosis together with an understanding of the fracture depth. Asymptomatic fractures in teeth with normal clinical and radiographic findings are assumed to be shallow. These teeth may be monitored for progression with annual visual exams. Photographs should be considered as a means to document the fracture status. If a new or enlarging fracture line is seen, even if the tooth remains asymptomatic without signs of endodontic disease, full-coverage restorative care is recommended. Additionally, in patients with risk factors for fracture progression, like bruxism, full-coverage restorative care can be considered.

Symptomatic fractures often initially present with cold and biting sensitivity, though symptoms may be intermittent and difficult to replicate. Historically, the term *cracked tooth syndrome* was used to describe these symptomatic fractures.[30] However, this term is no longer recommended given its incompletely descriptive nature. Teeth with symptomatic fractures should undergo pulp sensitivity testing because treatment recommendations are impacted by the pulpal diagnosis. Teeth presenting with reversible pulpitis warrant consideration of a full-coverage restoration only because the majority of these teeth will not require endodontic therapy.[31,32] That said, restorative care should proceed cautiously in case the need for endodontic intervention arises. A temporary crown should be placed and symptoms and pulp sensitivity should be reassessed 2 to 3 weeks following temporization. If symptoms are absent and pulp sensitivity test results are normal, the definitive restoration can be placed. If symptoms remain despite temporization, nonsurgical endodontic therapy should be considered[33–36] (Fig 11-12).

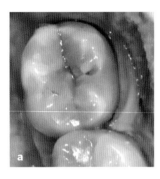 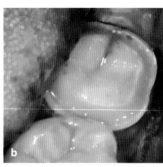

FIG 11-12 (a) Patients with unseparated fractures and symptoms of reversible pulpitis and biting discomfort often benefit from (b) full-coverage restorations. The tooth should be prepared and temporized and reassessed for symptom resolution. If symptoms resolve completely, no endodontic treatment is recommended. (Case courtesy of Dr Toby Kravitz.)

Teeth that present with symptomatic irreversible pulpitis or pulpal necrosis require NSRCT prior to placement of a full-coverage restoration, as long as the clinical and radiographic findings do not indicate fracture extension into root structure. The intraoperative use of a surgical operating microscope is advised for better visualization of the fracture and its extension because fractures crossing the pulpal floor and those greater than 5 mm beneath the canal orifice level have poorer prognoses.[26,27] Placement of an intraorifice barrier apical to the extent of the crack, the performance of occlusal reduction, and expedient placement of a full-coverage restoration are advised for the most favorable outcomes[27] (Fig 11-13).

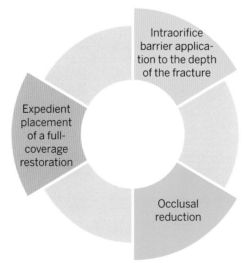

FIG 11-13 Factors associated with more favorable outcomes if intracoronal fractures are noted during endodontic treatment.

Cemental Tears

Cemental tears are localized infractions of the cementum overlying the root surface dentin without extension into pulpal structures (Fig 11-14). They develop most frequently in the incisors of older patients, most often due to occlusal trauma.[37,38] Cemental tears are often undetectable until secondary infection develops. Resultantly, symptoms typically include a localized area of swelling or drainage via a sinus tract. Pulp sensitivity tests, however, are frequently normal and indicative of vital tissue. In theory, cemental tears may be visible radiographically, particularly with the use of CBCT imaging, but limitations in resolution may make presurgical detection challenging (Fig 11-15). That said, radiographically detectable host-mediated bone loss due to infection is expected in these cases.

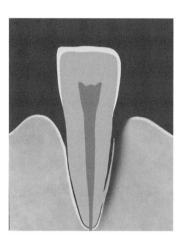

FIG 11-14 Cemental tears are localized infractions of the cementum overlying the root surface dentin without extension into pulpal structures

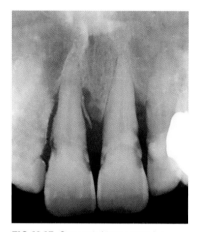

FIG 11-15 Cemental tears may be visible upon imaging, as in the case depicted here, though more frequently clinicians will notice only localized bony defects associated with the secondary infection of these tears. (Photo courtesy of Dr Jimmy Lu.)

Surgical access and visualization of the root surface is the most definitive means of diagnosing a cemental tear. Treatment aims to surgically remove the torn cementum. Regenerative periodontal therapy may be indicated in the presence of large defects. The prognosis is predicated on periodontal healing, with good success expected, particularly when the defects are noted in the apical or middle thirds of the root.[39]

References

1. Türp JC, Gobetti JP. The cracked tooth syndrome: An elusive diagnosis. J Am Dent Assoc 1996;127: 1502–1507.
2. Walton RE. Vertical root fracture: Factors related to identification. J Am Dent Assoc 2017;148:100–105.
3. Ricucci D, Siqueira JF Jr, Loghin S, Berman LH. The cracked tooth: Histopathologic and histobacteriologic aspects. J Endod 2015;41:343–352.
4. Glossary of Endodontic Terms, ed 10. American Association of Endodontists, 2020. https://www.aae.org/specialty/clinical-resources/glossary-endodontic-terms/. Accessed 3 April 2023.

5.   American Association of Endodontists. The Recommended Guidelines of the American Association of Endodontists for the Treatment of Traumatic Dental Injuries. 2013. https://www.aae.org/specialty/clinical-resources/treatment-planning/traumatic-dental-injuries. Accessed 3 April 2023.

6.   Bourguignon C, Cohenca N, Lauridsen E, et al. International Association of Dental Traumatology guidelines for the management of traumatic dental injuries: 1. Fractures and luxations. Dent Traumatol 2020;36:314–330.

7.   Friedman J, Marcus MI. Transillumination of the oral cavity with use of fiber optics. J Am Dent Assoc 1970;80:801–809.

8.   Wright HM Jr, Loushine RJ, Weller RN, Kimbrough WF, Waller J, Pashley DH. Identification of resected root-end dentinal cracks: A comparative study of transillumination and dyes. J Endod 2004;30:712–715.

9.   Rud J, Omnell KA. Root fracture due to corrosion. Diagnostic aspects. Scand J Dent Res 1970;78:397–403.

10.   Talwar S, Utneja S, Nawal RR, Kaushik A, Srivastava D, Oberoy SS. Role of cone-beam computed tomography in diagnosis of vertical root fractures: A systematic review and meta-analysis. J Endod 2016;42:12–24.

11.   Fayad MI, Ashkenaz PJ, Johnson BR. Different representations of vertical root fractures detected by cone-beam volumetric tomography: A case series report. J Endod 2012;38:1435–1442.

12.   Brady E, Mannocci F, Brown J, Wilson R, Patel S. A comparison of cone beam computed tomography and periapical radiography for the detection of vertical root fractures in nonendodontically treated teeth. Int Endod J 2014;47:735–746.

13.   Tsai YL, Liao WC, Wang CY, et al. Horizontal root fractures in posterior teeth without dental trauma: Tooth/root distribution and clinical characteristics. Int Endod J 2017;50:830–835.

14.   Clarkson RM, John K, Moule AJ. Horizontal palatal root fracture in a vital upper first premolar. J Endod 2015;41:759–761.

15.   Tsesis I, Rosen E, Tamse A, Taschieri S, Kfir A. Diagnosis of vertical root fractures in endodontically treated teeth based on clinical and radiographic indices: A systematic review. J Endod 2010;36:1455–1458.

16.   Chan CP, Tseng SC, Lin CP, Huang CC, Tsai TP, Chen CC. Vertical root fracture in nonendodontically treated teeth—A clinical report of 64 cases in Chinese patients. J Endod 1998;24:678–681.

17.   Cohen S, Blanco L, Berman L. Vertical root fractures: Clinical and radiographic diagnosis. J Am Dent Assoc 2003;134:434–441.

18.   Berman LH, Kuttler S. Fracture necrosis: Diagnosis, prognosis assessment, and treatment recommendations. J Endod 2010;36:442–446.

19.   Rivera E, Walton RE. Cracking the cracked tooth code: Detection and treatment of various longitudinal tooth fractures. Endodontics: Colleagues for Excellence, Summer 2008.

20.   Tamse A, Kaffe I, Lustig J, Ganor Y, Fuss Z. Radiographic features of vertically fractured endodontically treated mesial roots of mandibular molars. Oral Surg Oral Med Oral Pathol Oral Radiol Endod 2006;101:797–802.

21.   Tamse A, Fuss Z, Lustig J, Kaplavi J. An evaluation of endodontically treated vertically fractured teeth. J Endod 1999;25:506–508.

22.   Liao WC, Tsai YL, Wang CY, et al. Clinical and radiographic characteristics of vertical root fractures in endodontically and nonendodontically treated teeth. J Endod 2017;43:687-693.

23.   Neves FS, Freitas DQ, Campos PSF, Ekestubbe A, Lofthag-Hansen S. Evaluation of cone-beam computed tomography in the diagnosis of vertical root fractures: The influence of imaging modes and root canal materials. J Endod 2014;40:1530–1536.

24.   Kajan ZD, Taromsari M. Value of cone beam CT in detection of dental root fractures. Dentomaxillofac Radiol 2012;41:3–10.

25.   Alaugaily I, Azim AA. CBCT patterns of bone loss and clinical predictors for the diagnosis of cracked teeth and teeth with vertical root fracture. J Endod 2022;48:1100–1106.

26.   Sim IGB, Lim TS, Krishnaswamy G, Chen NN. Decision making for retention of endodontically treated posterior cracked teeth: A 5-year follow-up study. J Endod 2016;42:225–229.

27.   Davis MC, Shariff SS. Success and survival of endodontically treated cracked teeth with radicular extensions: A 2- to 4-year prospective cohort. J Endod 2019;45:848–855.

28.   Kang SH, Kim BS, Kim Y. Cracked teeth: Distribution, characteristics, and survival after root canal treatment. J Endod 2016;42:557–562.

29.   Krell KV, Caplan DJ. 12-month success of cracked teeth treated with orthograde root canal treatment. J Endod 2018;44:543–548.

30.   Cameron CE. Cracked-tooth syndrome. J Am Dent Assoc 1964;68:405–411.

31.   Guthrie RC, DiFiore PM. Treating the cracked tooth with a full crown. J Am Dent Assoc 1991;122:71–73.

32.   Krell KV, Rivera EM. A six year evaluation of cracked teeth diagnosed with reversible pulpitis: Treatment and prognosis. J Endod 2007;33:1405–1407.

33.   Yavorek A, Bhagavatula P, Patel K, Szabo A, Ibrahim M. The incidence of root canal therapy after full coverage restorations: A 10-year retrospective study. J Endod 2020;46:605–610.

34. Valderhaug J, Jokstad A, Ambjørnsen E, Norheim PW. Assessment of the periapical and clinical status of crowned teeth over 25 years. J Dent 1997;25:97–105.
35. Saunders WP, Saunders EM. Prevalence of periradicular periodontitis associated with crowned teeth in an adult Scottish subpopulation. Br Dent J 1998;185:137–140.
36. Kontakiotis EG, Filippatos CG, Stefopoulos S, Tzanetakis GN. A prospective study of the incidence of asymptomatic pulp necrosis following crown preparation. Int Endod J 2015;48:512–517.
37. Haney JM, Leknes KN, Lie T, Selvig KA, Wikesjö UM. Cemental tear related to rapid periodontal breakdown: A case report. J Periodontol 1992;63:220–224.
38. Lin HJ, Chang SH, Chang MC, et al. Clinical fracture site, morphologic and histopathologic characteristics of cemental tear: Role in endodontic lesions. J Endod 2012;38:1058–1062.
39. Lin HJ, Chang MC, Chang SH, et al. Treatment outcome of the teeth with cemental tears. J Endod 2014;40:1315–1320.

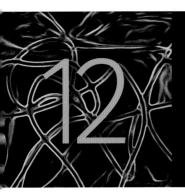

12

Resorption

Resorptive dental diseases encompass a heterogenous group of clinical entities that share a common histopathogenesis.[1] All involve the loss of the protective cellular layer lining the root structure. Internally, this structure is called *predentin* and contains odontoblasts. Externally, it is referred to as *precementum* and contains cementoblasts. When this protective cellular layer is lost, the underlying dentin or cementum is placed in direct contact with the adjacent pulp or periodontium. If the pulp or periodontium becomes inflamed, clastic cells may become activated. Without the protective cellular layer, dentin or cementum is degraded by the clastic cells[1] (Fig 12-1). While resorptive diseases share this common histopathology, their etiologies and the specific tissues involved vary. While some resorptive dental diseases are endodontically mediated and therefore respond to endodontic treatment, others are not. Therefore, accurate diagnosis is paramount. CBCT imaging is often the only way to differentiate among the many resorptive dental diseases. This chapter describes the resorptive dental diseases and their specific management strategies (Fig 12-2).

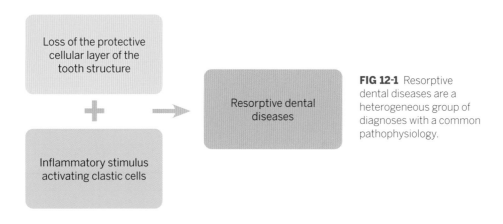

FIG 12-1 Resorptive dental diseases are a heterogeneous group of diagnoses with a common pathophysiology.

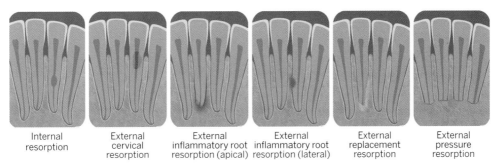

| Internal resorption | External cervical resorption | External inflammatory root resorption (apical) | External inflammatory root resorption (lateral) | External replacement resorption | External pressure resorption |

FIG 12-2 Types of resorptive dental diseases.

Internal Root Resorption

Internal root resorption (IRR) is the only resorptive dental disease that develops exclusively within the pulp space. IRR develops in response to some degree of coronal trauma to a tooth. Potential etiologic factors include deep caries, fracture, traumatic dental injury, vital pulp therapy, and drilling for restorative care without adequate coolant spray. This trauma causes direct or indirect damage to both the predentin and the adjacent pulp.[2,3] The pulpal damage often causes localized pulp necrosis, leading to inflammation of the adjacent vital tissues. This inflammatory stimulus activates clastic cells that degrade the now unprotected adjacent dentin. As the necrotic front advances, resorption will cease.[1] IRR is a common histologic finding, even when not clinically or radiographically detectable.[4]

The pulpal diagnosis of a tooth with IRR will be either irreversible pulpitis or pulp necrosis, depending on whether the lesion is active or arrested. Historically, pink discoloration of the crown was reported in IRR cases, but with the advent of CBCT imaging, this is now recognized as an attribute of external cervical resorption (ECR). Radiographically, IRR often appears contiguous and symmetric within the pulp space, though some degree of asymmetry can be expected in many cases (Fig 12-3). Late-stage lesions may perforate the external root structure. CBCT imaging is the most useful diagnostic tool to detect IRR, differentiate it from other types of resorption, and assess its level of root involvement (Fig 12-4).

FIG 12-3 *(a)* 2D radiographs of teeth with IRR will depict a radiolucency that appears contiguous and symmetric within the pulp space, though some degree of asymmetry can be expected in many cases. *(b)* Obturation material will fill the resorptive defects after nonsurgical root canal therapy (NSRCT).

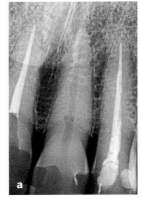
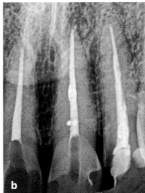

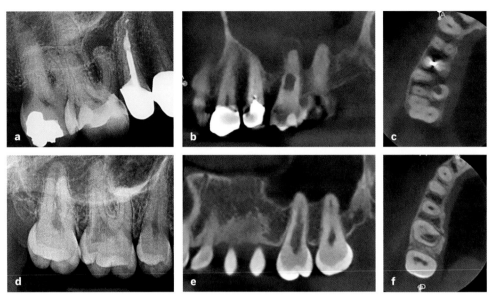

FIG 12-4 CBCT imaging is the only radiographic means available to accurately differentiate IRR from other resorptive diagnoses. *(a and d)* Both of these patients were referred for evaluation of suspected IRR in the maxillary right first molar. *(b and c)* CBCT imaging confirmed IRR in the first patient, and *(e and f)* ECR was diagnosed in the second.

Because IRR is pulpally mediated, nonsurgical root canal therapy (NSRCT) is the treatment of choice (Fig 12-5). Treatment is highly successful, especially for non-perforating IRR defects.[5] That said, consideration must be given to the thinness of the remaining dentin, which poses the risk of fracture or even root perforations and has a negative effect on prognosis. Certain unique treatment considerations arise for IRR. NSRCT techniques are limited by the reduced ability of chemomechanical methodologies to fully debride the unusual architecture of resorptive defects. To combat this, it is advised to use sonic or ultrasonic-activated irrigation with sodium hypochlorite[6] and provide treatment as two-visit root canal therapy using calcium hydroxide as an interappointment medication in order to maximize tissue dissolution.[3,7] Thermoplasticized gutta-percha allows for the most complete fill of the resorptive defect.[8,9] Compressible alternatives, such as bioceramics, resin-modified glass-ionomer cements, and composites, may be placed alongside traditional obturation materials used to fill the canal spaces apical to the defect. In sum, clinicians should take a case-specific approach to managing defects secondary to IRR.

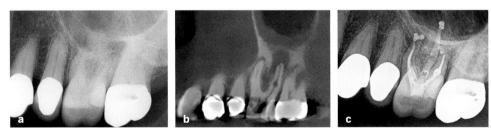

FIG 12-5 *(a to c)* NSRCT used to treat IRR.

Perforating lesions are more complex to treat due to the need to repair the perforation, and studies on the success of bioceramics in the management of non-iatrogenic perforations, such as those secondary to IRR, are limited. Of course, the unequivocal success of bioceramics in the repair of iatrogenic lateral and furcal perforations,[10,11] as well as their biocompatibility and osteoconductive properties,[12] make them the ideal materials to consider even in the presence of perforating IRR. Alternative methods, including incorporation of surgical access for external repair[13] and the use of regenerative endodontic techniques, have also been proposed.[14] That said, extraction may be warranted for teeth with a poor prognosis or when a patient desires the most reliable treatment outcome.

External Inflammatory Root Resorption

External inflammatory root resorption (EIRR) results from the activation of periapical cementoclasts following loss of the precementum due to trauma or apical periodontitis. Based on its location, it is diagnosed as either apical EIRR or lateral EIRR. Apical EIRR is a common finding in conjunction with apical periodontitis.[15] Lateral EIRR develops from severe dental trauma, such as luxation, or avulsive injuries wherein the precementum and periodontal ligament (PDL) structures undergo direct damage. If the area of damage is limited and the pulp remains vital, this condition may be transient and self-limiting and is referred to as *surface resorption*.[16,17] If pulp necrosis occurs, resulting in a continued source of inflammation through the infected dentinal tubules, resorption progresses.

Clinically, both apical and lateral EIRR are associated with a pulpal diagnosis of necrosis. Radiographically, EIRR will appear as a moth-eaten area of root structure on both 2D and CBCT images (Fig 12-6). In cases of either apical or lateral EIRR that are sustained by necrotic pulp tissue remnants activating cementoclasts, removal of the necrotic pulp tissue via NSRCT is the treatment of choice[15] (Fig 12-7). Two-visit therapy with interappointment calcium hydroxide left in place for 4 weeks is advised due to its antiresorptive properties.[18,19] Though this will halt the progression of disease in most cases, it may be ineffective in cases of extensive lateral EIRR, which may in turn progress to replacement resorption (RR) (Fig 12-8). It is important to note that resorbed dentin or cementum will not reform.

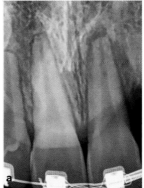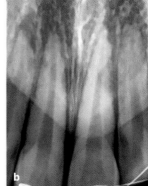

FIG 12-6 *(a and b)* Radiographically, EIRR will appear as a moth-eaten area of root structure on the lateral or apical root surface on both 2D and CBCT images.

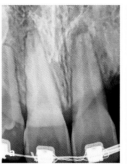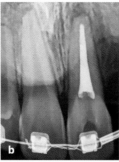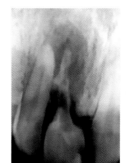

FIG 12-8 Even with NSRCT, extensive lateral EIRR cases may not resolve and may progress irrespective of treatment.

FIG 12-7 *(a)* In cases of either lateral or apical EIRR that are sustained by necrotic pulp tissue remnants activating cementoclasts, *(b)* removal of the necrotic pulp tissue via NSRCT represents the treatment of choice.

Replacement Resorption

RR is characterized by direct resorption and the replacement of cementum and dentin with bone.[17] RR develops when lateral EIRR becomes progressive and osteoclasts from the adjacent bone directly contact cementum. It is associated with severe dental trauma. In certain cases, such as the replantation of avulsed teeth in children where PDL death is certain (eg, the tooth was improperly stored or the extraoral dry time was greater than 60 minutes), RR is an expected outcome that will eventually result in tooth loss. That said, replantation is still preferred over immediate extraction because it allows for bone retention until implant replacement is achievable.

Clinically, particularly in extensive cases in young patients, RR is characterized by infrapositioning of the tooth, lack of physiologic mobility, and a metallic tone on percussion[1] (Fig 12-9). Radiographically, RR is associated with the loss of the lamina dura and root structure that appears continuous with bone (Fig 12-10). That said, RR may occur simultaneously with lateral EIRR and may involve some or all of the root structure, resulting in a mixed radiographic appearance.

No known intervention will halt the process of progressive RR. A decoronation procedure is advised as opposed to extraction for bone preservation related to replacement.[20] Once the tooth becomes infrapositioned more than 1 mm as compared to neighboring teeth, the crown is removed by sectioning. Any endodontic obturation material should

Infrapositioning of the tooth

A metallic tone on percussion

Lack of physiologic mobility

FIG 12-9 Clinical findings associated with progressive RR.

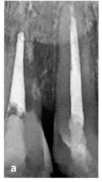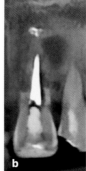

FIG 12-10 *(a and b)* Radiographically, RR is associated with the loss of the lamina dura and root structure, appearing continuous with bone on both periapical radiographs and CBCT.

be removed and the root left in place until complete bone fill occurs and implant replacement can be considered (Fig 12-11).In adults, composite buildups may instead be used to correct infrapositioning.[21]

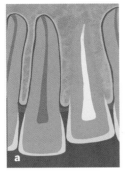 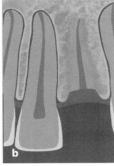 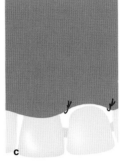 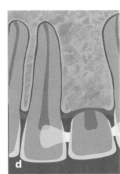

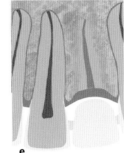 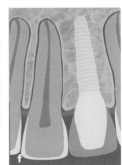

FIG 12-11 *(a)* Decoronation may be considered for infrapositioned teeth secondary to severe RR. *(b)* The crown should be sectioned and prior root canal filling materials removed. *(c)* Appropriate soft tissue management should be performed to attempt primary closure. *(d and e)* The remaining root structure may be left submerged to allow for *(f)* full bone replacement prior to implant replacement.

Pressure Resorption

Pressure resorption (PR) is caused by direct damage to the external root surfaces by forces including orthodontic movement, misaligned tooth eruption, and slow-growing tumors or cysts.[1] PR can be differentiated from EIRR by the presence of vital pulp tissues as well as an obvious agent of resorption. Orthodontic PR can be found at the apex or on lateral root surfaces, depending on the vector of orthodontic force. It is exceedingly common,[22,23] and its severity is correlated with intrusive or rotational movements[24] as well as orthodontic therapy of long duration[25] (Fig 12-12). Orthodontic PR is no more likely in endodontically treated versus non-endodontically treated teeth.[26,27] That said, teeth with untreated, active pulpal and periapical pathology are at a high risk of developing resorption.[28] PR may also develop secondary to misaligned eruption patterns, similar to the histopathogenesis of primary tooth exfoliation. Expansile, space-occupying lesions such as jaw cysts and benign tumors may also cause PR (Fig 12-13).

FIG 12-12
Orthodontic tooth movements, particularly intrusive and rotational movements, are associated with the development of PR.

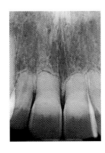

FIG 12-13
Misaligned eruption of teeth and benign cysts and tumors may cause PR, and removal of the stimulus will halt the resorptive process.

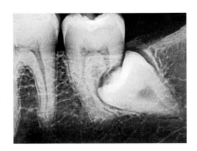

Understanding the etiology and type of resorption is crucial in differentiating PR from endodontically derived resorption because PR is treated by removing the source of pressure and not by NSRCT. Pauses in orthodontic movement[25] and delays in resuming orthodontic movement following traumatic dental injuries (eg, from 3 months to 1 year depending on their severity)[29] have been proposed to reduce the likelihood of orthodontic PR. Similarly, removal of the causative tooth or lesion will halt progressive PR. It is important to recognize that lost cementum and dentin cannot be replaced.[1] Therefore, teeth with extensive PR may ultimately be lost.

External Cervical Resorption

External cervical resorption (ECR) originates from inflamed junctional epithelial tissues at the base of the periodontal attachment adjacent to damaged precementum, typically in vital teeth.[30,31] Although ECR is the most current diagnostic term for this entity, it has historically been referred to as *invasive cervical root resorption*, among other terms.[30] Common etiologies for ECR include orthodontics, restorative care, periodontal surgery or dentoalveolar surgeries, nonvital bleaching (particularly with the use of Superoxol or heat), traumatic injuries, parafunction, certain medications, and certain viruses[32–40] (Fig 12-14).

Dental treatment	Trauma	Medical
• Orthodontics • Restorative care • Dentoalveolar surgery • Periodontal surgery	• Parafunction • Traumatic dental injuries	• Medications • Viruses

FIG 12-14 Etiologies of ECR.

Frequently, ECR is an asymptomatic condition most often identified incidentally. That said, because ECR destruction will eventually approach the pulp, its degree of severity must be considered during both diagnosis and management. Clinically, ECR can be difficult to detect. A subgingival cavitation containing soft tissue within may be detectable for more coronally located lesions. If bacteria invade the lesion, secondary caries or localized periodontal abscesses may develop. Supragingival ECR defects are associated with pink discoloration of the crown[30] (Fig 12-15). ECR lesions cause pulpal disease in very late stages or following treatment in which a lesion is excised with damage to the adjacent pulp tissue; therefore, symptoms are often absent.[30,31]

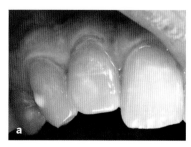 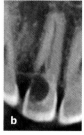

FIG 12-15 *(a and b)* Pink coronal discoloration is associated with ECR lesions wherein the resorptive tissues extend intracoronally.

Radiographically, ECR appears as a cavitation in its early stages. Lesions on the mesial or distal aspects of a tooth may be visible with periapical imaging, though they can easily be confused with cervical burnout or root caries. More likely, early ECR lesions will only be visible with CBCT imaging (Fig 12-16). As the pathology progresses, the defect will extend toward pulpal tissues and down root structures. The same cellular layer that protects root structure from invading IRR lesions exists to protect the pulp from lesions moving from the outside in. In reference to ECR, this cellular layer has been called the *pericanalar resorption-resistant sheet*. It appears as a radiopaque line surrounding the pulp tissue, and its presence is pathognomonic for ECR[30,31] (Fig 12-17). If the area remains free from infection and soft tissue ingrowth, advanced ECR lesions may exhibit a form of osseous repair, whereby osteoblasts lay down bone to create an RR-like condition[31,41,42] (Fig 12-18). ECR lesions can be classified based on their extent, as seen radiographically (Fig 12-19).[43]

FIG 12-16 *(a to c)* Early ECR lesions can be detectable with periapical imaging, particularly if located on the mesial or distal root surfaces, but may only be visible with CBCT.

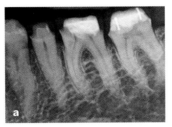 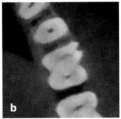 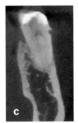

FIG 12-17 *(a and b)* Radiopaque lines surrounding the pulp tissue are pathognomonic for ECR lesions and represent the pericanalar resorption-resistant sheet.

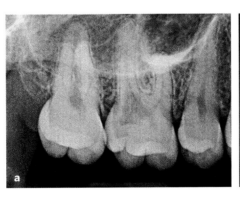 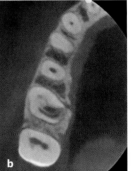

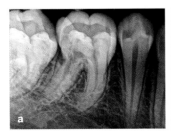 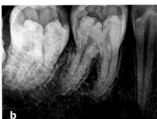 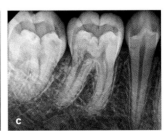

FIG 12-18 Osseous ingrowth may be noted in late-stage ECR lesions that remain free of infection. *(a)* The mandibular right first molar was asymptomatic when incidental class 4 ECR was noted on its distal aspect during a routine radiographic exam. *(b)* The lesion remained clinically undetectable and radiographically stable, at 1 year and *(c)* 4 years, with evidence of osseous ingrowth within.

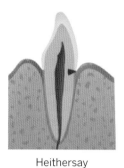
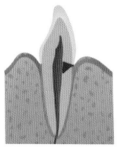
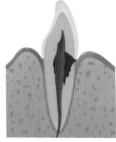
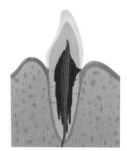

| Heithersay Class 1 | Heithersay Class 2 | Heithersay Class 3 | Heithersay Class 4 |

Class 1: Small, well-defined lesions localized to the cervical area and involving dentin only.

Class 2: Slightly larger, well-defined lesions localized to the cervical area but penetrating further into dentin and approximating the coronal pulp.

Class 3: Larger, less defined lesions extending into the coronal third of the root.

Class 4: Large lesions extending beyond the coronal third of the root.

FIG 12-19 Heithersay's classification system is the most widely used for ECR.[43]

A variety of means exist for the management of ECR.[43,44] Like PR, it does not result from endodontic pathology, and thus endodontic treatment will not alleviate the condition. Class 1 lesions that are accessible are best treated surgically in what is termed an *external repair*.[43] Flap design should allow for full exposure and debridement of the lesion. Full treatment involves application of 90% trichloroacetic acid for 1 to 4 minutes, followed by a rinse with sterile water or saline. A tissue-friendly restorative material, such as a resin-modified glass-ionomer cement or an insoluble bioceramic filling material, should be placed to fill the lesion prior to flap closure. Class 2 and 3 lesions that are accessible can be treated similarly, with the addition of vital pulp therapy or NSRCT in cases with pulpal involvement as evidenced by preoperative signs and symptoms of pulpitis or pulpal exposure[43,44] (Fig 12-20).

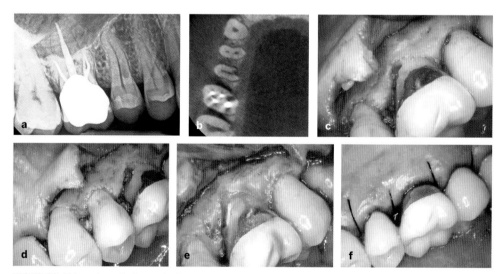

FIG 12-20 External repair via surgical treatment is indicated for many ECR lesions, with the potential need for NSRCT or vital pulp therapy for lesions that encroach on the pulp space. *(a)* Class 1 ECR was noted on the maxillary right second premolar with periapical imaging, and *(b)* a second class 2 ECR lesion was found incidentally on the maxillary right first molar with CBCT imaging. Resultantly, external surgical repair was completed to repair the palatal lesions found on both the first molar and second premolar with *(c)* exposure, *(d)* debridement, and *(e)* restoration of the defects using a bioceramic putty (EndoSequence BC Root Repair Material Fast Set Putty, Brasseler USA) prior to *(f)* flap reapproximation and suturing. (Surgical photos courtesy of Dr Stephen Fucini.)

Surgically inaccessible lesions, such as those located below the alveolar crest, may be treated using an internal approach in conjunction with NSRCT.[44] Following endodontic access and debridement of any overlying tissues, the ECR lesion can be located, debrided, and treated internally with the trichloroacetic acid solution (Fig 12-21). The area can be restored with a resin-modified glass-ionomer cement or bioceramic material, followed by completion of NSCRT. Given the presence of perforating resorption and the associated risks, irrigation with sodium hypochlorite is not advised until the defect is restored. Alternative treatments involving orthodontic extrusion and intentional replantation can be considered on a case-by-case basis.

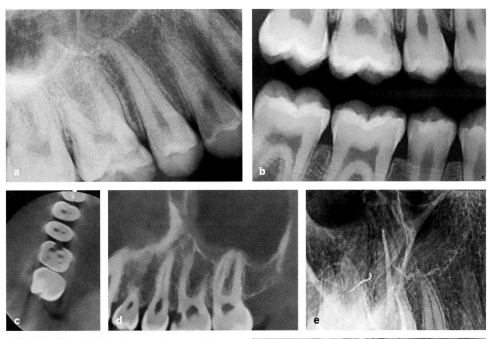

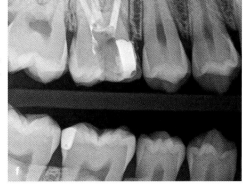

FIG 12-21 When ECR lesions are inaccessible externally, an internal approach may be taken instead. The maxillary right first molar had class 2 ECR noted on its mesial interproximal surface as seen on *(a)* periapical and *(b)* bitewing radiographs, as well as *(c)* axial and *(d)* sagittal sections of CBCT. *(e and f)* External repair was deemed infeasible; therefore, an internal approach was taken during delivery of NSRCT. The ECR lesion was treated with 90% trichloroacetic acid and repaired with a resin-modified glass-ionomer cement.

Considerations of restorability and accessibility may limit treatment options for larger class 3 and 4 lesions. That said, extraction of teeth with a poor prognosis is not always immediately warranted. Untreatable lesions may be carefully monitored for the long term, with interventions performed only if signs or symptoms of progressive disease develop (Fig 12-22). Empirically, experts advise periodic monitoring at 12-month inter-vals. Of course, untreatable lesions with signs and symptoms of pulpitis or periodontal infection should be considered for immediate extraction to minimize bone loss that could negatively affect future replacement options.[43,44]

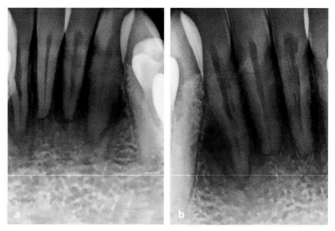

FIG 12-22 Untreatable lesions may be carefully monitored for the long-term, with interventions only if signs or symptoms of progres-sive disease develop. *(a)* The initial periapical radiograph showing an untreatable lesion. *(b)* The same lesion at the 3-year follow-up.

In sum, resorption represents a group of diagnoses with similar pathophysiology but differing etiologies, affected tissues, and treatment management strategies. A summary of resorptive dental disease diagnoses and treatments is presented in Table 12-1.

TABLE 12-1 Summary of resorptive dental diseases, including their origins, presentation, and management

Resorption type	Etiology	Tissues involved	Anticipated pulpal diagnosis	Treatment
IRR	Deep caries, fracture, traumatic dental injury, vital pulp therapy, or drilling without adequate coolant spray	Damage to predentin, odontoclasts from pulp tissue	Irreversible pulpitis (if active resorption), pulpal necrosis (if arrested)	NSRCT
EIRR	Traumatic dental injuries, apical periodontitis	Damage to precementum, odontoclasts from PDL	• If following trauma: normal pulp (transient form only), irreversible pulpitis, or pulp necrosis • If due to apical periodontitis: pulp necrosis	NSRCT
RR	Progressive EIRR	Osteoclasts and osteoblasts replace the odontoclasts from external inflammatory resorption	Pulp necrosis or previously endodontically treated teeth	No known treatment halts the progression of RR; decoronation may be required
PR	Orthodontics, slow-growing cysts and tumors, misaligned tooth eruption	Damage to precementum, odontoclasts from PDL	Normal pulp	Remove the causative factor (eg, halt orthodontics, excise cysts or tumors, extract offending tooth)
ECR	Orthodontics, restorative care, periodontal surgery, dentoalveolar surgery, nonvital bleaching, traumatic injuries, parafunction, medications, viruses	Damage to precementum, odontoclasts from junctional epithelium	Normal pulp in early lesions, potential for irreversible pulpitis or necrosis with advanced lesions	External (surgical) or internal repair; possible NSRCT or vital pulp therapy if pulp tissues are secondarily involved

References

1. Tronstad L. Root resorption—Etiology, terminology and clinical manifestations. Endod Dent Traumatol 1988;4:241–252.
2. Wedenberg C, Lindskog S. Experimental internal resorption in monkey teeth. Endod Dent Traumatol 1985;1:221–227.
3. Patel S, Ricucci D, Durak C, Tay F. Internal root resorption: A review. J Endod 2010;36:1107–1121.
4. Gabor C, Tam E, Shen Y, Haapasalo M. Prevalence of internal inflammatory root resorption. J Endod 2012;38:24–27.
5. Calişkan MK, Türkün M. Prognosis of permanent teeth with internal resorption: A clinical review. Endod Dent Traumatol 1997;13:75–81.
6. Andersen M, Lund A, Andreasen JO, Adreasen FM. In vitro solubility of human pulp tissue in calcium hydroxide and sodium hypochlorite. Endod Dent Traumatol 1992;8:104–108.
7. Türkün M, Cengiz T. The effects of sodium hypochlorite and calcium hydroxide on tissue dissolution and root canal cleanliness. Int Endod J 1997;30:335–342.
8. Gencoglu N, Yildirim T, Garip Y, Karagnec B, Yilmaz H. Effectiveness of different gutta-percha techniques when filling experimental internal resorptive cavities. Int Endod J 2008;41:836–842.
9. Goldberg F, Massone EJ, Esmoris M, Alfie D. Comparison of different techniques for obturating experimental internal resorptive cavities. Dent Traumatol 2000;16:116–121.
10. Main C, Mirzayan N, Shabahang S, Torabinejad M. Repair of root perforations using mineral trioxide aggregate: A long-term study. J Endod 2004;30:80–83.
11. Siew K, Lee AHC, Cheung GSP. Treatment outcome of repaired root perforation: A systematic review and meta-analysis. J Endod 2015;41:1795–1804.
12. Mitchell PJ, Pitt Ford TR, Torabinejad M, McDonald F. Osteoblast biocompatibility of mineral trioxide aggregate. Biomaterials 1999;20:167–173.
13. Patel S, Durack C, Ricucci D, Bakhsh AA. Root resorption. In: Berman LH, Hargreaves KH (eds). Cohen's Pathways of the Pulp, ed 12. St Louis: Elsevier, 2021:711–736.
14. Kaval ME, Güneri P, Çalişkan MK. Regenerative endodontic treatment of perforated internal root resorption: A case report. Int Endod J 2018;51:128–137.
15. Vier FV, Figueiredo JA. Prevalence of different periapical lesions associated with human teeth and their correlation with the presence and extension of apical external root resorption. Int Endod J 2002;35:710–719.
16. Hammarström L, Pierce A, Blomlöf L, Feiglin B, Lindskog S. Tooth avulsion and replantation—A review. Endod Dent Traumatol 1986;2:1–8.
17. Andreasen JO, Kristerson L. The effect of limited drying or removal of the periodontal ligament. Periodontal healing after replantation of mature permanent incisors in monkeys. Acta Odontol Scand 1981;39:1–13.
18. Bourguignon C, Cohenca N, Lauridsen E, et al. International Association of Dental Traumatology guidelines for the management of traumatic dental injuries: 1. Fractures and luxations. Dent Traumatol 2020;36:314–330.
19. Trope M, Moshonov J, Nissan R, Buxt P, Yesilsoy C. Short vs. long-term calcium hydroxide treatment of established inflammatory root resorption in replanted dog teeth. Endod Dent Traumatol 1995;11:124–128.
20. Malmgren B. Ridge preservation/decoronation. Pediatr Dent 2013;35:164–169.
21. Patel S, Krastl G, Weiger R. ESE position statement on root resoprtion. Int Endod J 2023;56:792–801.
22. Massler M, Malone AJ. Root resorption in human permanent teeth. Am J Orthod 1954;40:619–633.
23. Cwyk F, Scat-Pierre F, Tronstad L. Endodontic implications of orthodontic tooth movement. J Dent Res 1984;63:1039.
24. Zahrowski J, Jeske A. Apical root resorption is associated with comprehensive orthodontic treatment but not clearly dependent on prior tooth characteristics or orthodontic techniques. J Am Dent Assoc 2011;142:66–68.
25. Roscoe MG, Meira JBC, Cattaneo PM. Association of orthodontic force system and root resorption: A systematic review. Am J Orthod Dentofacial Orthop 2015;147:610–626.
26. Mattison GD, Delivanis HP, Delivanis PD, Johns PI. Orthodontic root resorption of vital and endodontically treated teeth. J Endod 1984;10:354–358.
27. Esteves T, Ramos AL, Pereira CM, Hidalgo MM. Orthodontic root resorption of endodontically treated teeth. J Endod 2007;33:119–122.
28. Brin I, Ben-Bassat Y, Heling I, Engelberg A. The influence of orthodontic treatment on previously traumatized permanent incisors. Eur J Orthod 1991;13:372–377.
29. Kindelan SA, Day PF, Kindelan JD, Spencer JR, Duggal MS. Dental trauma: An overview of its influence on the management of orthodontic treatment. Part 1. J Orthod 2008;35:68–78.
30. Heithersay GS. Clinical, radiologic, and histopathologic features of invasive cervical resorption. Quintessence Int 1999;30:27–37.

31. Patel S, Mavridou AM, Lambrechts P, Saberi N. External cervical resorption. Part 1: Histopathology, distribution and presentation. Int Endod J 2018;51:1205–1223.

32. Heithersay GS. Invasive cervical resorption: An analysis of potential predisposing factors. Quintessence Int 1999;30:83–95.

33. Harrington GW, Natkin E. External resorption associated with bleaching of pulpless teeth. J Endod 1979;5:344–348.

34. Rotstein I, Friedman S, Mor C, Katznelson J, Sommer M, Bab I. Histological characterization of bleaching-induced external root resorption in dogs. J Endod 1991;17:436–441.

35. Mavridou AM, Bergmans L, Barendregt D, Lambrechts P. Descriptive analysis of factors associated with external cervical resorption. J Endod 2017;43:1602–1610.

36. Patel S, Saberi N. External cervical resorption associated with the use of bisphosphonates: A case series. J Endod 2015;41:742–748.

37. Llavayol M, Pons M, Ballester ML, Berástegui E. Multiple cervical root resorption in a young adult female previously treated with chemotherapy: A case report. J Endod 2019;45:349–353.

38. von Arx T, Schawalder P, Ackermann M, Bosshardt DD. Human and feline invasive cervical resorptions: The missing link? Presentation of four cases. J Endod 2009;35:904–913.

39. Patel K, Schirru E, Niazi S, Mitchell P, Mannocci F. Multiple apical radiolucencies and external cervical resorption associated with varicella zoster virus: A case report. J Endod 2016;42:978–983.

40. Kumar V, Chawla A, Kaur A. Multiple idiopathic cervical root resorptions in patients with hepatitis B virus infection. J Endod 2018;44:1575–1577.

41. Mavridou AM, Hauben E, Wevers M, Schepers E, Bergmans L, Lambrechts P. Understanding external cervical resorption in vital teeth. J Endod 2016;42:1737–1751.

42. Mavridou AM, Hauben E, Wevers M, Schepers E, Bergmans L, Lambrechts P. Understanding external cervical resorption patterns in endodontically treated teeth. Int Endod J 2017;50:1116–1133.

43. Heithersay GS. Treatment of invasive cervical resorption: An analysis of results using topical application of trichloracetic acid, curettage, and restoration. Quintessence Int 1999;30:96–110.

44. Patel S, Foschi F, Condon R, Pimentel T, Bhuva B. External cervical resorption. Part 2: Management. Int Endod J 2018;51:1224–1238.

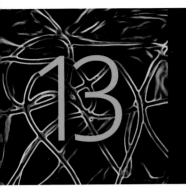

Periodontal-Endodontic Infections

D ue to their anatomical proximity, pathologies affecting the periodontium and pulp may impact one another, resulting in combined periodontal-endodontic infections. Disease processes may spread from one structure to another via anatomical or pathologic structures. Anatomical communications include the apical foramen, lateral canals, furcal canals, and dentinal tubules.[1] Additional anatomical communications may be created by grooves in the root structure, which can propagate the spread of periodontal disease apically. Pathologic communications include root fractures, perforating internal root resorption, perforating external cervical resorption (ECR), and iatrogenic perforations (Fig 13-1). When evidence of combined periodontal-endodontic infections is present, careful diagnostics are key to establishing the true etiology and pathogenesis of the condition at hand prior to planning for management. Periodontal-endodontic pathology can mimic pathology secondary to vertical root fractures and rare nonodontogenic pathology, including malignancies.[2]

Anatomical	**Pathologic**
• Apical foramen • Lateral canals • Furcal canals • Dentinal tubules • Longitudinal grooves	• Root fractures • Perforating resorption • Iatrogenic perforations

FIG 13-1 Communication points between the pulp and periodontium.

The most widely accepted diagnostic classification system of periodontal-endodontic infections was proposed by Simon et al in 1972.[3] Diagnoses are based on the presumed etiology of the presenting lesion. Categories include primary endodontic, primary endodontic/secondary periodontal, primary periodontal, primary periodontal/secondary endodontic, and true combined lesions (Fig 13-2).

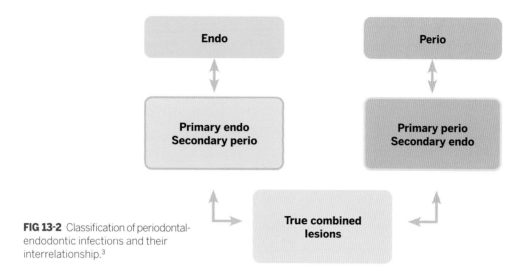

FIG 13-2 Classification of periodontal-endodontic infections and their interrelationship.[3]

Primary endodontic pathology originates from the dental pulp. It is characterized by necrotic pulp tissue, and the periodontal probing depths are normal. If present, sinus tracts or swelling are located adjacent to the periapex. There is no periodontal attachment loss, and radiographic findings of bone loss are confined to the apical tissues. The recommended treatment is nonsurgical root canal therapy (NSRCT).

Primary endodontic/secondary periodontal lesions also originate from a necrotic pulp[3] (Fig 13-3). Longstanding lesions can result in destruction along the periodontal ligament (PDL) with associated periodontal attachment loss and drainage through the periodontal sulcus. These lesions are also characterized by necrotic pulp tissue, but localized and deep periodontal probing defects are expected. Swelling or sinus tracts may be more coronally positioned. Apicomarginal bony defects are expected to be visible with 2D radiographs or CBCT. NSRCT is the primary treatment, and adjunctive periodontal treatment may be indicated for more extensive periodontal defects (Fig 13-4).

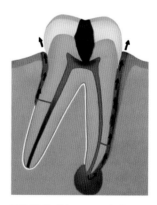

FIG 13-3 Primary endodontic/secondary periodontal infections are characterized by pulp necrosis and localized probing defects. The originating infection is the necrotic pulp tissue.

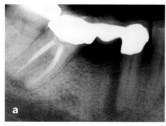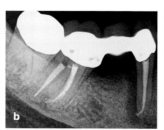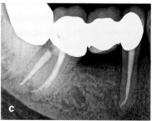

FIG 13-4 (a) This primary endodontic/secondary periodontal lesion on the mandibular right second premolar presented with a wide 13-mm probing depth on the distal aspect under the bridge. (b) NSRCT was completed, and (c) complete radiographic healing was apparent at the 1-year follow-up.

Primary periodontal lesions originate from the marginal periodontium. Clinical findings typically include more generalized periodontal attachment loss than seen in primary endodontic/secondary periodontal pathology, as well as mobility, fremitus, and bleeding on probing. Plaque and calculus buildup may be present both locally and generally because periodontitis is commonly found throughout the mouth. The pulp tissue of a tooth affected by periodontitis is typically vital. Radiographic findings include horizontal bone loss and intrabony defects that spare the apical tissues (Fig 13-5). Management involves periodontal therapies, usually beginning with scaling and root planing.

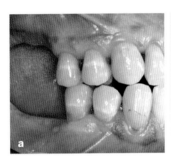 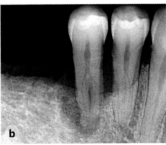

FIG 13-5 *(a)* The mandibular right second premolar with a primary periodontal lesion responded normally to pulp sensitivity tests. Clinically, grade 3 mobility, probing defects of 9 mm on the distal aspect of the tooth, and a sinus tract with purulent drainage were noted. *(b)* Radiographically, an angular bony defect was noted. (Case courtesy of Dr Yichu Wu.)

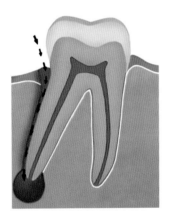

FIG 13-6 Primary periodontal/secondary endodontic lesions originate from periodontal attachment loss extending to the apical foramina or lateral canals and resulting in endodontic involvement.

Primary periodontal/secondary endodontic lesions originate from periodontal attachment loss extending apically to involve the apical foramina or lateral canals and resulting in endodontic involvement (Fig 13-6). Because periodontal disease that is severe enough to expose the apical termini of root canals is often severe enough that these teeth may already be lost, some argue that this diagnosis is a theoretical construct or at least extremely rarely encountered clinically. Clinical findings are similar to those of primary periodontal pathology. Pulp tissue may exhibit signs of inflammation, including pulpal diagnoses of reversible pulpitis to symptomatic irreversible pulpitis, or pulpal necrosis may be observed. Radiographically, apicomarginal bony defects are expected. Periodontal management of these cases may necessitate scaling and root planing or surgical intervention. Endodontic management of primary periodontal/secondary endodontic lesions depends upon the stage of endodontic disease. If reversible pulpitis is diagnosed, periodontal therapy should resolve the pulpal symptoms. If symptomatic irreversible pulpitis or pulpal necrosis is present, endodontic therapy should precede periodontal management. The prognosis for these teeth is primarily related to the periodontal condition.

True combined endodontic and periodontal lesions develop from coalescing primary endodontic and periodontal lesions (Fig 13-7). Clinically, these lesions mimic primary periodontal/secondary endodontic lesions, with nonvital pulp tissue and wider areas of periodontal attachment loss. Radiographic findings include apicomarginal bony defects. Management must address both endodontic and periodontal pathoses. Multidisciplinary procedures may include root amputation and hemisection, so careful consideration should be given to the resulting prognosis when deciding whether to maintain or extract a tooth with combined periodontal-endodontic pathology.

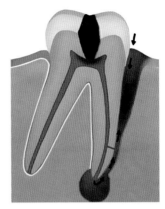

FIG 13-7 True combined endodontic and periodontal lesions develop from coalescing primary endodontic and periodontal lesions.

References

1. De Deus QD. Frequency, location, and direction of the lateral, secondary, and accessory canals. J Endod 1975;1:361–366.
2. Levi PA Jr, Kim DM, Harsfield SL, Jacobson ER. Squamous cell carcinoma presenting as an endodontic-periodontic lesion. J Periodontol 2005;76:1798–1804.
3. Simon JH, Glick DH, Frank AL. The relationship of endodontic-periodontic lesions. J Periodontol 1972;43:202–208.

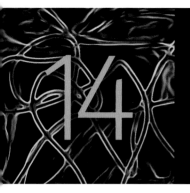

Traumatic Dental Injuries

ental trauma is common, especially in childhood. While injuries in the primary dentition are best managed by pediatric dental specialists,[1] injuries in both the immature and mature permanent dentition can be managed in general dental or endodontic settings. Clear, evidence-based guidelines exist from both the American Association of Endodontists (AAE) and, more recently, from the International Association of Dental Traumatology (IADT), and these should be used to establish a diagnosis, guide management in the acute stage, and develop a long-term follow-up plan.[2-5] As guidelines are periodically updated, clinicians must stay abreast of changes and follow the latest guidelines relevant to their location of practice.

Traumatic dental injuries rarely occur in isolation. Other bodily injuries may occur concomitantly, and more serious conditions, such as head trauma, take precedence for management over the dental injury. Therefore, a comprehensive primary and secondary assessment (detailed in chapter 1) is advised prior to the work-up of dental trauma if dental practitioners are the first medical providers to evaluate trauma patients.[6] The primary patient assessment follows the acronym **ABCDE**, which refers to appropriate **airway maintenance**, adequate **breathing and ventilation**, intact **circulation** without evidence of shock, evaluation for neurologic **disability**, and **exposure** of the patient for a comprehensive examination[7] (Fig 14-1). Neurologic disability can be assessed using the Glasgow Coma Scale (see chapter 1). Any aberrant findings in the primary assessment warrant emergency medical referral. The secondary survey follows the acronym **SAMPLE**, which stands for **signs and symptoms** associated with the condition, **allergies**, **medications**, **past illnesses**, **last meal eaten**, and the **events and environment** leading up to the trauma (Fig 14-2). A patient's tetanus vaccination status should also be reviewed because a booster may be necessary following avulsions.

Primary Assessment

A	**A**irway maintenance
B	Adequate **B**reathing and ventilation
C	Intact **C**irculation without evidence of shock
D	Evaluation for neurologic **D**isability
E	**E**xposure of the patient for a comprhrehensive examination

FIG 14-1 Components of the primary assessment following dental trauma.

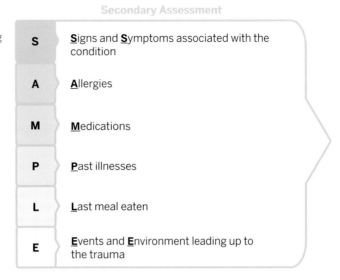

FIG 14-2 Components of the secondary assessment following dental trauma.

Secondary Assessment

S	**S**igns and **S**ymptoms associated with the condition
A	**A**llergies
M	**M**edications
P	**P**ast illnesses
L	**L**ast meal eaten
E	**E**vents and **E**nvironment leading up to the trauma

Once the patient is determined to be medically stable, an immediate and comprehensive endodontic work-up is advised. This should include a subjective and objective exam, with particular attention given to pulp sensitivity testing, periapical testing, and assessment for mobility and soft tissue injuries.[8] That said, neural injury secondary to dental trauma can result in transient loss of normal pulp sensitivity responses for up to 3 months.[2,4,9,10] Consequently, a lack of response to thermal or electric pulp sensitivity testing should not be used as the sole basis for pulpal diagnosis during this time period. Percussion sensitivity may be due to inflammation following an acute injury, the mobility of fractured segments, or the development of apical periodontitis. Manual palpation can detect apical displacement of luxated roots, associated discomfort, and developing apical periodontitis. Mobility can suggest a wide variety of traumatic injuries. Single tooth mobility may reflect loosening caused by a luxation injury or a cervically located horizontal root fracture. Mobility of several teeth in concert suggests an alveolar fracture. A lack of physiologic mobility, particularly when associated with a characteristic metallic tone on percussion, may indicate a lateral or intrusive luxation injury or, in late stages, developing replacement resorption (RR). Intraoral photographs are suggested to monitor for soft tissue healing and coronal discoloration, as well as re-eruption patterns of intruded teeth.[4]

Radiographs are also a crucial component of the comprehensive endodontic work-up following dental trauma. Minimally, multiple angles of periapical radiographs are advised following traumatic injuries.[2,4] Additionally, periapical images of the socket are advised following avulsive injuries prior to replantation. While some guidelines recommend occlusal radiographs, their utility is disputed due to significant anatomical noise found in these images, particularly when CBCT images are available. If soft tissue lacerations are present, radiographs of the affected areas are advised to assess for the presence of tooth fragments or radiopaque material within the soft tissues. CBCT imaging is routinely advised when available because it is able to detect root and alveolar fractures and visualize the displacement of luxation injuries.[2,4,11–13]

As with any endodontic work-up, the clinical and radiographic findings are evaluated together to develop a pulpal and periapical diagnosis, as well as the adjunctive trauma diagnosis. Traumatic dental injuries can be categorized as *(1)* those that result in tooth or jaw fracture, *(2)* luxation-type injuries, and *(3)* avulsions (Fig 14-3). Clinicians must recognize that multiple injuries may be present within the same tooth or dental arch, and treatment may be prioritized based on the trauma diagnosis.[14] Injuries with acute priority require management within hours. These include the repositioning of root or alveolar fractures or luxated teeth and the replantation of avulsed teeth.[14] Injuries with subacute priority may have management delayed for several hours. These include complicated crown fractures with pulp exposures, concussions, subluxations, and intrusions.[14] Delayed priority injuries include uncomplicated crown fractures, whose treatment can be delayed beyond 24 hours[14] (Fig 14-4).

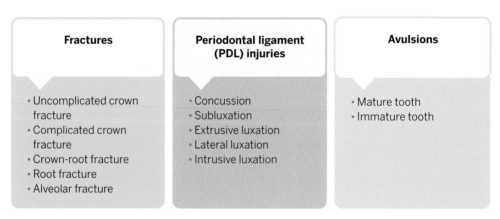

FIG 14-3 Categorization of traumatic dental injuries according to presentation and management.

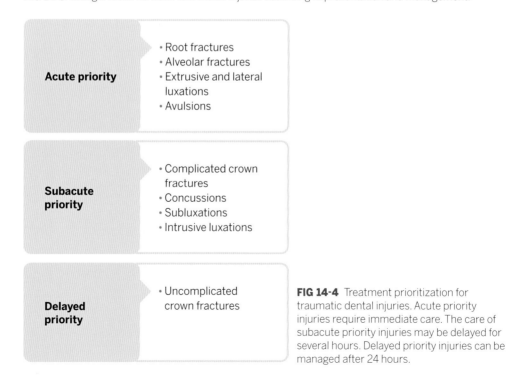

FIG 14-4 Treatment prioritization for traumatic dental injuries. Acute priority injuries require immediate care. The care of subacute priority injuries may be delayed for several hours. Delayed priority injuries can be managed after 24 hours.

Because traumatic dental injuries often occur in young patients with immature roots, endodontic interventions should prioritize continued root development for the best long-term outcomes. Thus, whenever possible, vital pulp therapy or regenerative endodontic procedures are preferred over apexification in the management of immature teeth. Even in mature roots, vital pulp therapy is the recommended first-line treatment following traumatic pulp exposures.[4] Treatment of traumatic injuries may involve splinting depending on the injury. When indicated, splinting can improve patient comfort and function and help to maintain tooth positioning.[4] Flexible splints are advised due to risks of periodontal ligament (PDL) damage and RR with rigid splinting.[15,16] Therefore, splinting should be performed with flexible wire or other material, such as fishing line, that is no greater than 0.4 mm in diameter.[2,4,5] In general, short-duration splinting is recommended, and appropriate splint timing is explicitly outlined in trauma guidelines[2,4,5] (Fig 14-5).

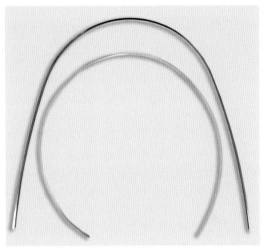

FIG 14-5 Splinting materials should be flexible to allow for physiologic movement of teeth. Acceptable splinting materials include up to 0.4-mm-diameter orthodontic wire, fishing line, and titanium mesh splints.

Generally, patients should eat a soft diet for 1 to 2 weeks following the diagnosis and treatment of traumatic dental injuries.[2] Oral hygiene should be maintained with a soft-bristled toothbrush and a prescribed 0.12% chlorhexidine mouth rinse. Contact sports should be avoided for at least 2 weeks following injury, and patients should be counseled on the importance of preventive measures like custom-fitted mouthguards when they are resumed[4,5] (Fig 14-6).

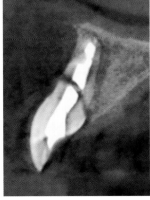

FIG 14-6 Trauma patients should be counseled on the use of athletic mouthguards to prevent further injuries. This patient developed pulp necrosis following a luxation injury and was successfully treated with a bioceramic apexification. Retraumatization 1 year later resulted in a horizontal root fracture that required tooth extraction.

Traumatic dental injuries pose a lifetime risk of pulpal and periapical pathology, including pulp necrosis, pulp canal obliteration, and resorptive dental diseases. Resultantly, these injuries should be followed closely and for an extended duration to evaluate them for late-stage complications.[2–5] Follow-up schedules are injury specific and are discussed in relation to the individual injuries described in the following sections. Resorption in particular is common following dental trauma, including lateral external inflammatory root resorption (EIRR), internal root resorption (IRR), and external cervical resorption (ECR) (see chapter 12) (Fig 14-7). Avulsions have an especially high likelihood of causing resorption. For this reason, intracanal calcium hydroxide and systemic doxycycline are often used for their antiresorptive properties.[17]

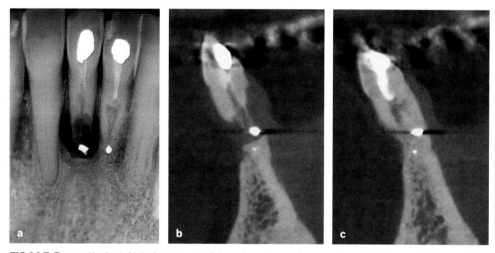

FIG 14-7 Traumatic dental injuries may result in various types of resorption, oftentimes as late sequelae. (a) This 62-year-old patient reported a history of trauma falling off his bicycle as a child. Incomplete endodontic care may have also contributed to IRR in the mandibular left central incisor (b) and EIRR in the mandibular right central incisor (c).

Fractures

Several classification systems describe dental fractures. Whereas the AAE Glossary of Endodontic Terms[18] was used to discussed fractures in chapter 11, the AAE trauma guidelines nomenclature will be used in this chapter to review the fractures originating from dental trauma.[2,4] The overlap between these classification systems is presented in Fig 14-8, and a summary of recommendations for the diagnosis and treatment of traumatic fractures is presented in Table 14-1.

FIG 14-8 Comparison of fracture nomenclature from the AAE trauma guidelines and the AAE Glossary of Endodontic Terms.

Uncomplicated crown fractures
- Infractions
- Enamel fractures
- Enamel-dentin fractures

Complicated crown fractures
- Enamel-dentin-pulp fractures

TABLE 14-1 Diagnosis and treatment of traumatic fractures

	Clinical findings	Management	Follow-up schedule
Uncomplicated crown fracture	• No pulpal exposure • No signs of pulpal or PDL inflammation	• Restorative care	• 6–8 weeks • 1 year
Complicated crown fracture	• Pulpal exposure • No signs of pulpal or PDL inflammation	• Direct pulp cap and restorative care	• 6–8 weeks • 3 months • 6 months • 1 year
Crown-root fracture	• If pulp exposed, abnormal response to pulp sensitivity testing • Percussion tenderness • Mobility of coronal segment	• Multidisciplinary, often requiring endodontic, surgical, or orthodontic exposure and restorative care versus extraction or root submergence	• 1 week • 6–8 weeks • 3 months • 6 months • 1 year • Yearly for 5 years
Horizontal root fracture	• Possible extrusive or lateral displacement and mobility • Percussion tenderness • Unreliable pulp sensitivity testing	• Splinting of the fractured segment for 4 weeks to 4 months • Sometimes nonsurgical root canal therapy (NSRCT) up to the fracture line or extraction	• 4 weeks • 6–8 weeks • 4 months • 1 year • Yearly for 5 years
Alveolar fracture	• Mobility of several teeth together • Change in occlusal plane	• Surgical repositioning • Splinting for 4 weeks	• 4 weeks • 6–8 weeks • 4 months • 1 year • Yearly for 5 years

Uncomplicated crown fractures

Crown fractures without pulp exposure, including infractions, enamel-only fractures, and enamel-dentin fractures, are termed uncomplicated crown fractures in the context of traumatic dental injuries[2,4] (Fig 14-9). Fractures may be completely or incompletely

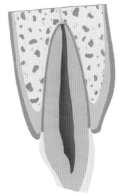

FIG 14-9 Uncomplicated crown fractures involve the loss of enamel and dentin without pulp exposure.

separated. If an uncomplicated crown fracture is the sole trauma-related diagnosis, no symptoms or signs of pulpal or periapical pathology are expected, including percussion or palpation tenderness or abnormal responses to pulp sensitivity testing. If pulpal and periapical signs and symptoms are present, a secondary trauma-related diagnosis, such as a luxation-type injury or root fracture, is suspected.

Management of uncomplicated crown fractures involves restorative care. If fractured fragments are available for reattachment, they may be bonded following soaking in water or saline for rehydration.[4] If the fragment is unavailable, bonded restorative materials are appropriate. A calcium hydroxide liner can be considered when fractures are less than 0.5 mm from the pulp.[4] Because 6% of crown fractures undergo pulp necrosis,[19] patients should be advised to monitor for signs and symptoms of developing pathology, including sensitivity, pain, and tooth discoloration. Clinical and radiographic follow-up is advised at 6 to 8 weeks and 1 year post injury to evaluate for asymptomatic pathology.[2,4]

Complicated crown fractures

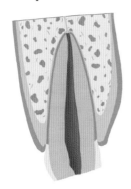

FIG 14-10 Complicated crown fractures involve the loss of enamel and dentin with pulp exposure.

Any crown fracture with pulp exposure is termed a complicated crown fracture according to the dental trauma guidelines.[2,4] These fractures involve enamel, dentin, and pulp (Fig 14-10). Fractures may be completely or incompletely separated. If the complicated crown fracture is the sole trauma-related diagnosis, signs and symptoms of pulpal disease may be absent. Teeth may, however, exhibit thermal sensitivity due to the pulp exposure. If periapical symptoms are present, especially tenderness to percussion or biting, a secondary trauma-related diagnosis, such as a luxation-type injury, should be ruled out.

Complicated crown fractures in immature and fully mature teeth should be treated with vital pulp therapy. Ideally, a bioceramic-based direct pulp cap should be placed within 48 hours of injury.[2,4] Calcium hydroxide may be used as an alternative in esthetically sensitive areas because bioceramics have the potential to cause coronal discoloration[20] (Fig 14-11). In mature teeth, treatment delays beyond 48 hours are associated with saliva and biofilm contamination, necessitating more invasive endodontic therapy such as pulpotomy or NSRCT.[21] Restoration of the missing tooth fragment can include reattachment of the fractured segment of tooth or bonded restorative materials. That said, when restorative needs indicate post placement, NSRCT may be required. As with uncomplicated crown fractures, 6% of teeth having undergone complicated crown fractures develop pulpal necrosis, and patients must monitor for signs and symptoms, including sensitivity, pain, and tooth discoloration.[19] Clinical and radiographic follow-up is advised at 6 to 8 weeks, 3 months, 6 months, and 1 year after injury to assess for asymptomatic disease.[4]

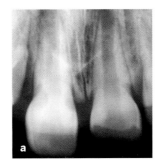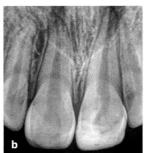

FIG 14-11 *(a)* Complicated crown fractures, like the one in this maxillary left central incisor, are best treated with vital pulp therapy. A pulp cap was placed, and the tooth was restored. *(b)* At the 3-year follow-up, the tooth remained vital, and complete apical closure was noted.

Crown-root fractures

Fractures extending from the crown to the root surface and involving enamel, dentin, and cementum are termed crown-root fractures. These fractures may or may not expose the pulp (Fig 14-12). Percussion sensitivity is often present, and mobility of fractured segments is likely. An exposed pulp may exhibit signs of inflammation, including thermal sensitivity. Crown-root fractures are best visualized with CBCT imaging, which can show not only the fracture itself but also its relationship to the periodontium, a key component in treatment planning (Fig 14-13).

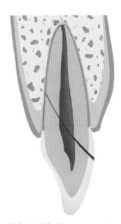

FIG 14-12 Crown-root fractures involve enamel, dentin, and cementum and may or may not expose the pulp.

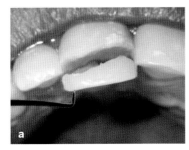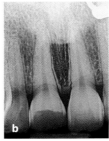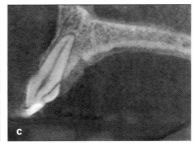

FIG 14-13 CBCT imaging was crucial in the work-up of this crown-root fracture on the maxillary right central incisor. *(a)* This patient fell, fracturing the tooth. *(b)* Periapical imaging showed structural loss. *(c)* The sagittal section of CBCT imaging showcased the full extent of the injury.

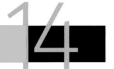

Interdisciplinary treatment planning and management is crucial for crown-root fractures. Maintenance of these teeth may require pre-prosthetic NSRCT if inadequate coronal structure remains and vital pulp therapy or NSRCT when the pulp is exposed. Depending on the extent of root involvement, crown-lengthening surgery or orthodontic extrusion may be required prior to restorative care. Given the complexity of some cases, root submergence, intentional replantation, or autotransplantation may be considered.[4] Extraction may also be the treatment of choice. Clinical and radiographic follow-up is advised at 1 week, 6 to 8 weeks, 3 months, 6 months, 1 year, and yearly for 5 years after injury.[4]

Root fractures

Trauma-associated root fractures are typically horizontally or obliquely oriented (Fig 14-14). Depending on the location and any dislocation resulting from the fracture, the coronal portion of the tooth may be mobile and possibly displaced or may remain normally positioned. The affected tooth is often sensitive to percussion. A transient loss of a pulp sensitivity response is common in teeth with root fractures. Radiographically, oblique fracture lines are difficult to visualize with periapical imaging, but CBCT images will show their location and extent clearly (Fig 14-15).

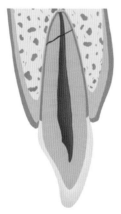

FIG 14-14 Root fractures that develop due to trauma can be oriented either horizontally or obliquely through the root structure.

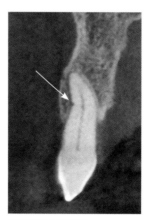

FIG 14-15 CBCT imaging, particularly sagittal sections of anterior teeth, provides the best means to assess the location and orientation of horizontal root fractures. This image very clearly depicts the horizontal root fracture located in the middle third of the root oriented obliquely.

The management and prognosis of root fractures depend on the location of the fracture, coronal mobility, and the amount of displacement of the coronal segment. Displaced segments must be expediently repositioned within hours of the injury, with radiographic confirmation of appropriate repositioning. A flexible splint should be placed for 4 weeks or up to 4 months in the case of cervically positioned fractures[4] (Fig 14-16).

FIG 14-16 Treatment for horizontal root fractures involves the repositioning and flexible splinting of the coronal fragment for 4 weeks in most patients and for up to 4 months in patients with more cervically positioned fractures.

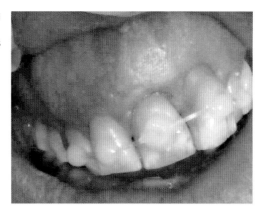

Pulp necrosis occurs in approximately 22% of root-fractured teeth.[22] Because the majority of cases undergo pulp necrosis in the coronal segment only,[22] when necrosis develops, root canal therapy should be completed with the fracture line as the apical terminus (Fig 14-17). When root canal therapy is completed in the coronal segment of a tooth with a horizontal root fracture, working length should be determined with the use of electronic apex locators (EALs) and radiography. Obturation can be performed with traditional gutta-percha–based systems or with bioceramic cements similar to the artificial barriers of apexification procedures, depending on the diameter of the apical preparation.[23,24] Should pathology develop in the apical segment of a horizontally fractured tooth, this fragment should be removed surgically due to a poor prognosis of orthograde endodontic treatment through a fracture line.[24] Clinical and radiographic follow-up is advised at 4 weeks, 6 to 8 weeks, 4 months, 1 year, and yearly for 5 years after injury.[2,4]

FIG 14-17 *(a)* When necrosis of the coronal fragment develops following a horizontal root fracture, *(b)* NSRCT should be completed to the fracture line as opposed to the apex. (Case courtesy of Dr David Baker.)

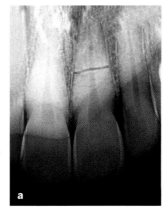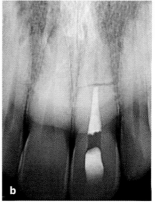

Alveolar fractures

Fractures of the alveolus may occur with severe traumatic injuries. Clinically, there may be mobility of several teeth together or changes to the occlusion may be noted (Fig 14-18). Pulp sensitivity tests may be unresponsive due to the severity of the injury, and percussion and palpation tenderness may be present. Panoramic and CBCT images are the best tools for visualizing alveolar fractures (Fig 14-19).

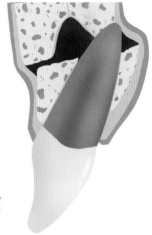

FIG 14-18 Alveolar fractures may be associated with the mobility of several adjacent teeth.

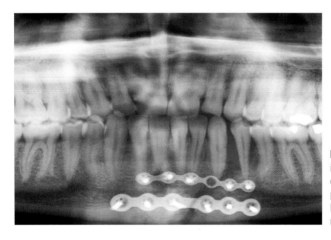

FIG 14-19 Panoramic and CBCT images are often best equipped to detect alveolar fractures, like the panoramic image of this mandibular alveolar fracture following open reduction and internal fixation.

If displacement is noted, management involves surgical repositioning of displaced teeth and bone and placement of a splint on the associated teeth for 4 weeks. Oral and maxillofacial surgeons may be best equipped to manage cases involving alveolar fracture.[4] Clinical and radiographic follow-up for affected teeth is advised at 4 weeks, 6 to 8 weeks, 4 months, 1 year, and yearly for 5 years after injury.[2,4]

PDL Injuries

Blunt force dental trauma can result in damage to the PDL and associated structures. PDL injuries may occur in an isolated fashion, among several teeth, or with comorbid fractures in an individual tooth or teeth. Clinically, these injuries can range in presentation from percussion sensitivity to mobility or displacement. Radiographically, they may present with a widened PDL on periapical films or tooth displacement on CBCT imaging. Diagnosis is based on clinical and radiographic findings, and both treatment and follow-up are dependent on the diagnosis. A summary of the diagnosis and management of PDL injuries is presented in Table 14-2.

TABLE 14-2 Diagnosis and management of PDL injuries

	Displacement	Pulpal response	Percussion	Mobility	Radiographic findings	Management	Follow-up schedule
Concussion	None	Normal	Sensitive	Physiologic	None/PDL widening	No immediate interventions	• 4 weeks • 1 year
Subluxation	None	Unreliable	Sensitive	Mobile	None/PDL widening	Splinting for 2 weeks for patient comfort	• 2 weeks • 12 weeks • 6 months • 1 year
Extrusive luxation	Extruded	Unreliable	Sensitive	Mobile	PDL widening, extrusive displacement	Immediate repositioning and splinting for 2 weeks (4 weeks if marginal bone breakdown)	• 2 weeks • 12 weeks • 6 months • 1 year
Lateral luxation	Horizontally	Unreliable	Sensitive	Immobile	PDL widening, lateral displacement	Immediate repositioning and splinting for 4 weeks	• 2 weeks • 4 weeks • 8 weeks • 12 weeks • 6 months • 1 year • Yearly for 5 years
Intrusive luxation	Intruded	Unresponsive	Sensitive	Immobile	Loss of apical PDL, shorter tooth than neighbors	• Depends on root maturity and the degree of displacement; monitoring for spontaneous re-eruption or orthodontic/surgical repositioning • Mature roots require NSRCT	• 2 weeks • 4 weeks • 8 weeks • 12 weeks • 6 months • 1 year • Yearly for 5 years

Concussion

The mildest PDL injury, a concussion, is characterized by percussion tenderness without mobility or displacement of the tooth. Pulp sensitivity testing is often normal. Radiographically, the tooth may appear normal or present with a widened PDL (Fig 14-20). Though no acute management is required, concussed teeth have an elevated risk of developing pulp necrosis (estimated at 3% in the 10 years following the injury[25]) and should be monitored with clinical and radiographic examinations at 4 weeks and 1 year following the injury.[4] If signs and symptoms of pulp necrosis develop, NSRCT should be initiated.

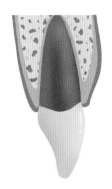

FIG 14-20 A concussion is a PDL injury characterized by percussion tenderness without mobility or displacement.

Subluxation

Subluxations are characterized by percussion tenderness and mobility without displacement of the tooth. Pulp sensitivity testing may be normal or abnormal due to either transient neural damage[9] or true pulpal degeneration. Consequently, the pulpal diagnosis cannot be based on this finding alone for up to 3 months following injury. Radiographically, the tooth may appear normal or have a widened PDL (Fig 14-21). A passive and flexible splint may be placed for up to 2 weeks following the injury if desired for patient comfort.[4] Following subluxation injuries, teeth have an elevated risk of pulp necrosis (estimated at 6%[25]) and should be followed with clinical and radiographic examinations at 2 weeks, 12 weeks, 6 months, and 1 year following the injury.[4] If signs and symptoms of pulp necrosis develop, NSRCT should be initiated.

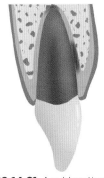

FIG 14-21 A subluxation is a PDL injury characterized by percussion tenderness and mobility without displacement of the tooth. Radiographs often appear normal, or PDL widening may be present.

Extrusive luxation

Extrusive luxation is characterized by coronal dislocation of the tooth, resulting in an elongated appearance of the affected tooth (Fig 14-22). Percussion tenderness and clinical mobility are often present. Pulp sensitivity testing may or may not be normal due to either transient neural damage [9] or true pulpal degeneration. Consequently, a pulpal diagnosis cannot be determined based on this finding alone for up to 3 months following injury. Radiographically, generalized PDL widening will be present, and either periapical or CBCT imaging will show the coronal displacement of the tooth (Fig 14-23).

The extruded tooth should be repositioned as soon as possible following the injury. A passive and flexible splint should be

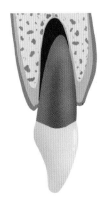

FIG 14-22 An extrusive luxation is a PDL injury characterized by displacement of the tooth out of the socket. The tooth is often mobile, and percussion tenderness is often noted.

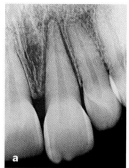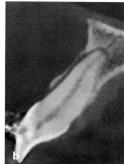

FIG 14-23 *(a and b)* Periapical radiographs and CBCT images for extrusive luxations will display PDL widening and the coronal displacement of the crown compared to neighboring teeth.

placed for 2 weeks, or up to 4 weeks if the marginal bone is broken down or fractured.[4] Following extrusive luxations, teeth have an elevated risk of developing pulp necrosis (estimated at 26%[25]) and should be followed with clinical and radiographic examinations at 2 weeks, 4 weeks, 8 weeks, 12 weeks, 6 months, 1 year, and yearly for 5 years following the injury.[4] If signs and symptoms of pulp necrosis develop, NSRCT should be initiated.

Lateral luxation

Lateral luxation refers to the horizontal displacement of a tooth in either the buccal/facial or lingual/palatal direction. Percussion tenderness is often present, and as a result of the tooth being wedged within the alveolar bone housing, the laterally luxated tooth is often immobile (Fig 14-24). Pulp sensitivity testing may or may not be normal due to either transient neural damage [9] or true pulpal degeneration. Consequently, a pulpal diagnosis cannot be based on this finding alone for up to 3 months following injury. Radiographically, generalized PDL widening may be present, and CBCT imaging will show the lateral displacement of the root (Fig 14-25).

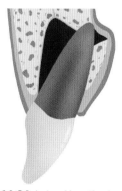

FIG 14-24 Lateral luxation is a PDL injury characterized by horizontal displacement of the crown and displacement of the root structure in the opposite direction. The tooth will be percussion tender and immobile because the apex is frequently locked in the alveolar bone.

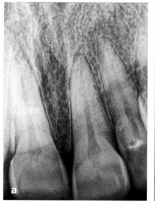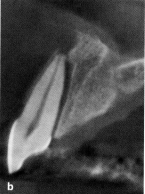

FIG 14-25 *(a)* Periapical images of laterally luxated teeth may show PDL widening, and *(b)* CBCT images will show the displacement of the crown and root structure.

The tooth should be repositioned as soon as possible following the injury, which may require the use of forceps and local anesthesia. Alternatively, if the apical end of the root is palpable, one finger can be used to push down on the root apex while the tooth is manually pushed back into the socket. A passive and flexible splint should be placed for 4 weeks following injury.[4] Teeth suffering lateral luxation injuries have an elevated risk of developing pulp necrosis (estimated at 58%[25]) and should be followed with clinical and radiographic examinations at 2 weeks, 4 weeks, 8 weeks, 12 weeks, 6 months, 1 year, and yearly for 5 years following the injury.[4] If signs and symptoms of pulp necrosis develop, NSRCT should be initiated.

Intrusive luxation

Intrusive luxation refers to the displacement of a tooth into the socket. Because the apical tissues are crushed during intrusions, these teeth suffer significant pulpal damage (Fig 14-26). Clinically, teeth will appear shorter than counterparts. Percussion tenderness is often present, and the tooth is often immobile due to its locked position in the alveolar bone. The tooth may be initially nonresponsive to pulp sensitivity testing given the severity of the injury leading to pulpal degeneration. Radiographically, the tooth will appear apically displaced as compared to its neighbors, and the apical PDL will be obliterated from view.

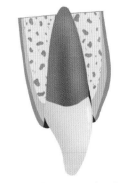

FIG 14-26 An intrusive luxation is a PDL injury characterized by displacement of the tooth into the socket. The tooth will be percussion tender and immobile because the root is locked in the alveolar bone.

Management of intrusive luxation injuries depends upon the stage of root maturation, patient age, and the degree of intrusion. Mature teeth intruded less than 3 mm should be allowed to spontaneously re-erupt. If spontaneous re-eruption has not occurred within 8 weeks of the injury, surgical or orthodontic repositioning should commence before replacement resorption develops. When intrusion is between 3 and 7 mm, surgical or orthodontic repositioning is immediately indicated. For intrusions greater than 7 mm, teeth should undergo surgical repositioning followed by 4 weeks of splinting.[4] That said, severe intrusions may require tooth extraction (Fig 14-27). Immature permanent teeth should be allowed to spontaneously re-erupt, irrespective of the amount of intrusion. If re-eruption has not occurred within 4 weeks of the injury, orthodontic repositioning should be initiated.[4] Treatment recommendations for intrusive luxations are presented in Table 14-3.

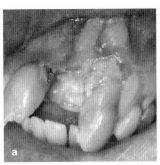 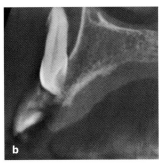 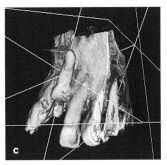

FIG 14-27 *(a to c)* In cases of severe intrusive luxations, like for this patient, extraction may be the treatment of choice.

TABLE 14-3 Treatment recommendations for intrusive luxations based on root maturity and the degree of intrusion

Mature apices	
< 3 mm intrusion	Allow for spontaneous re-eruption. If no movement is noted after 4 weeks, initiate surgical or orthodontic repositioning.
3–7 mm intrusion	Surgical or orthodontic repositioning should be initiated.
> 7 mm intrusion	Surgical repositioning.
Immature apices	
Any degree of intrusion	Allow for spontaneous re-eruption. If no movement is noted after 4 weeks, initiate orthodontic repositioning.

Because mature teeth suffering intrusive luxation injuries have a high risk of pulp necrosis (estimated at 85%[25]), endodontic intervention is routinely advised. NSRCT should be initiated in mature teeth within 2 weeks of the intrusive luxation. Two-visit therapy with placement of intracanal, interappointment calcium hydroxide for 4 weeks is advised prior to obturation to maximize antiresorptive properties.[4] Immature teeth are better able to heal due to the robust apical blood supply, and endodontic therapy either by apexification or regenerative endodontic procedures is advised only if signs and symptoms of pulpal degeneration occur.[4] Clinical and radiographic follow-up is advised at 2 weeks, 4 weeks, 8 weeks, 12 weeks, 6 months, 1 year, and yearly for 5 years following the injury.[4]

Avulsions

Avulsion involves the complete loss of the tooth from the alveolar housing.[2,5] As a result, the pulpal blood supply is completely severed, and the PDL is severely damaged (Fig 14-28), with sequelae including pulpal necrosis and associated periapical disease, as well as EIRR. Successful avulsion management involves prompt replantation of the tooth, immediately or within 1 hour of the injury to minimize PDL cell death. If immediate replantation is not possible, the tooth must be stored in a physiologic solution such as milk, saline, saliva, or a proprietary tooth saver solution to maintain the vitality of the PDL[26–28] (Fig 14-29).

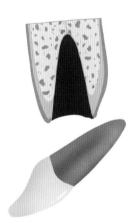

FIG 14-28 Avulsion involves the complete loss of the tooth from the alveolar housing.

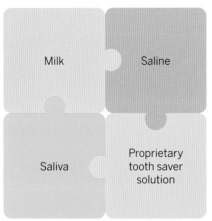

FIG 14-29 If an avulsed tooth cannot be immediately replanted, it should be stored in a physiologic storage medium, such as one of those listed here. Water is not an acceptable storage medium because it will lead to PDL cell lysis and death.

Milk

Saline

Saliva

Proprietary tooth saver solution

Teeth with mature apices will inevitably undergo pulp necrosis following avulsions. Consequently, NSRCT is always indicated following their replantation. Immature teeth with an apical diameter of at least 1 mm may undergo spontaneous revascularization.[29] Resultantly, NSRCT should be delayed in these teeth to allow for potential revascularization and continued root development. Generally, even in situations where replanted teeth have poor prognoses, current guidelines advise replantation in every case possible. Even in the presence of delays and/or inappropriate storage, replantation ensures that the patient has all options available to them, including extraction or retention.[5]

Because teeth undergoing replantation encounter many potential sources of bacterial contamination, antibiotics are recommended for patients following avulsions. Doxycycline is the drug of choice for patients over 12 years old, whereas amoxicillin is advised for younger patients.[2] A 7-day course is advised, with dosages tailored to patient weight. Antibiotics, particularly doxycycline, possess antiresorptive properties, which is desirable in these teeth with extremely damaged roots where resorptive complications are common, if not imminent.[18,30]

Treatment guidelines for teeth with mature apices

Teeth replanted prior to the office visit

The area should be gently rinsed with water, saline, or chlorhexidine, and the tooth position should be confirmed clinically and radiographically. Minor discrepancies in positioning may be corrected using manual repositioning under local anesthesia. More significant discrepancies may require surgical repositioning within 48 hours of the injury. Whenever local anesthetic is used for replantation, vasoconstrictors are contraindicated due to the possible effects on blood flow and healing.[5] A passive and flexible splint should be placed for 2 weeks, though more rigid splinting for up to 4 weeks may be indicated with comorbid alveolar or jaw fractures. Associated soft tissue lacerations may require suturing. NSRCT should be initiated within 2 weeks with the use of intracanal, interappointment calcium hydroxide for 4 weeks prior to obturation.[5]

Teeth stored in physiologic storage medium and/or with an extraoral dry time less than 60 minutes

The root surface should be handled as little as possible, and the tooth should be kept in the storage medium until the moment of replantation. A pre-replantation radiograph is advised to assess for comorbid injuries or alveolar fracture within the socket. Following administration of local anesthesia without vasoconstrictor, the root and socket may be rinsed with saline and the tooth gently replanted, with its position confirmed clinically and radiographically. Any alveolar fractures within the socket will require correction if they impinge upon full replantation. A passive and flexible splint should be placed for 2 weeks, or up to 4 weeks with concomitant alveolar or jaw fracture.[5] Soft tissue lacerations should be sutured. NSRCT should be initiated within 2 weeks with the use of intracanal, interappointment calcium hydroxide for 4 weeks prior to obturation.[5]

Teeth with an extraoral dry time greater than 60 minutes

The prognosis for maintaining the tooth in these cases is poor. Typically, RR develops and results in tooth loss. However, tooth replantation is still advised to maintain esthetics and function in the short term and to maintain bone for future replacement options. Necrotic tissue from the root should be removed gently with gauze, and replantation, splinting, and NSRCT can otherwise be performed as described for properly stored teeth.[5] Careful follow-up is key in these cases of delayed replantation because poor outcomes are expected. A decoronation procedure may be considered if RR results in greater than 1 mm of infrapositioning of the tooth from its neighbors, as may occur in patients who are still growing.

Treatment guidelines for teeth with immature apices

Teeth replanted prior to the office visit

The area should be rinsed with water, saline, or chlorhexidine. The tooth position should be confirmed clinically and radiographically. If malpositioning is noted, efforts to reposition can occur as with the mature tooth. A passive and flexible splint should be placed for 2 weeks, though associated alveolar or jaw fractures warrant rigid splinting for up to 4 weeks.[5] Soft tissue lacerations should be sutured. Endodontic therapy is not indicated unless signs and symptoms of pulp degeneration occur at follow-up. If these signs and symptoms are noted, regenerative endodontic treatment or apexification is the treatment of choice.[5]

Teeth stored in physiologic storage medium and/or with an extraoral dry time less than 60 minutes

The tooth should be left in the physiologic storage medium until the examination is complete. Following administration of vasoconstrictor-free local anesthesia, the root and socket should be rinsed with saline. Alveolar fractures within the socket may require correction, and any coagulum within the socket may require removal to completely seat the tooth within the socket. The tooth must be replanted with gentle pressure and its position confirmed clinically and radiographically. A passive and flexible splint should be placed for 2 weeks, though associated alveolar or jaw fractures warrant rigid splinting for up to 4 weeks.[5] Soft tissue lacerations should be sutured. Endodontic therapy, namely regenerative endodontic procedures or apexification, is not indicated unless signs and symptoms of pulp degeneration are present at the follow-up.[5]

Teeth with an extraoral dry time greater than 60 minutes

For immature teeth with an extraoral dry time longer than 60 minutes, the prognosis is poor. These teeth typically undergo RR, resulting in tooth loss. However, tooth replantation is still advised for esthetic, functional, and psychologic reasons and to maintain the alveolar contour in young patients for as long as possible to aid in implant placement. Necrotic tissue from the root should be removed gently with gauze, and replantation and splinting can otherwise be performed as previously described.[5] Endodontic therapy is not indicated unless signs and symptoms of pulp degeneration are present at the follow-up. If endodontic intervention does become necessary, care should be taken to use resorbable root filling materials to aid in the decoronation procedures required once RR occurs.

Follow-up

Whether the avulsed teeth are mature or immature, clinical and radiographic follow-up should be performed at 2 weeks (for splint removal), 1 month, 2 months, 3 months, 6 months, 1 year, and yearly for 5 years following the injury.[5] As with all traumatic injuries, patients should be informed from the beginning of the lifetime of increased risk for potential complications in these severely traumatized teeth. Commonly, RR occurs, which will result in infrapositioning of the tooth in a growing patient (Fig 14-30) and potential tooth loss in its latest stages. Treatment recommendations for avulsions are presented in Table 14-4.

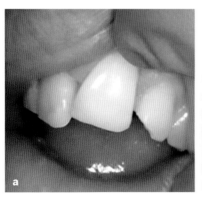 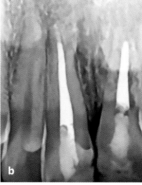

FIG 14-30 *(a and b)* RR is common following avulsions and will result in infrapositioning of the tooth in growing patients.

TABLE 14-4 Recommended treatment strategies for the management of avulsions

Stage	Prior to office visit	Replant-ation	Splinting	Endodontic treatment	Follow-up
Mature	Already replanted	NA	2 weeks flexible (4 weeks rigid with alveolar fractures)	NSRCT	2 weeks 1 month 2 months 3 months 6 months 1 year Yearly for 5 years
	Proper storage and/or EDT < 60 mins	Yes			
	Improper storage	Yes			
Immature	Already replanted	NA	2 weeks flexible (4 weeks rigid with alveolar fractures)	Not unless signs/symptoms of endodontic disease develop (if so, apexification or REP)	2 weeks 1 month 2 months 3 months 6 months 1 year Yearly for 5 years
	Proper storage and/or EDT < 60 mins	Yes			
	Improper storage	Yes			

EDT = extraoral dry time; REP = regenerative endodontic procedure

References

1. Day PF, Flores MT, O'Connell AC, et al. International Association of Dental Traumatology guidelines for the management of traumatic dental injuries: 3. Injuries in the primary dentition. Dent Traumatol 2020;36:343–359.
2. American Association of Endodontists. The Recommended Guidelines of the American Association of Endodontists for The Treatment of Traumatic Dental Injuries. 2013. https://www.aae.org/specialty/clinical-resources/treatment-planning/traumatic-dental-injuries/. Accessed 5 April 2023.
3. Levin L, Day PF, Hicks L, et al. International Association of Dental Traumatology guidelines for the management of traumatic dental injuries: General introduction. Dent Traumatol 2020;36:309–313.
4. Bourguignon C, Cohenca N, Lauridsen E, et al. International Association of Dental Traumatology guidelines for the management of traumatic dental injuries: 1. Fractures and luxations. Dent Traumatol 2020;36:314–330.
5. Fouad, AF, Abbott PV, Tsilinigaridis G, et al. International Association of Dental Traumatolody Guidelines for the management of traumatic dental injuries: 2. Avulsion of permanent teeth. Dent Traumatol 2020;36:331–342.
6. Steelman R. Rapid physical assessment of the injured child. J Endod 2013;39(3, suppl):S9–S12.
7. Myers GL. Evaluation and diagnosis of the traumatized dentition. J Endod 2019;45(12S):S66–S71.
8. Levin LG. Pulp and periradicular testing. Pediatr Dent 2013;35:113–119.
9. Bhaskar SN, Rappaport HM. Dental vitality tests and pulp status. J Am Dent Assoc 1973;86:409–411.
10. Ozçelik B, Kuraner T, Kendir B, Aşan E. Histopathological evaluation of the dental pulps in crown-fractured teeth. J Endod 2000;26:271–273.
11. Special Committee to Revise the Joint AAE/AAOMR Position Statement on use of CBCT in Endodontics. AAE and AAOMR joint position statement: Use of cone beam computed tomography in endodontics 2015 update. Oral Surg Oral Med Oral Pathol Oral Radiol 2015;120:508–512.
12. Fayad MI, Ashkenaz PJ, Johnson BR. Different representations of vertical root fractures detected by cone-beam volumetric tomography: A case series report. J Endod 2012;38:1435–1442.
13. Patel S, Brown J, Semper M, Abella F, Mannocci F. European Society of Endodontology position statement: Use of cone beam computed tomography in endodontics: European Society of Endodontology (ESE) developed by. Int Endod J 2019;52:1675–1678.

14. Bakland LK, Andreasen JO. Dental traumatology: Essential diagnosis and treatment planning. Endod Topics 2004;7:14–34.

15. von Arx T, Filippi A, Buser D. Splinting of traumatized teeth with a new device: TTS (titanium trauma splint). Dent Traumatol 2001;17:180–184.

16. Nasjleti CE, Castelli WA, Caffesse RG. The effects of different splinting times on replantation of teeth in monkeys. Oral Surg Oral Med Oral Pathol 1982;53:557–566.

17. Hammarström L, Blomlöf L, Feiglin B, Andersson L, Lindskog S. Replantation of teeth and antibiotic treatment. Endod Dent Traumatol 1986;2:51–57.

18. Glossary of Endodontic Terms, ed 10. American Association of Endodontists, 2020. https://www.aae.org/specialty/clinical-resources/glossary-endodontic-terms/. Accessed 5 April 2023.

19. Ravn JJ. Follow-up study of permanent incisors with enamel fractures as a result of an acute trauma. Scand J Dent Res 1981;89:213–217.

20. Beatty H, Svec T. Quantifying coronal tooth discoloration caused by Biodentine and Endosequence root repair material. J Endod 2015;41:2036–2039.

21. Cvek M, Cleaton-Jones PE, Austin JC, Andreasen JO. Pulp reactions to exposure after experimental crown fractures or grinding in adult monkeys. J Endod 1982;8:391–397.

22. Andreasen FM, Andreasen JO, Bayer T. Prognosis of root-fractured permanent incisors—Prediction of healing modalities. Endod Dent Traumatol 1989;5:11–22.

23. Kim D, Yue W, Yoon TC, Park SH, Kim E. Healing of horizontal intra-alveolar root fractures after endodontic treatment with mineral trioxide aggregate. J Endod 2016;42:230–235.

24. Cvek M, Mejàre I, Andreasen JO. Conservative endodontic treatment of teeth fractured in the middle or apical part of the root. Dent Traumatol 2004;20:261–269.

25. Andreasen FM, Pedersen BV. Prognosis of luxated permanent teeth—The development of pulp necrosis. Endod Dent Traumatol 1985;1:207–220.

26. Blomlöf L. Milk and saliva as possible storage media for traumatically exarticulated teeth prior to replantation. Swed Dent J Suppl 1981;8:1–26.

27. Trope M, Friedman S. Periodontal healing of replanted dog teeth stored in Viaspan, milk and Hank's balanced salt solution. Endod Dent Traumatol 1992;8:183–188.

28. Van Hassel HJ, Oswald RJ, Harrington GW. Replantation 2. The role of the periodontal ligament. J Endod 1980;6:506–508.

29. Kling M, Cvek M, Mejare I. Rate and predictability of pulp revascularization in therapeutically reimplanted permanent incisors. Endod Dent Traumatol 1986;2:83–89.

30. Sae-Lim V, Wang CY, Choi GW, Trope M. The effect of systemic tetracycline on resorption of dried replanted dogs' teeth. Endod Dent Traumatol 1998;14:127–132.

Glossary

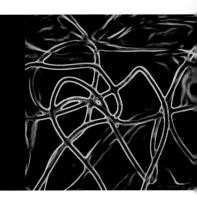

Diagnostic Terms

Pulpal diagnoses[1]

Asymptomatic irreversible pulpitis: An asymptomatic vital inflamed pulp due to caries, caries excavation, or trauma presumed incapable of healing without appropriate endodontic intervention, which may include vital pulp therapy. The tooth may respond normally to pulp sensitivity testing or may be associated with mild sensitivity to thermal stimuli.

Normal pulp: The pulp is free of symptoms and responds normally to sensitivity testing.

Previously initiated therapy: This diagnosis indicates endodontic treatment has been initiated but obturation material is absent.

Previously treated: This diagnosis indicates prior endodontic treatment with evidence of obturation material within the canals.

Pulp necrosis: This diagnosis indicates degeneration of the dental pulp. The pulp is nonresponsive to sensitivity testing.

Reversible pulpitis: The pulp has evidence of inflammation that is expected to return to normal following removal of the inciting stimulus. Symptoms include non-lingering sensitivity to thermal stimuli without spontaneous pain.

Symptomatic irreversible pulpitis: A symptomatic vital inflamed pulp that is incapable of healing without endodontic intervention. Symptoms include lingering pain in response to thermal stimuli, spontaneous pain, or radiating/referred pain.

Periapical diagnoses[1]

Acute apical abscess: Swelling of the soft tissues that is secondary to pulpal necrosis; the acute apical abscess is often characterized by rapid onset and pain, worsened by pressure.

Asymptomatic apical periodontitis: Though neither signs nor symptoms of inflammation of the apical periodontium are present, an apical radiolucency is indicative of inflammation and destruction of the apical periodontium that is of pulpal origin.

Chronic apical abscess: A sinus tract with intermittent discharge of pus secondary to pulpal necrosis and associated apical inflammation and destruction; because the infection is draining, discomfort may be minimal or absent.

Condensing osteitis: A localized bony reaction presenting as a radiopacity adjacent to the apex of a tooth, presumed to be due to a low-grade inflammatory stimulus originating in the pulp. These lesions should not be confused with radiopacities not associated with signs of pulpal inflammation, termed *enostoses* or *dense bone islands*.

Normal apical tissue: Clinical signs and symptoms are absent, and the teeth are not sensitive to percussion, palpation, or biting; radiographically, the periodontal ligament and lamina dura are intact and are uniform in appearance.

Symptomatic apical periodontitis: Inflammation of the apical periodontium is apparent based on clinical symptoms and signs, including a painful response to percussion, palpation, and/or biting; an apical radiolucency may or may not be present.

Other diagnostic terminology

ALARA: "As low as reasonably achievable," used in reference to dental radiography in which the fewest images with the lowest radiation exposure should be used to avoid the known and unknown risks associated with radiation exposure.

Periapical tests: Diagnostic tests aimed at elucidating the health or diseased state of periapical tissues as measured by percussion, palpation, or biting.

Pulp sensitivity tests: Diagnostic tests aimed at elucidating the pulpal status (normal, inflamed, necrotic); currently available options include cold, heat, and electric testing modalities.

Treatment Terminology

Dental anatomy

Apical: Relating to the apex of the tooth.

Apical constriction: The area of the root canal with the smallest diameter, generally located 0.5 to 1.5 mm from the apical foramen. The apical constriction is the point at which most clinicians terminate shaping and obturation. It is otherwise known as the *minor apical diameter*.

Apical foramen: The most apical opening of the root canal, which may or may not coincide with the anatomical or radiographic apex. It is otherwise known as the *major apical diameter*.

Coronal: Relating to the crown of the tooth.

Orifice: The coronal opening of the root canal space visible along the pulpal floor.

Nonsurgical endodontics

Access: The opening created in the occlusal surface of the tooth to gain entry into the root canal space.

Apical stop: A clinician-created barrier at the apical end of the canal preparation.

Cold lateral condensation: Method of obturation involving gutta-percha mechanically packed within the canal space via the sequential placement of cones in a space created by a spreader device and seared off at the canal orifice.

Coronal disassembly: The removal of restorative material from the crown of the tooth during nonsurgical root canal therapy or retreatment.

Coronal flaring: The instrumentation of the coronal portion of the root canal space to permit the introduction of other rotary and hand files to the working length.

Dental dam isolation: A latex rubber or non-latex dam used for isolation during nonsurgical endodontics and restorative care. Dental dam isolation is the standard of care during nonsurgical endodontic care.

Glide path: A smooth pathway created within the canal space to the working length.

Flare-up: An acute exacerbation of periradicular pathology after the initiation or continuation of root canal treatment.[1]

Intracanal medicament: A material placed into the instrumented canal spaces in lieu of obturation material when endodontic treatment is completed in two or more visits. In the United States, intracanal medicaments can include calcium hydroxide or antibiotic pastes.

Intraorifice barrier: A bonded restorative material, often comprised of resin-modified glass ionomers or flowable resins, placed over the obturated canal orifices and sometimes across the chamber floor to provide an enhanced barrier against coronal leakage that might occur if temporary restorative materials break down,[2,3] if restorative procedures are completed without the use of dental dam isolation,[4] or in teeth with coronally derived root fractures.[5]

Irrigant: A liquid used during nonsurgical endodontic treatment to flush the canal system of debris. Irrigants may possess other properties including antimicrobial effects, the ability to dissolve organic tissue, and the ability to dissolve hard tissue components of smear layers. Common irrigants include sodium hypochlorite, ethylenediaminetetraacetic acid (EDTA), and chlorhexidine.

Instrumentation: The process of physical debridement of the root canal system. Instrumentation can be performed with hand instruments like K files or Hedstrom files or with motor-driven rotary instruments.

Obturation: The process of filling the instrumented and disinfected root canal spaces. Obturation techniques include warm vertical condensation and cold lateral condensation.

Pulpectomy: Removal of the entirety of the pulp tissue from the root canal spaces.

Recapitulation: The reintroduction of a small hand file to the working length, often between rotary instruments, to prevent blockage of the canal.

Smear layer: Debris that accumulates on the canal walls and is packed into dentinal tubules during cleaning and shaping. The smear layer consists of dentin shavings, cell debris, and pulp remnants, along with potential microbial contamination.[6]

Solvent: A liquid used to dissolve obturation material during nonsurgical retreatment procedures. The most commonly used solvent is chloroform, as it is most effective in dissolving gutta-percha. Alternative solvents include isopropyl alcohol, orange solvent, xylene, and eucalyptol.

Straight-line access: The ability of a file to reach the apical foramen or the first point of canal curvature undeflected.

Ultrasonics: A specialized drill that uses ultrasonic energy and tips of various shapes, sizes, and coatings with a myriad of applications in nonsurgical and surgical endodontics. Nonsurgical applications include the ability to aid in locating small and calcified canals and utility in removing blockages within canal spaces.

Warm vertical condensation: Method of obturation involving gutta-percha condensed into the canal space with a heated element followed by gutta-percha backfill from a heated device dispensing flowable material.

Working length: The distance from the apical terminus to an established coronal reference point.

Restorative care

Coronal leakage: Entry of saliva and associated infectious agents and irritants into the root canal space via the coronal access. Coronal leakage is a contributing factor to the development of recurrent or persistent apical periodontitis.

Coronal seal: Restorative material used to prevent coronal leakage by temporary or definitive means.

Direct restoration: A restoration shaped within the mouth and bonded directly to the tooth that does not require additional laboratory fabrication.

Ferrule: Vertical wall of the tooth structure that supports fracture resistance.

Full-coverage restoration: A type of restoration that covers all cusps of a tooth.

Indirect restoration: A restoration formed outside the oral cavity (ie, based on an impression) and then cemented into the mouth as opposed to being shaped directly within the tooth.

Intracoronal restoration: A restoration surrounded by more than one remaining natural wall of a tooth; in the context of endodontics, this generally refers to fillings removed as part of the endodontic access or to restorations placed within the access opening.

Intraorifice barrier: A bonded restoration placed over the pulpal floor and into the canal orifice to protect endodontically treated canals from coronal leakage in case of breakdown of the temporary coronal seal.

Surgical endodontics

Bioceramics: Calcium silicate cements with documented biocompatibility and the ability to induce hard tissue formation and periodontal ligament (PDL) regeneration and maintain pulp vitality. The materials are antimicrobial and set in the presence of moisture, including blood. Research supports their first-line use for vital pulp therapy, including direct pulp caps and pulpotomy procedures, as well as in regenerative endodontic procedures and apexification in immature permanent teeth, for the repair of root perforations, and as root-end fillings for apical microsurgery.

Chlorhexidine: Chlorhexidine is an effective disinfectant that can be used as an oral rinsing agent or irrigant during operative procedures. In endodontics, it is mostly used as an oral rinsing agent to reduce bacterial or viral loads prior to treatment or perisurgically to maintain the health of periodontal tissues.

Full-thickness incision: The creation of an opening through all layers of the mucosa and periosteum to facilitate access to bony pathology.

Intrasulcular incision: A horizontal incision made through the gingival sulcus that splits the interdental papilla.

Osteotomy: The production of an opening through the alveolar bone to facilitate access to the root and any associated apical pathology.

Papilla-preserving incision: A horizontal incision made through the gingival sulcus that spares the papilla.

Resection: The removal of the root apex during apical microsurgery. At least 3 mm of the apex should be removed to address the majority of lateral and accessory canals within the root structure. Additional resection may be necessary if apical fractures or other defects are visible.

Retrofilling: The placement of a restoration, typically a bioceramic material, into the prepared apical canal space.

Retropreparation: The act of preparing the apical canal space. Retropreparation involves the removal of gutta-percha and any tissue via microsurgical ultrasonic instrumentation.

Submarginal incision: A horizontal incision made through the attached gingiva as opposed to through the gingival sulcus.

Suture: The materials and techniques used to close the incision following apical microsurgery. Common suture materials include silk and synthetic filaments, among others. Common suture techniques include simple interrupted sutures, sling sutures, and both vertical and horizontal mattress sutures.

Ultrasonics: A specialized drill powered by ultrasonic energy that accommodates tips of various shapes, sizes, and coatings, with myriad applications in nonsurgical and surgical endodontics. A mainstay of surgical endodontic therapy for creating conservative and accurate retropreparations.

Vital pulp therapy and immature dentition management

Apexification: A procedure performed on necrotic immature permanent teeth aimed at developing an apical barrier to house compacted obturation material within the canal space. Procedures involve either the use of long-term calcium hydroxide or immediate placement of bioceramic materials to form an artificial barrier.

Apexogenesis: A procedure performed on vital immature permanent teeth wherein vital pulp tissue is left in the canal space to promote continued root development. Treatments include direct pulp capping and pulpotomy procedures.

Bioceramics: Calcium silicate cements with documented biocompatibility and the ability to induce hard tissue formation and periodontal ligament (PDL) regeneration and maintain pulp vitality. The materials are sterile and set in the presence of moisture, including blood. Research supports their first-line use for vital pulp therapy, including direct pulp caps and pulpotomy, as well as in regenerative endodontic procedures and apexification in immature permanent teeth, for the repair of root perforations, and as root-end fillings for apical microsurgery.

Pulp cap: Placement of a restorative material over an exposed pulp.

Pulpotomy: Removal of the coronal portion of the pulp, preserving the vital radicular pulp. May take the form of a *full pulpotomy*, wherein all chamber pulp tissue is removed to the level of canal orifices, or a *partial* or *Cvek pulpotomy*, in which only the inflamed portion of coronal pulp is removed.

Regenerative endodontic procedure: An endodontic procedure performed on necrotic immature permanent teeth wherein the necrotic pulp is disinfected and stem cells from the apical papilla are introduced so that continued root development can occur alongside apical healing.

Complications

Apical zipping: The creation of an oval- or elliptical-shaped apical foramen because of file overextension and transportation of the outer wall. Zip perforation typically develops due to aggressive instrumentation with larger hand instruments or inflexible nickel-titanium (NiTi) rotary instruments.

Flare-up: An acute exacerbation of periradicular pathology after the initiation or continuation of root canal treatment.[1]

Ledging: The iatrogenic development of a hard stop in a previously patent canal space due to aggressive instrumentation short of the working length.

Paresthesia: Altered sensation, namely "pins and needles," pricking, or tingling, in the distribution of an injured nerve.

Perforation: A communication between the canal space and external tooth structure. Perforations may occur iatrogenically or can be caused by caries or resorptive defects.

Persistent pain: Pain following endodontic treatment that lasts beyond normal postoperative soreness, defined as more than 7 days after treatment.

Separation: The fracture of a portion of a root canal instrument in the canal space.

Transportation: An instrumentation error marked by the removal of root structure on the outer canal curvature in the apical half of the canal. May be prevented by precurving the tips of hand instruments and using flexible rotary instruments within canal spaces.

Adjunctive Terms

Fractures

Cemental tear: A type of root fracture characterized by the complete or partial detachment of cementum from the underlying dentin.

Crown-root fractures: These fractures involve enamel, dentin, and cementum, with or without pulp exposure.

Enamel fractures: These limited fractures, also referred to as *uncomplicated crown fractures*,[7,8] are defined by a loss of enamel only.

Enamel-dentin fractures: Also called *uncomplicated crown fractures*,[7,8] these are marked by loss of enamel and dentin.

Enamel-dentin-pulp fractures: Also called *complicated crown fractures*,[7,8] these involve the loss of enamel and dentin with concomitant pulp exposure.

Horizontal root fractures: Also called oblique root fractures, these run in the transverse or axial plane of the root, splitting it into apical and coronal halves that may be complete or incomplete in their separation.

Infractions: Also called *craze lines*, infractions are cracks in the enamel without associated loss of tooth structure.

Longitudinal root fractures: Fractures extending through the vertical plane of the tooth that can be further distinguished based on their extension into vertical root fractures or split roots.

Unseparated coronal fractures: A crown fracture of unknown depth wherein the fractured portions of tooth structure remain approximate to one another.

Resorptive diagnoses

External cervical resorption (ECR): Resorption derived from clastic cells in the periodontium that erode the cementum and dentin externally in vital teeth.

External inflammatory root resorption (EIRR): Resorption derived from clastic cells in the periodontium that erode the cementum and dentin externally following dental trauma or in necrotic teeth.

Internal root resorption (IRR): Resorption derived from clastic cells in the pulp space that erode the dentin in teeth with irreversibly inflamed pulps during their progression to necrosis.

Pressure resorption (PR): Resorption caused by pressure from orthodontic tooth movement, misaligned tooth eruption, or benign cysts or tumors that leads to loss of the dental hard tissues, typically in vital teeth.

Resorption: The physiologic or pathologic loss of dentin, cementum, or bone not otherwise attributable to caries, trauma, or fracture.

Traumatic dental injuries

Alveolar fracture: Fracture of the alveolus, which may result in displacement of the fractured segments or the mobility of several teeth in concert.

Avulsion: The complete displacement of a tooth out of its alveolar housing.

Complicated crown fracture: Complete or incomplete fracture of enamel and dentin with pulp exposure.

Concussion: An injury to the periodontal ligament (PDL) resulting in percussion tenderness without associated mobility or displacement.

Crown-root fracture: Complete or incomplete fracture of enamel, dentin, and cementum. The pulp may or may not be exposed.

Horizontal root fracture: Fracture of cementum, dentin, and pulp that may result in displacement of the coronal fragment of the tooth structure.

Luxation: An injury to the periodontal ligament (PDL) resulting in displacement of the tooth, though not its complete loss. Luxation injuries may result in lateral, intrusive, or extrusive displacement and may be associated with mobility and percussion tenderness, though luxated teeth may also lack mobility if "locked into" fractured bone.

Subluxation: An injury to the periodontal ligament (PDL) resulting in percussion tenderness and mobility of the tooth without displacement.

Uncomplicated crown fracture: Complete or incomplete fracture of enamel and/or dentin without pulp exposure.

References

1. Glossary of Endodontic Terms, ed 10. American Association of Endodontists, 2020. https://www.aae.org/specialty/clinical-resources/glossary-endodontic-terms. Accessed 11 April 2023.
2. Swanson K, Madison S. An evaluation of coronal microleakage in endodontically treated teeth. Part I. Time periods. J Endod 1987;13:56–59.
3. Madison S, Wilcox LR. An evaluation of coronal microleakage in endodontically treated teeth. Part III. In vivo study. J Endod 1988;14:455–458.
4. Goldfein J, Speirs C, Finkelman M, Amato R. Rubber dam use during post placement influences the success of root canal-treated teeth. J Endod 2013;39:1481–1484.
5. Davis MC, Shariff SS. Success and survival of endodontically treated cracked teeth with radicular extensions: A 2- to 4-year prospective cohort. J Endod 2019;45:848–855.
6. Mader CL, Baumgartner JC, Peters DD. Scanning electron microscopic investigation of the smeared layer on root canal walls. J Endod 1984;10:477–483.
7. Bourguignon C, Cohenca N, Lauridsen E, et al. International Association of Dental Traumatology guidelines for the management of traumatic dental injuries: 1. Fractures and luxations. Dent Traumatol 2020;36:314–330.
8. American Association of Endodontists. Recommended Guidelines of the American Association of Endodontists for The Treatment of Traumatic Dental Injuries. https://www.aae.org/specialty/wpcontent/uploads/sites/2/2019/02/19_TraumaGuidelines.pdf. Accessed 13 Oct 2023.

Index

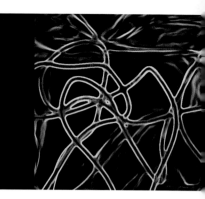

Page numbers followed by "t" denote tables; those followed by "f" denote figures.

Index

Index

Index

Index